PSYCHIATRY - THEORY, APPLICATIONS AND TREATMENTS

# PSYCHOSIS

## CAUSES, DIAGNOSIS AND TREATMENT

# Psychiatry - Theory, Applications and Treatments

Additional books in this series can be found on Nova's website
under the Series tab.

Additional e-books in this series can be found on Nova's website
under the e-books tab.

PSYCHIATRY - THEORY, APPLICATIONS AND TREATMENTS

# PSYCHOSIS

## CAUSES, DIAGNOSIS AND TREATMENT

XENIA ANASTASSIOU-HADJICHARALAMBOUS
EDITOR

Nova Biomedical
*New York*

For permission to use material from this book please contact us:
Telephone 631-231-7269; Fax 631-231-8175
Web Site: http://www.novapublishers.com

## NOTICE TO THE READER



**LIBRARY OF CONGRESS CATALOGING-IN-PUBLICATION DATA**

ISBN: 978-1-62081-516-8

LCCN: 2012940132

*Published by Nova Science Publishers, Inc. † New York*

# Contents

# PREFACE

*'severe mental illness like Psychosis can lead to a tragedy like this -- that people can see things that aren't real and hear things that aren't real and believe things that aren't real, and act in that distorted reality'.*
~ Andrea Yates

Psychosis is considered the most debilitating psychiatric condition. It presents an enormously heavy burden of suffering in terms of its prevalence, morbidity, and potentially high personal, familial and social costs. In effect, along the passage of time there has been substantial accumulation of research on this puzzling disorder. Despite the continually accumulating research that focuses on Psychosis, its precise nature remains poorly understood. Consequently there is a need for systematic review of the lines of inquiry along the many dimensions of the very diverse psychiatric condition of Psychosis.

Having this in mind, this edited volume attempts to provide to interested researchers and clinicians an up-to-date, systematic, and integrative review of the clinically relevant empirical evidence on the causes, diagnosis and treatment of Psychosis. Beyond the chapters that provide systematic reviews of the theoretical framework and the research evidence across critical dimensions of Psychosis, several experts in the field present their own findings of their very recent investigations. Finally via these systematic reviews and empirical reports new lines of inquiry are identified which the contributors hope would prove academically valuable thought-provoking and stimulating towards an integrative view of the nature of Psychosis.

Chapter 1 covers the clinical features, assessment, and differential diagnosis of Psychosis. Successful management of patients with Psychosis requires accurate identification of the condition underlying their symptoms. Psychotic symptoms, however, not only overlap with a wide array of conditions, but, can also be attributable to the use of substances. The clinical approach to the diagnosis of Psychotic Disorders is a multifaceted procedure involving the consideration of a broad differential diagnosis. In effect, the introductory chapter of this volume provides an overview of current assessment principles for patients who present with symptoms of Psychosis. This introductory chapter, aims at illustrating the various conditions that commonly co-occur with Psychosis, or of which Psychosis is a symptom in order to inform diagnostic decisions.

Chapter 2 reviews the up to date state empirical literature on Pediatric Psychosis, an understudied disorder that is cumbersome to diagnose, differentiate and treat. The chapter begins with a brief overview of the diagnostic features of Paediatric Psychosis and the factors implicated in making the diagnosis elusive and at times inaccurate. It continues with the differential diagnoses that are often implicated in the misdiagnosis of psychotic symptomatology in children. The next section, covers the sparse epidemiological data on the prevalence followed by the factors implicated in the aetiology of the disorder. The developmental considerations of the disorder are covered next. The final section reports on the evidence-based status of the treatment approaches for Paediatric Psychosis and identifies future directions of research.

Chapter 3 reviews early neurodevelopmental risk factors for Psychosis, with consideration of the modulating role of neurohormones and one's biological sex. Genetic factors (e.g., candidate genes, modifier genes, epigenetics) and adverse pre-/peri- natal events (such as obstetric complications) are the initial focus, given they exert effects (though not exclusively) during early development. Deficits in sensory processing and sensoriomotor gating are then reviewed as one among several cognitive and behavioral domains that may represent early developmental putative indicators of Psychosis risk, that are not as yet clearly linked with prenatal influences. Throughout, putative risk factors are contextualized with respect to sex differences, the potential modulating role of neurohormones, and synergistic effects towards bolstering current theoretical models of Psychosis proneness.

Chapter 4 constitutes an empirical prospective survey examining the occurrence of Psychotic Disorders (i.e. Schizophrenia, Schizotypal Disorder, Delusional Disorders and/or Psychotic Mood Disorders) in childhood, adolescence and their outcome in adulthood in a group of former Swedish child and adolescent psychiatric patients.

Early studies documented that many patients with psychotic symptoms had experienced childhood traumas, but, because of methodological weaknesses no causal link could be established. Over the last decades, large-scale studies aimed to clarify the link between childhood trauma and Psychosis in a more accurate and methodologically rigorous manner. Chapter 5 reports on the evidence-based status of the link between childhood trauma and Psychosis.

Identifying Psychosis in early stages is of major importance in terms of treatment. The onset of Psychosis may be unexpected or insidious, but in the majority of individuals there is some type of prodromal phase marked by the slow and gradual development of a variety of signs and symptoms. The chapter 6, covers the stages, the course and prognosis of Psychosis.

Chapter 7 reviews the past twenty years of research on semantic memory function in schizophrenia and the possible links with psychotic symptoms.

Chapter 8 presents a new study examining semantic memory and the relationship with symptomatology in 73 community-based patients with schizophrenia and 71 healthy controls. This new study reports a specific semantic memory impairment that shows stronger links with negative than positive symptomatology. The implications are discussed.

Family psycho-education is an evidence-based treatment for Psychotic Disorders. Chapter 9 outlines a service delivery protocol for a modified version of family psycho-education designed specifically for individuals with first-episode Psychosis.

Chapter 10 addresses fundamental considerations when developing routine and formal family interventions services. It provides a comprehensive overview, including the rationale, evidence-base and service models; it defines formal and routine family interventions; and describes a model which integrates research into the family emotional climate, attributions and interactions.

Chapter 11 reviews recent developments concerning clinical care for Psychosis. The new focus on violence, duration of untreated Psychosis and insight are deeply influencing the way psychiatry and society consider the person suffering from Psychosis. In particular, coercion into treatment gains a new legitimacy. Chapter 11, concludes by noting the stigmatizing effects of these trends.

Psychosis has been described to occur between 11-18% of Systemic lupus erythematosus (SLE) patients, both at disease onset and during follow-up period. It is essential to differentiate primary Psychotic Disorders unrelated to SLE from substance or drug-induced Psychotic Disorders and psychologically mediated reactions to SLE as a major stressor. Chapter 12 reviews the prevalence, etiology and clinical presentation of Psychosis in SLE. In addition it discusses treatment protocol for this serious manifestation in SLE.

This edited volume is conceptualized as a useful tool for advanced clinical psychology students, researchers, and other mental health professionals for whom a tool on Psychosis could prove useful in their scientific inquiry, and/or evidence-based professional practice. Researchers and students will find this book useful due to its wide coverage of factors implicated in the aetiology, diagnosis and treatment of Psychosis. Last but not least, the clinically relevant material that is cited in this volume makes it a useful tool for clinicians that base their practice on treatment approach that is empirically supported.

Without the thorough and systematic work of the contributors this volume would have been impossible. I therefore wish to acknowledge the level of their cooperation, commitment, and dedication they showed throughout the hard at times, but, yet challenging process of writing for this volume. My thanks also go to the staff of NOVA for their constant support throughout the process. To my close collaborator and co-author in this volume, Professor Cecilia Essau for her thought-provoking comments in the course of the writing up of the chapter of this volume.

Last but not least, my gratitude goes to my beloved partner in this life Marios whose flourished love and constant support through the many years of our life together has been amazingly beneficial to my scientific inquiry. My very special thanks to my inspiration in this life, the light of my life, my adorable -and adored- kids Manos and Nefeli ; and to the kids of all contributing authors, who like my own kids, had to be particularly patient with their parents in the course of the writing process of this volume. My deepest appreciation to my mum, for her constant support through the years, and, for providing a safe base for my kids while I was spending endless time in my office working on compiling the work of this volume.

Xenia Anastassiou-Hadjicharalambous
Nicosia, Cyprus
November, 2011

In: Psychosis: Causes, Diagnosis and Treatment
Editor: Xenia Anastassiou-Hadjicharalambous
ISBN: 978-1-62081-516-8


*Chapter 1*

# PSYCHOTIC SYMPTOMATOLOGY: CLINICAL FEATURES, ASSESSMENT AND DIFFERENTIAL DIAGNOSIS

***Maria-Eva Tsola and Xenia Anastassiou-Hadjicharalambous****
University of Nicosia, Cyprus

## ABSTRACT

Successful management of patients with psychosis requires accurate identification of the condition underlying their symptoms. Psychotic symptoms, however, not only overlap with a wide array of medical and neurological conditions but can also be attributable to the use of substances. The clinical approach to the diagnosis of psychotic disorders is a multifaceted procedure involving the consideration of a broad differential diagnosis. This chapter is an overview of current assessment principles for patients who present with symptoms of psychosis. By illustrating different conditions that commonly co-occur with psychosis, or of which psychosis is a defining symptom, it aims to inform diagnostic decisions.

## INTRODUCTION

The term psychosis has been defined, historically, in a number of different ways, none of which has gained universal acceptance [1, 2, 3]. In general, psychosis describes a mental state characterized by a broad-spectrum impairment of reality testing. Hallucinations and delusions are the two distinctive psychiatric features of psychosis, the presence of which typically indicates that the patient has either distorted or lost contact with reality. Hallucinations, which are sensory perceptions in the absence of an external source, can occur in any sensory modality and may take the form of voices, visions, odors, or even complex tactile perceptions [4]. Delusions are firmly held false beliefs that can range from ideas that are plausible, albeit

* E-mail address: *hadjicharalambous.x@unic.ac.cy.*

unlikely, to bizarre convictions. Psychosis is also marked by the presence of thought disorder which is defined as a broad disruption in the form, or organization, of thinking. In the DSM-IV-TR [1], the significance of the term psychosis varies from disorder to disorder: for certain psychotic disorders, broader definitions apply, whereas for others, narrower definitions are more appropriate [3]. In delusional disorder, for example, the psychotic symptoms are restricted to prominent delusions, whereas the psychotic symptoms of substance-induced psychosis and psychosis secondary to a general medical condition are delusions or hallucinations about which the person lacks insight. Schizophrenia and schizoaffective disorder are based on the broader definition of psychosis which includes delusions, any prominent hallucinations, as well as disorganized speech, and catatonic or disorganized behavior.

Psychosis is not a single and uniform disability. Psychotic symptoms may emerge in isolation from other disturbances, be an associated feature of other disturbances, or be a substantial component of a major psychotic disorder. In the DSM-IV-TR [1], those disorders that require the presence of psychosis as a defining feature include schizophrenia, substance-induced psychotic disorder, schizophreniform disorder, schizoaffective disorder, delusional disorder, brief psychotic disorder, shared psychotic disorder, and psychotic disorder due to a general medical condition. Disorders in which psychotic symptoms may be present but are not required for the diagnosis include mood disorders with psychotic features as well as several cognitive disorders such as dementia of the Alzheimer's type.

Psychosis is a phenomenon with a variety of differing etiologies found in many conditions. As a result, while typical symptoms of psychosis (delusions, hallucinations, disorganized speech and behavior, and inappropriate or blunted affect) are commonly associated with the diagnosis of schizophrenia, the occurrence of psychotic symptoms does not always indicate that a primary psychiatric disorder like schizophrenia is present [3, 4, 5, 6, 7, 8, 9, 10, 11, 12]. Different types of medical and neurological conditions, including brain tumors, Huntington's disease, epilepsy, and endocrine disorders can present with psychotic symptoms. Symptoms of psychosis can also be caused by the effects of intoxication with or withdrawal from substances of abuse or prescribed and non-prescribed medications. Regardless of etiology, psychotic illness is a severe condition that affects virtually all aspects of a person's life and carries with it an elevated risk of chronicity and social disability [9, 11, 13]. Accurate identification of the condition underlying these symptoms is critically important for selecting treatment and predicting outcome. A common difficulty experienced by clinicians when a patient presents with psychosis is determining whether psychotic symptoms correspond to a primary psychiatric disorder or are secondary to a medical or neurological condition, intoxication, or the side effects of medication [14].

## Diagnostic and Assessment Issues

The objective in the early phase of assessment is to assess danger and stabilize the crisis rather than to establish a final diagnosis [9, 14, 15]. For example, patients who appear agitated, frightened or paranoid, or are verbally aggressive and threatening, may require immediate behavioral and/or pharmacological intervention [15]. The diagnostic evaluation of the psychotic patient begins once the basic safety precautions have been taken and the patient is adequately capable of cooperating with the professional.

The diagnostic impression obtained in the first episodes of mental disorders has, nevertheless, important therapeutic and prognostic implications. Based on this first diagnostic impression, decisions are taken concerning the selection of treatment to be implemented and the service that the patient is to be referred to, and parameters are set to outline the expected evolution of each case. Consequently, the purpose of the initial assessment is to formulate a comprehensive reconstruction of the development of the psychotic disorder in the context of the individual patient's life story.

An initial, complete diagnostic evaluation for a person presenting with psychotic symptoms generally includes a comprehensive history (psychiatric; general medical; psychosocial, and family, including perinatal and developmental history) and a mental status examination that is primarily focused on eliciting psychotic symptoms from the patient [12, 15]. Psychotic and related disorders are considered diagnoses of exclusion because their symptoms overlap with a wide array of psychiatric, neurological, and general medical disorders but can also be attributable to the use of substances. Evaluating a patient with a first episode of psychosis, therefore, requires consideration of a broad differential diagnosis.

In order to facilitate the diagnostic procedure, the etiology of psychosis is commonly divided into two separate categories: primary psychiatric disorders (i.e., schizophrenia and other psychiatric disorders) and secondary psychoses [8]. Secondary psychoses consist of delirium, dementia, medical and neurological conditions, and abuse of substances. The first step in the differential diagnosis of psychosis is to exclude medically related or substance-induced psychotic disorders [16]. The second step is to differentiate psychosis caused by schizophrenia from psychosis associated with affective and other disorders that may present with psychotic features [16]. In spite of this useful classification, differentiating primary from secondary psychoses exclusively on the basis of psychopathology remains a diagnostic challenge, as psychotic states with differing etiologies may present with phenomenologically similar symptoms. The final diagnosis is, for this reason, often best determined during a multiple-contact, longitudinal assessment process [14, 17] throughout which psychotic symptoms in secondary conditions are excluded before entertaining the diagnosis of schizophrenia [12]. All assessments consist of direct client interviews, collateral data, client observations, and a review of available documented history [10, 11, 14, 15, 17].

As a rule, clinical features that are not characteristic of primary psychiatric disease commonly point toward the presence of secondary psychosis. Such atypical features include absence of a family history of major mental illness; lack of prior episodes of psychosis; an acute illness onset; an age at onset beyond the middle 30s; clouding of consciousness (i.e., confusional states); focal neurological abnormality; non-auditory hallucinations; co-existing deficit syndromes such as delirium, dementia, aphasia, amnesia; atypical clinical course or atypical response to treatment; as well as psychosis in a patient undergoing treatment in an emergency, general medical, or intensive care unit [4, 5, 7, 11, 18, 19].

In view of the multitude of alternative etiological factors of psychosis and in order to avoid the mistaken attribution of psychosis to a psychiatric disorder, a comprehensive physical examination is considered an essential assessment component, along with the history taking and mental status examination. For new-onset cases of psychosis in particular, a thorough history and physical examination with emphasis on the neurological and cognitive parts are the starting point for the initial approach to psychosis [4, 8, 9, 10, 11]. Routine laboratory tests that may facilitate the detection of possible organic factors and/or covert substance abuse include a complete blood count (CBC); hematocrit and hemoglobin; renal and metabolic panels; liver enzymes; thyroid function tests; determination of electrolyte levels; and HIV serological tests. Additional investigations, such as magnetic resonance imaging (MRI), or computed tomography (CT) and electrophysiological studies (EEG) may be indicated when the history suggests the need to rule out a space-occupying lesion or developmental malformation as the potential cause of the psychosis [4, 5, 6, 8, 9, 11, 15, 19, 20, 21].

# Differential Diagnosis: Exclusion of Secondary Psychoses

## 1. Secondary Psychosis Due to a General Medical Condition

Psychotic symptoms have been described in many neurological and general medical disorders [11, 12, 18, 21]. The fact that medical conditions represent potentially reversible causes of psychotic symptoms, along with the multitude of negative consequences of failing to make a diagnosis of such a condition, represent the primary reasons for medically examining patients who present with symptoms of psychosis [10, 15].

In order to assess potential medical and/or neurological causes of the presenting psychosis, a thorough history is taken from the patient and other informants (i.e., the patient's relatives), and a standard physical, mental status, and neurological examination is carried out. Clinical presentations that are characterized by an acute onset, features of delirium (i.e., clouding of consciousness), disorientation in time and place, disturbance of memory, impaired attention, fluctuation of conscious awareness, and visual hallucinations [11, 19] are generally indicative of an underlying medical or neurological cause. When the clinical picture is marked with such atypical features, complementary laboratory and neuroimaging investigations may be required, depending on the hypothesized diagnosis. If no medical or neurological cause of psychosis becomes evident following the standard clinical process (i.e., absence of focal neurological signs and symptoms), it is typically assumed that the symptoms of psychosis are most likely caused by a primary psychiatric disorder [12, 19]. Importantly, presence of a medical or neurologic disorder does not preclude the possibility of a comorbid psychiatric disorder.

### *Endocrine Diseases*

*Thyroid Disorders.* Hypofunction of hyperfunction of the thyroid gland can result in florid psychosis. In the form of hypothyroidism, psychosis may present with both auditory hallucinations and paranoia (typically characterized by delusions of persecution and reference) in a condition known as 'myxedema madness' [19, 22, 23, 24]. In severe cases of autoimmune hyperthyroidism ('thyrotoxicosis 'or 'thyrotoxic storm'), a patient may present with psychotic symptoms such as prominent hallucinations and delusions of paranoid type, as well as symptoms of depression and mania [23, 24].

*Adrenal Disorders.* Hyperadrenalism (Cushing's syndrome) most commonly results from exogenous corticosteroids, but may also be the result of adrenocorticotropic hormone

(ACTH) secretion by a pituitary tumor (Cushing's disease), or corticosteroid secretion by an adrenal tumor [23]. These endocrine disorders may present with symptoms of psychosis, along with other psychiatric symptoms, including anxiety, depression, and cognitive disturbances [8, 22, 23, 24].

### *Autoimmune Diseases*

*Systemic Lupus Erythematosus (SLE)* is a connective tissue, systemic autoimmune disease that affects small blood vessels and is marked by multiple abnormalities of the immune system including a diverse array of neurological and psychiatric manifestations that may affect either the central or peripheral nervous systems in individual patients [25, 26]. The neuropsychiatric complications of SLE, include seizures, stroke, cognitive impairment and psychiatric disorders, and may be among some of the earliest symptoms of the disease, becoming evident even prior to the manifestation of gross peripheral organ pathology. Psychosis has been well documented to occur in a significant minority of patients as a result of the immune disease itself, unrelated to medical treatment [8, 25, 26]. Symptoms of psychosis in SLE patients typically present in the form of delirium with psychotic features and tend to peak with disease relapses and quickly disappear with remissions [26].

*Hashimoto's encephalopathy (HE)*, a relatively very rare condition that appears in all age groups [27], is an association of autoimmune thyroiditis (thyrotoxicosis) with encephalopathy. The condition presents with a great variety of neuropsychiatric symptoms [27] including focal or generalized seizures; confusion; headaches; choroid movements; stroke-like episodes, as well as recurrent symptoms of psychosis, the most common of which are hallucinations [8, 22, 27]. HE is corticosteroid-responsive, and prompt treatment typically leads to rapid recovery [8, 27].

### *Infections*

Although most infectious causes of psychosis have viral etiologies resulting in encephalitis, a variety of other infectious agents such as bacteria, fungi, and parasites may also invade the nervous system and produce symptoms of psychosis [28]. Clinical features that are suggestive of viral encephalitis encephalitic psychoses are headache, lethargy, and fever, and in some cases psychosis [8, 22]. Human Immunodeficiency Virus (HIV) infection and neurosyphilis can present with psychosis and should specifically be considered in all patients with psychosis [8, 22]. Delusions with persecutory, grandiose, or somatic components are the most prominent psychotic symptom in HIV infection. Hallucinations, disorders of thought processes, disturbances of affect, and bizarre behavior also commonly coexist with the psychosis [28].

### *Seizures*

The relationship between seizures, particularly temporal lobe epilepsy, and psychosis is well established, with epidemiological studies indicating elevated rates of schizophrenia in patients with epilepsy and vice versa [8]. Even though the hallucinatory states of epilepsy are almost always accompanied by additional epileptic features such as confusion or altered awareness, the clinical phenomenology of epileptic states is often indistinguishable from that of primary psychosis [29]. Typically, the psychotic symptoms in patients with epilepsy are described as episodic rather than continuing, with normal functioning between episodes [19].

In view of the fact that clinical seizures are the outstanding feature of epilepsy, psychotic symptoms that occur in the context of seizures have traditionally been classified according to their temporal relationship to these events, into ictal, postictal (or peri-ictal), and interictal categories [8, 19, 29, 30, 31]. Ictal psychosis can occur in a non-convulsive state ('complex partial status epilepticus'), and is immediately suggested by its paroxysmal onset and brief duration, lasting from minutes to hours [8, 22, 30]. This epileptic state may result in mental states remarkably similar to those seen in primary psychosis, characterized by restless, fearful, and agitated behavior with delusions and hallucinations, ideas of reference, paranoia, and thought disorder [11, 29]. Hallucinations that take place in the ictal state tend to be brief and stereotyped visual experiences [32]. Postictal psychosis emerges close to the seizure and while it can last several days or weeks, it rarely develops into a chronic psychosis. Psychotic symptoms typical of this epileptic state are noted for their similarity to schizophrenia-like/paranoid and affective psychoses [29]. Chronic interictal psychosis typically occurs in the setting of a chronically uncontrolled seizure disorder, such as chronic epilepsy [22, 31], and is marked by hallucinatory and other psychotic features occurring in clear consciousness [29] and intense dysphoric affect [8, 22]. Because frontal lobe seizures can be very difficult to diagnose, serial EEGs improve the possibility of making a diagnosis of epilepsy. Further assistance in diagnosis may also come from the examination of serum prolactin levels which increase following epileptic seizures [30].

### *Cerebral Tumors*

Even though psychosis secondary to a brain tumor is rare [19], psychotic symptoms are one of the most basic, and sometimes the single manifestation of an intracranial tumor. Even though secondary to brain tumor, these symptoms may be indistinguishable from the typical symptoms of primary psychotic disorders. The diagnostic possibility of a brain tumor should, in consequence, always be considered in patients with new-onset psychosis [22, 33, 34], and in elderly patients, particularly if persistent headaches or other neurological signs (i.e., seizures), or certain focal signs (i.e., aphasia) are present [8, 34]. Psychotic symptoms may follow seizures, which are common with brain tumors, especially if located in the temporal lobes but can also be caused by tumors in other regions including the frontal and parietal lobes and the corpus callosum [19, 22]. Various general differences have been noted when comparing the psychotic symptoms secondary to brain tumor to those of schizophrenia. The onset of psychotic symptoms is typically subacute or gradual [22] and formal thought disorder and catatonia in cases of psychosis secondary to brain tumor are rare. Hallucinations secondary to brain tumors are most commonly visual and tend to be less complex than in patients with schizophrenia [19]. Delusions in brain tumors are generally of paranoid or persecutory type and simpler in nature compared to the systematized delusions of schizophrenia [19, 33, 34]. Patients with psychosis secondary to brain tumors may present with signs of delirium (i.e., clouding of consciousness, confusional states, disorientation) as a result of diffuse impairment of brain tissue [19].

### *Traumatic Brain Injury*

Although psychosis is a relatively uncommon psychiatric consequence following brain injury [22, 35], a history of head injury is a risk factor for the development of a chronic psychotic syndrome that can be clinically indistinguishable from schizophrenia [8, 35, 36]. The type (open or closed brain injury); the severity of brain injury, usually evidenced by EEG and neuroimaging abnormalities (e.g., focal lesions in the frontal and temporal lobes) and a family history of psychosis are strongly associated with the emergence of psychosis following head injury [8, 35, 36, 37, 38]. Psychosis secondary to traumatic brain injury is typically delusional-hallucinatory in nature, and negative symptoms of schizophrenia are generally less common [35, 36, 37, 38].

***Demyelinating Diseases***

Diseases that disrupt the integrity of white matter tracts in the brain can lead to psychosis, likely to be caused by the functional disconnectivity of critical brain regions. The clinical consequences of this 'disconnection' depend on the localization of the white-matter pathology, whether it is in the brain, spinal cord, or brain stem [39].

*Multiple sclerosis (MS)* is the most common demyelinating disease, and is associated with psychosis more often than can be expected by chance [8, 40], although the rate of psychosis is low [19, 22]. The psychiatric clinical picture of MS patients is primarily characterized by the presence of positive psychotic symptoms, generally accompanied by signs suggestive of disseminated lesions (e.g., concurrent with nystagmus) [22], with relative preservation of affective responses [40].

*Inherited leukodystrophies*, such as metachromatic leukodystrophy (MLD) and adrenoleukodystrophy (ALD) are associated with a high prevalence of neuropsychiatric symptoms, including psychosis. While inherited leukodystrophies are usually diagnosed during childhood when systemic and neurological symptoms emerge, adult-onset cases can present with a predominantly psychiatric picture [22, 39]. MLD in particular is associated with a very high rate of psychosis, perhaps as high as 50% in the adult age group [8, 41]. MLD is a rare, recessively inherited disorder that occurs secondary to mutations in the gene for aryl sulfatase A (ASA), predominantly affecting white matter, and resulting in the accumulation of sulfatides in the brain, peripheral nerves, kidneys, and gallbladder [22]. In MLD, psychotic symptoms, which very closely resemble those of schizophrenia [22], may be a result of impaired central nervous system (CNS) function during a critical period of development of the CNS [41]. A number of further symptoms and signs, such as ataxia, spasticity, seizures, or a peripheral neuropathy may also constitute presenting features, or may emerge in the context of psychosis, personality change or dementia [22]. ALD is an X-linked disorder in which very long- chain fatty acids accumulate as a result of defective beta-oxidation within the peroxisome [8, 39]. Even though the disorder typically afflicts young boys, less severe forms of the illness have their onset during adolescence or adulthood [39]. In adult-onset ALD, where disruptions to myelination predominantly affect posterior zones, mood disorders with psychotic symptoms (e.g., mania, or affective psychosis) occur more commonly than psychotic symptoms that resemble schizophrenia [41]. The diagnosis of a demyelinating disorder is suggested by abnormal findings on MRI scans, such as diffuse, symmetric, and confluent demyelination [39]. As the disease progresses, the extensive loss of white matter causes a significant enlargement of the ventricles. For inherited leukodystrophies in particular, clinical symptoms distinctive of these conditions consist of progressive cognitive decline, other neurological findings (e.g., seizures or a neuropathy), or other systemic findings (e.g., adrenal insufficiency in patients with ALD) [8, 39].

***Basal Ganglia Disorders***

*Wilson's disease (WD),* also known as hepatolenticular degeneration, is an autosomal recessive disorder involving multiple mutations of the gene ATP7B which is critical to hepatic copper excretion [42, 43]. The initial presentation of Wilson's disease may be with psychotic symptoms, with a movement disorder appearing only much later [22, 43]. The disorder leads to an accumulation of copper deposits throughout the body, including the liver, brain, musculoskeletal system, heart, kidneys, endocrine system, red blood cells, skin, and other tissues [42]. Copper deposition occurs for the most part in the liver and the basal ganglia lenticular nucleus of the brain [8, 42]. Early recognition of WD is of critical importance since the disorder responds well to treatment with decoppering agents [42]. WD is diagnosed by determining low blood ceruloplasmin and is confirmed by elevated copper levels on liver biopsy [8, 15, 42]. Clinical clues that suggest the need of a diagnostic workup to exclude WD include the manifestation of hepatic, neurological (i.e., mild tremor, speech difficulties), or psychiatric symptoms, mainly when accompanied by a family history of WD or the existence of Kayser-Fleischer rings (KFRs) on slit lamp exam [4, 8, 42].

*Huntington's Disease (HD)* is a progressive neurodegenerative disease with a classical autosomal dominant pattern of inheritance [30]. The disease tends to be more severe if the onset is early, and premonitory psychiatric features are more common in such cases [35]. Even though choreiform movements are typically the first behavioral manifestation of the disorder, psychiatric symptoms may sometimes precede the movement disorder or cognitive dysfunction of Huntington's disease and, as a result, delay its recognition [8, 35], particularly because the syndrome of psychosis and chorea may appear indistinguishable from schizophrenia when complicated from tardive dyskinesia [22]. Psychiatric symptoms presenting in patients with HD, often collectively referred to as alterations in personality, generally consist of increased suspiciousness, ideas of reference, impulsivity, eccentricity, and irritability [35]. Prominent psychotic symptoms secondary to HD are typically hallucinations and delusions of persecutory, referential, or grandiose nature [35]. Symptoms of psychosis may gradually fade away as the cognitive impairment progresses [43]. The diagnosis of HD is strongly suggested by the characteristic clinical features and family history, and established by genetic testing [8, 35]. Neuroimaging (CT, MRI, and SPECT) may play a role in determining the severity of cerebral involvement [35].

*Fahr's disease (FD)* is described as symmetrical, bilateral basal ganglia calcification (BGC) without parathyroid dysfunction or physical abnormalities, generally hereditary with an autosomal dominant pattern of inheritance [8, 22, 44]. Although the condition presents most commonly with motor deficits, approximately 40% of FD patients present with primarily cognitive and other psychiatric symptoms [44]. Onset between the ages of 20 and 40 has been associated with schizophreniform psychoses and catatonic symptoms, whereas onset between the ages of 40 and 60 has been associated with dementia and choreoathetosis [43]. The course of FD is characteristically slow and progressive. Neurological or psychiatric symptoms such as psychosis tend to precede cognitive decline [44] and include auditory and visual hallucinations, paranoid delusions or paranoid trends, ideas of reference, ideas of influence, catatonia, fugue states, and atypical features such as complex perceptual distortions [44]. Even though the condition is rare, the diagnosis of FD should be considered in patients who present with the characteristic triad of neurological, cognitive, and psychiatric symptoms [43, 44]. Diagnosis is based on family history information and results obtained from brain CT scan, which is sensitive in demonstrating minimal basal ganglia calcification [44].

*Parkinson's disease (PD).* Psychosis is a common neuropsychiatric complication of PD, affecting nearly 50% of all patients over the course of the disease [45, 46]. Psychosis associated with PD is characterized by a temporal and clinical profile of hallucinations and delusions that differs from the typical pattern of primary psychotic disorders. In general, PD-related psychosis emerges as a complication of anti-parkinsonian therapy in advanced stages of the disease [45, 46, 47] and in susceptible individuals [48]. Early onset of psychosis following the initiation of dopaminergic therapy, (i.e., within the first 3 months), is atypical for PD and is usually indicative of alternative diagnoses, such as dementia with Lewy bodies and Alzheimer's disease [45, 46, 47]. Psychotic symptoms in PD include hallucinations and delusions of variable range and severity [45]. Even though hallucinations can take place in any sensory modality, and at any time during the course of PD, visual hallucinations are the most common element of psychosis in PD [45, 46, 47, 48]. Hallucinations in PD are usually fully formed and characterized by stereotyped and recurrent themes [45, 46, 47, 48]. In contrast to the auditory hallucinations typical of schizophrenia, auditory hallucinations in PD variably co-occur with visual hallucinations, and are less likely to be seen in isolation [46]. The hallucinatory experience tends to be typically brief, lasting seconds to minutes at a time, with variable frequency and generally occurs in a clear sensorium [46]. Although each hallucinatory episode is brief, the hallucinatory state, once established, is a chronic one and symptoms may continue or re-emerge among patients treated with antipsychotics [46]. In PD, delusions are less common, with a prevalence ranging from 3% to 30% [45]. When delusions are present in patients with PD, they are typically of paranoid nature [45, 46, 48] and are characterized by well-systematized ideas that focus on a single theme [45]. In contrast to the delusions of schizophrenia, PD-related delusions most often occur in a clear sensorium and do not include further elements of a thought disorder [48].

## 2. Secondary Psychosis Due to Substance Abuse

A variety of psychoactive substances, such as alcohol, marijuana, cocaine, hallucinogens, and amphetamine, can induce transient psychotic states that are not indicative of an underlying primary psychotic disorder [5, 8, 11, 12, 13, 18, 20, 21, 22, 49, 50, 51, 52]. With variations related to the pharmacological effects of different categories of substances, psychotic symptoms are typically experienced in the contexts of acute intoxication, withdrawal, delirium (related to either intoxication or withdrawal), substance-induced mood disorder (with psychotic symptoms), or substance-induced psychosis [50, 53, 54, 52]. Numerous commonly prescribed medications can also evoke psychotic symptoms, particularly those with direct effects on the brain, such as anticholinergics, corticosteroids, anti-parkinsonian medications, and anticonvulsants [5, 51, 55, 56, 57]. Toxins reported to induce psychotic symptoms include carbon monoxide, heavy metals (i.e., arsenic, manganese, mercury, and thallium), organophosphate insecticides, and volatile substances such as fuel or paint [57].

The diagnostic distinction between a substance-induced psychosis and a primary psychotic disorder that co-occurs with drug use is critically important in planning for appropriate treatment [11, 12, 15, 50, 53, 58]. The issues of assessment and treatment planning are primarily significant in the early stages of psychotic disorder when the symptom picture is usually unclear and an error in diagnosis can result in medical mismanagement [9,

13, 15, 54, 57, 59], in particular when the substance abuse is covert, denied, or not reported accurately [20]. Diagnosis depends on the collection of evidence which must support the position that the psychotic symptomatology is substance induced. The co-occurrence of psychosis and substance use is challenging diagnostically because persons with primary psychotic disorders who use psychoactive substances frequently present for treatment with signs and symptoms similar to those whose psychosis resulted from the use of drugs alone [13, 58]. Further complicating matters, the use of substances with psychotomimetic properties can exacerbate already existing psychotic symptoms and in many cases lead to a return of acute psychosis [9, 10, 18, 20, 43, 49, 50, 60, 61]. Consequently, when patients with a history of substance abuse present with psychotic symptoms, their symptoms can be diagnosed as either an independent psychiatric disorder that is not substance induced; identified as manifestations of use, intoxication, or withdrawal, or attributed to the combined effects or the interaction of both conditions [17, 20, 54, 57, 60, 62].

Diagnosis largely depends on recognition of a temporal relationship between the ingestion of the suspect substance and the onset of psychotic symptoms, clinical presentation and a thorough medical and medication history. Because patients with acute psychosis are often excessively disorganized to provide an accurate history, and because substance-abusing patients often minimize their use and try to keep their problems hidden, consultation with family, friends, and other reliable informants (i.e., health care providers) is valuable in understanding any pre-existing mental health issues and recent changes in behavior or medical treatment. Medication history should include the patient's use of prescription, non-prescription, and illicit drugs, as well as any herbal products or nutritional supplements being ingested, and recent discontinuation of any medication. Laboratory monitoring regularly complements the assessment procedure and typically includes a complete blood cell count (CBC), serum electrolytes, urine toxicology screening, and liver-function tests [5, 9, 10, 15, 51, 56, 57].

The chronology-based timeline method is a useful approach for distinguishing between substance-induced and independent psychiatric conditions [9, 12, 54, 57]. First, the age at which the patient developed dependence and fulfilled criteria for substance abuse should be noted [57]. Determining the chronology of symptoms is facilitated by establishing the patient's age at major life events (i.e., graduation, marriage), and then determining whether the criterion of interest (i.e., tolerance) occurred previous to or following a particular event. The second step involves the consideration of psychiatric symptomatology during the course of substance abuse, or before the onset of the dependence syndrome. This procedure can help establish whether an acute or chronic substance use disorder caused the onset of the psychosis; whether use of substances only forced the re-emergence of psychiatric symptoms or a disorder that had occurred earlier in the lifetime of the patient, or whether the substance use disorder intensified the severity of the underlying psychiatric disorder [54]. An equally important third step is the review of psychiatric symptomatology in the context of abstinence of several months (when intoxication or withdrawal effects can no longer account for psychotic symptoms). If major psychiatric symptoms occurred before the onset of substance abuse or during periods of sustained abstinence, the individual most likely suffers from two independent disorders [57]. If no major psychiatric symptoms can be demonstrated either before or in the prolonged absence of substance abuse, the psychosis is probably secondary to the substance abuse [57]. The fourth and final step is the most critical, and involves observation of the patient over a month of abstinence to determine whether the symptoms of psychosis improve sufficiently or drop below the diagnostic threshold. DSM-IV [1] diagnosis of primary psychotic disorder is encouraged when psychotic features last for more than a month with sustained abstinence. Improvement of psychiatric symptoms following abstinence usually indicates that the psychosis was secondary to substance abuse. In the same way, relapse of psychotic symptoms upon re-exposure to the offending substance (or withdrawal) further supports the diagnosis of substance-induced psychosis [50, 54, 62]. Even though long-term follow-up is recognized as the most definitive method for making a diagnostic distinction between substance-induced and independent or primary psychotic symptoms [20, 54, 62], establishing a causal link between psychotic symptoms and the ingested drug is particularly difficult when the drugs of abuse are illicit [8, 53, 60] and when patients abuse multiple substances, each with a differing profile of psychotogenic effects and duration of withdrawal syndromes.

## Differentiating between Primary Psychoses and Mental Disorders that May Present with Psychotic Features

### 1. Mood Disorders

Schizophrenia overlaps more prominently with the major mood disorders than any other psychiatric disorder [20, 51, 63, 64]; with schizophrenia patients being at increased risk of developing depression relative to the already high lifetime prevalence of depression in the general population [51, 60, 64]. Importantly, the advent of depression along the course of the illness is associated with an increased rate of relapse; more frequent and longer duration of hospitalizations; poor response to pharmacological treatments; as well as increased rates of substance abuse and suicide/suicide attempts [51, 65, 66]. Differentiating the two syndromes is imperative not only for the aforementioned reasons, but also because the disorders respond to different treatments, particularly pharmacological interventions [20, 51, 67].

The diagnostic distinction between schizophrenia and a major mood disorder is based on determining whether active psychotic symptoms occur in the absence of mood symptoms, or conversely, whether affective symptoms are present in the context of chronic psychotic disorders [68, 69]. This assessment is typically complicated by the fact that mood symptoms are commonly present in all phases of schizophrenia (prodrome, acute, and remission), or may be superimposed on the symptoms of residual schizophrenia ('post-psychotic depression'), and psychotic symptoms are frequently reported by persons with severe mood disorders [5, 9, 18, 20, 65, 66, 69]. Further complicating the clinical picture are patients who display signs of depressive or manic symptoms, but do not meet the full syndromal criteria for an affective disorder [18, 51, 69]. One additional complexity involves the difficulty to establish the chronological relationship between the onset of mood symptoms and psychotic symptoms- a requirement of many classification systems [18]. Finally, in the context of a chronic psychotic disorder, several of the symptoms that typically constitute a depressive syndrome may in fact be negative symptoms of schizophrenia or side effects of antipsychotic medication, or may occur in a prodrome to a psychotic relapse [11, 68].

The DSM-IV-TR [1], distinguishes between schizophrenia and psychotic mood disorders, mainly based upon psychosis being the core-defining feature of the schizophrenia diagnosis, whereas in mood disorders it is considered a secondary clinical phenomenon [70]. In patients with affective disorders, psychotic symptoms, if they occur, typically coincide with the mood disturbance, and a recurrent pattern of depressive or manic episodes (or both) is usual. In contrast, in patients with schizophrenia, mood disturbances are not necessarily present, but if they are, a recurrent pattern is uncommon, and the mood symptoms have a duration that is brief in relation to the total duration of the disturbance, or do not meet full criteria for a mood episode. The diagnostic criterion that is of most importance in differentiating between schizophrenia and a mood disorder is, therefore, the context in which psychotic symptoms occur. When psychotic symptoms occur only after a patient has begun a mood episode, but disappear once the mood is stable, the patient's diagnosis is either bipolar disorder or major depressive disorder with psychotic features [4, 11, 20, 68, 69]. When psychotic symptoms that are typical of schizophrenia have been present for at least two weeks in the absence of mood symptoms, they usually suggest the presence of either schizophrenia or schizoaffective disorder [4, 11, 20, 68]. Significantly, a diagnosis of schizophrenia does not preclude a secondary diagnosis of a mood syndrome [68, 69].

### *Differentiating between Major Depressive Disorder with Psychotic Features and Schizophrenia*

Depressive episodes in patients with schizophrenia generally occur along with other symptoms of schizophrenia and within the context of an otherwise typical symptom pattern for schizophrenia [11]. The negative symptom syndrome of schizophrenia, however, shares many clinical similarities with some of the major psychological features of primary depressive illness [4, 65, 66, 68] and may cause particular problems when these symptoms are viewed upon as a possible differential diagnostic criterion. Relevant overlapping features between the two syndromes include lack of energy, anhedonia and social withdrawal, diminished interest, pleasure, energy, or motivation along with psychomotor retardation, insomnia, and impaired ability to concentrate [11, 65, 66, 69]. In differentiating the two syndromes, blunted affect which suggests negative symptoms and prominent subjectively low mood or cognitive features such as guilt or suicidal thoughts, which suggests depression, are the two most helpful distinguishing symptoms [65, 66]. An emphasis on the patient's internal subjective states may, in consequence, be a useful approach in detecting important aspects of depressive symptomatology in schizophrenia [65]. Onset of depressive symptoms following a clear psychosocial stressor is an additional clue to diagnosing depressive symptoms in a patient who has schizophrenia [68]. The gradual development of the disease apart from a mood disorder, incomplete remission between psychotic episodes, prolonged social and occupational impairments, and characteristic symptoms further contribute to a diagnosis of schizophrenia [16].

Patients with psychotic depression are typically severely behaviorally disturbed [69]. The hallucinations experienced by patients with major depression, are typically of shorter duration and fragmented compared to those of schizophrenia; they occur within the context of predominantly affective symptoms [11], and patients usually attach delusional interpretations to them, such as infestation, poisoning, or spying [69]. Delusional themes in the psychotic subtype of major depression tend to be mood congruent, usually reflecting ruminative concerns about guilt, worthlessness, nihilism, and physical decay [4, 69]. Conversely, in schizophrenia the delusions tend to be bizarre and generally unrelated to the mood. When mood incongruent delusions (i.e., persecutory delusions) are experienced in the context of a major depressive episode, these must be accompanied by more typical depressive symptoms for a diagnosis of mood disorder with psychotic features to be considered [11]. Despite the strong similarity to the affective disorders, schizoaffective disorder and affective disorders are not identical [71]. Schizoaffective episodes are, by definition, always psychotic whereas affective episodes are not. They are also typically more severe than affective episodes [72] and the clinical presentation of depression is less typical compared to that of psychotic depression [73]. Some schizoaffective episodes ('schizo-dominant type') have a strong relation to schizophrenia, with a higher incidence of schizophrenia in the family history [71].

### *Differentiating between Bipolar Disorder with Psychotic Features and Schizophrenia*

Bipolar affective disorder is characterized by episodes of psychosis during both high ("manic") and low (depressive) relapses [21]. Making the differential diagnosis between schizophrenia and bipolar disorder is most problematic in patients presenting with a first episode of psychosis because at that point, the longitudinal course of illness which best distinguishes these disorders, is not clinically observable. Viewed cross-sectionally, symptoms that characteristically accompany the height of a manic episode, such as irritability, anger, paranoid delusions, formal thought disorder, and catatonic-like excitement cannot distinguish manic states from schizophrenia [11, 67, 74]. In patients with schizophrenia, these symptoms are typically secondary to an exacerbation of positive symptoms, whereas in manic states, they typically correspond to the euphoria, grandiosity, and increase in goal-directed activities that are typical of the characteristic expansive and elated affect of this condition [11, 67, 68]. Because presenting symptoms can be similar in mania and schizophrenia, in distinguishing between bipolar illness and psychotic disorders, attention must be given to the clustering of symptoms, rather than individual symptoms [67]. Level of premorbid functioning, family history of psychiatric illness, sequence and patterning of symptoms, and the character of any prior episodes including functioning during inter-episode periods are important in differentiating between the two conditions [74]. Even though not diagnostically specific, a family history of bipolar disorder and a history of episodic illness with good inter-episode functioning [67, 74], as well as sudden onset of symptoms and a prevalence of affective symptoms [11] generally point toward the presence of bipolar mood disorder with psychotic features. Prominence of affective symptoms is the criterion which generally makes possible differentiating mood disorders with psychotic features from schizophrenia. Thus, the presence of psychotic symptoms, including bizarre or mood incongruent delusions and Schneiderian first rank symptoms, is consistent with a diagnosis of mania as long as these are accompanied by substantial affective symptoms most of the time [74]. A diagnosis of schizophrenia or schizoaffective disorder is considered when the delusions or hallucinations are experienced in the absence of affective episodes for a period of time that exceeds two weeks. Schizophrenia is diagnosed if the patient manifests continuous overt signs of psychosis for at least six months and the manic symptoms are brief relative to the durations of the symptoms of schizophrenia. Schizoaffective disorder, manic type, is diagnosed if the criterion of 6 months of continuous psychotic illness is not met, but the patient exhibits more than 2 weeks of delusions and hallucinations in the absence of mood symptoms.

## 2. Personality Disorders

Psychotic disorders (i.e., schizophrenia) and psychotic symptoms (i.e., hallucinations and delusions) co-occur more significantly with the personality disorders of cluster A (paranoid, schizoid, and schizotypal) [11, 75]. Cluster A personality disorders are frequently referred to as 'schizophrenia spectrum disorders' and are thought to represent clinical variants of severe psychotic disorders [75] due to the presence of chronic, bizarre, or idiosyncratic thoughts or behaviors that are analogous to those of schizophrenia. Symptoms of reduced affective experience or expression (i.e., social withdrawal, anhedonia, and flat affect) are also comparatively similar to the negative symptoms of schizophrenia, but are experienced at a substantially lesser degree [4, 5, 76]. Thus, even though the typical features of schizophrenia are present, they are not of sufficient magnitude in either severity or degree of social /occupational impairment to constitute schizophrenia [11]. In the DSM-IV [1] paranoid personality disorder is defined as a pattern of suspiciousness whereby others' motives are interpreted as hostile or malevolent; schizoid personality disorder is defined as a pattern of social detachment or indifference with a restricted range of affect; and schizotypal personality disorder is defined as a pattern of cognitive and perceptual distortions, interpersonal deficits, and odd behavior.

Of the Cluster A personality disorders, schizotypal personality disorder presents a psychotic-like dimension that is more symptomatically and genetically related to schizophrenia [11, 77, 78, 79, 80, 81]. More specifically, schizotypal personality disorder patients have a profile of cognitive impairment and structural brain abnormalities, particularly in the temporal cortex, similar to that found in patients with schizophrenia [77, 78]. Schizotypal personality disorder, like schizophrenia, is set apart by the presence of positive symptoms (including ideas of reference, cognitive/perceptional distortions, and magical thinking) and negative symptoms (i.e., cognitive disorganization). Despite their phenol-menological similarity, however, the deficits of schizoaffective personality disorder patients are more circumscribed and selective compared to those of schizophrenia, which is characterized by severe, generalized deterioration across a variety of domains [81]. The more subtle cognitive impairments of patients with schizotypal personality disorder are reflected in their eccentricity and interpersonal disengagement but do not reach the threshold of overt psychosis [80]. The patient with schizotypal personality disorder may, as a result, appear suspicious and superstitious; complain of vague ideas of reference and have few social contacts; as well as report vague hallucinatory experiences, although none of these symptoms reaches the level of those required to meet the symptoms listed in criterion A of schizophrenia [11]. Thus, compared with schizophrenia, schizotypal personality disorder involves more subtle positive symptoms, whereas the negative symptoms of withdrawal and blunting may be as pronounced as those typical of schizophrenia [77, 79, 80]. Consequently, the severity of the positive signs is the primary factor distinguishing between schizotypal personality disorder and schizophrenia. Even though differentiation from schizophrenia may not be possible on the basis of cross-sectional data, the course of the illness generally enables a differential diagnosis: the patient with schizotypal personality disorder presents a stable clinical picture over time, whereas the patient with schizophrenia presents a clinical picture marked by progressive deterioration.

## DIFFERENTIATING AMONG PRIMARY PSYCHOTIC DISORDERS

### Schizophrenia

The DSM-IV [1] diagnostic criteria for schizophrenia require the presence of characteristic positive, negative, and/or disorganized symptoms (active phase symptoms) for a significant portion of time for the duration of at least one month. Impairment in psychosocial function and continuous signs of the disturbance must be evident for at least six months, including at least one month of active phase symptoms but may include periods of prodromal or residual symptoms. The longitudinal course of schizophrenia is classified as episodic, continuous, or single episode, with remission, residual symptoms, and prominent negative symptoms further specified. In addition, based on the constellation of symptoms present, subtypes are specified as paranoid, disorganized, catatonic, undifferentiated, and residual.

The symptoms of schizophrenia overlap with a wide range of other disorders that also may involve psychotic symptoms as defining features. Establishing a diagnosis of schizophrenia, therefore, requires particularly close consideration of other overlapping disorders of which psychosis is a defining symptom, including schizophreniform disorder; schizoaffective disorder; delusional disorder; brief psychotic disorder, and shared psychotic disorder [5, 15, 20, 60, 63]. These disorders share various features of schizophrenia, tend to be more common in the relatives of schizophrenia patients, and are treated with similar medications. These diagnoses are distinguished from one another by history obtained from the patient and collateral information about time, course, presence or absence of mood symptoms, and presence or absence of stressors. Nevertheless, the symptoms of schizophrenia are in general not sufficiently specific to make a definitive diagnosis, and it is important to follow the longitudinal clinical course in making a differential diagnosis [11, 16, 70].

### Schizophreniform Disorder

Schizophreniform disorder is a psychotic illness characterized by a symptomatic presentation that is equivalent to schizophrenia but without the chronic course of that disorder. To satisfy the diagnostic criteria for schizophreniform disorder, the patient must display psychotic symptoms sufficient to meet DSM-IV criteria for the active phase of schizophrenia, but returns to baseline functioning within six months [82]. Social or occupational dysfunction is not required to meet the diagnosis, although it may occur at some point in the illness [1]. Thus, schizophreniform disorder is likely to be the diagnosis in patients who have an abrupt, rather than an insidious onset and who have a good premorbid adjustment [11]. DSM-IV [1] describes two possible conditions for this diagnosis: (1) when an individual has recovered from their symptoms within the six-month period (the "pure" form of schizophreniform disorder) and (2) when six months have not yet elapsed since the original symptoms began, hence, the patient does not meet the diagnostic criteria for schizophrenia. For this latter condition, the term "provisional" is used. The distinction between schizophrenia and schizophreniform disorder is based on the presence of a prodromal syndrome [73], mode of onset, the shorter course of the disorder (less than six months for prodromal, active, and residual symptoms combined) and by the absence of deterioration from previous levels of functioning with a gradual return into the normal spectrum of behavior [11, 73, 82].

## Schizoaffective Disorder

Schizoaffective disorder (SAD) represents an association between schizophrenic and affective symptoms [66, 72, 83]. The disorder is characterized by persistent psychotic symptoms and episodic mood disturbances of the depressive, manic, and/or mixed type. For a diagnosis of schizoaffective disorder to be made, patients must, therefore, fulfill the criteria of a major mood (depressive, manic or mixed manic) episode and present symptoms of schizophrenia [67, 84]. Schizoaffective disorder differs from schizophrenia in that both affective symptoms and the features of schizophrenia are equally prominent and occur together [11, 67, 73, 82]. In contrast to schizophrenia, in schizoaffective disorder significant mood symptoms as stated in the DSM-IV [1] must be present for "a substantial portion of the total duration of the disturbance". The mood symptoms in schizophrenia, on the other hand, may have a duration that is brief comparative to the total duration of the disturbance; occur only during the prodromal or residual phases, or do not meet full criteria for a mood episode [11]. The delusions and hallucinations experienced in schizoaffective disorder, in addition, tend to be less bizarre and less severe than those typical of schizophrenia [73]. Patients with schizoaffective disorder may also have a relatively abrupt onset of illness and fail to meet the six-month-duration criterion for schizophrenia [11]. In addition patients with schizophrenia are more likely to exhibit loosening of associations and a blunted or inappropriate affect than patients with schizoaffective disorder [73]. Since it is the temporal relationship between psychotic and mood symptoms that distinguishes schizoaffective disorder from schizophrenic and mood disorders, the differential diagnosis requires access to longitudinal clinical data, which need to be assessed for temporal overlap and relative distribution over time [73, 82, 87].

## Delusional Disorder

The diagnosis of delusional disorder is made when the patient exhibits non-bizarre (plausible) delusions of at least one month's duration that cannot be attributed to other psychiatric disorders, and the patient's condition does not meet the criteria for schizophrenia or schizophreniform disorder [1, 4, 5, 63]. Delusions are categorized according to their content, and the predominant type (grandiose, erotomanic, jealous, persecutory, somatic, mixed, or unspecified) is specified when the diagnosis is made. Of the subtypes of delusional disorder, the persecutory type is the most common. Delusional disorder, persecutory subtype, may be particularly difficult to differentiate from the paranoid type of schizophrenia [11, 82]. A distinguishing characteristic of patients with delusional disorder is that impairment of functioning is limited to the circumscribed delusional system [1, 4, 22, 63] in which only a single, well-encapsulated, non-bizarre delusional system is present [11], and personality deterioration is minimal. Hallucinations, incoherence, disorganized behavior, fragmented delusions and negative symptoms are not included in the diagnosis of delusional disorder, as in typical schizophrenia [11]. When such symptoms occur in patients with delusional disorder, they are not prominent and their themes tend to be congruent with the delusional belief [22, 63], whereas in paranoid schizophrenia the delusions tend to be bizarre and are accompanied by other clinical features of schizophrenia, such as prominent auditory hallucinations, thought disorder, and deterioration of psychosocial functioning. Finally, age of onset of delusional disorder is later than for schizophrenia, often over 50 years [11].

### Brief Psychotic Disorder

A diagnosis of brief psychotic disorder requires the presence of delusions, hallucinations, disorganized speech or grossly disorganized or catatonic behavior, with duration of at least one day, but less than one month [1]. Symptoms are often dramatic and florid and are often thematically related to precipitating circumstances [82]. An acute onset with a rapid transition from a non-psychotic state to florid psychosis is characteristic of brief and acute psychosis, and an important element in the distinction from schizophrenia [84], which typically develops gradually. Prompt recovery with a full return to premorbid level of functioning within a month is dictated by definition.

### Shared Psychotic Disorder

In this disorder, an individual who is not otherwise psychotic acquires a significant other's established delusional beliefs in the context of a close relationship and often in isolation. The dominant partner ('primary case') is typically more seriously ill and suffers from a delusional psychosis, usually schizophrenia or delusional disorder [82]. A characteristic feature of shared psychotic disorder is a pattern of dominance and submission. Since the similarity of delusions between the two individuals is unique to shared psychotic disorder, the primary issue in the differential diagnosis is ruling out the presence of schizophrenia or other psychosis in the submissive partner ('secondary case') [82].

## CONCLUSION

Given the etiological heterogeneity of psychosis, the possibility of psychotic symptoms representing an underlying non-psychiatric condition should be considered from the outset. Even though primary psychiatric disorders with no identifiable biological etiology are often accountable for the advent of psychosis, neurological, medical, and substance-related disorders are often accompanied by symptoms of psychosis that are indistinguishable from those seen in primary psychiatric disorders. The differential diagnosis of psychosis must, therefore, be informed by a careful and thorough consideration of the multitude of secondary conditions that can account for the clinical presentation of the client under evaluation.

During the initial phase of assessment, when the clinical picture is commonly unclear, there is a heightened risk of failure to recognize the possibility of a secondary psychosis, or, to mistakenly attribute the symptoms of a non-psychiatric condition to a primary psychiatric disorder. Lack of familiarity with such complex clinical presentations can result in patients receiving less than optimal management and care, with sometimes irreversible consequences. This point in itself emphasizes the importance for clinicians to have a good knowledge of the differential diagnosis of psychosis.

Even though the diagnosis of psychosis is not always definitive, the diagnostic approach to psychosis that appears to be most accurate is one that encompasses an array of other (possibly correctable) factors that might explain the symptoms. One essential element in the differential diagnosis of the psychotic patient is the recognition of the distinctive constellation of features of specific neurological and medical conditions of which psychosis is a symptom and sign. In view of the fact that final diagnosis mainly depends on the exclusion of various plausible etiological factors, knowledge about these conditions and the precise circumstances under which psychotic symptoms present in their context, considerably increases diagnostic accuracy. Correspondingly, given that psychotic states are frequently secondary to the use of psychoactive substances, knowledge concerning the psychiatric effects of substances significantly facilitates the assessment procedure and, thus, the formulation of the appropriate treatment plan. The decision to request laboratory tests and neurological examinations is based on history, clinical presentation, and the need to rule out any possible organic cause of psychosis, whether a medical condition or substance abuse disorder. Findings obtained from these examinations constitute important elements in the differential diagnosis of psychosis in providing further evidence of a causative relationship between the symptoms and a specific condition. Finally, diagnostic decisions concerning primary psychiatric disorders require a longitudinal observation of the psychotic symptoms and the course of illness, with a particular focus on their overlap with other disorders that may present with psychotic features.

## References


[1] American Psychiatric Association, *Diagnostic and statistical manual of mental disorders,* 4th Ed., Text Revision. Washington, DC: Author, 2000.

[2] M. Burgy, "The concept of psychosis: Historical and phenomenological aspects," *Schizophrenia Bulletin,* vol. 34, pp.1200-1210, 2008.

[3] J. Parnas, J. Nordgaard, and S. Varga, "The concept of psychosis: A clinical and theoretical analysis," *Clinical Neuropsychiatry,* vol.7, no. 2, pp.32-37, 2010.

[4] O. Freundenreich and D.C. Goff, "Psychotic patients," in *Massachussetts general hospital handbook of general hospital psychiatry,* 6th Ed., T.A. Stern and G.L. Fricchione, Eds. Philadelphia: Saunders Elsevier, 2010, pp.119-132.

[5] M. J. Minzenberg, J. H. Yoon, and C. S. Carter, "Schizophrenia," in *The American psychiatric publishing textbook of psychiatry,* 5th Ed., R. E. Hales, S. C. Yudofsky, and G.O. Gabbard, Eds. Arlington, VA: American Psychiatric Publishing, Inc., 2008, pp.407-456.

[6] J.W. Newcomer, P. Fahnestock, and D. Haupt, "Schizophrenia and related disorders," in *Adult Psychiatry*, 2nd Ed., E. H. Rubin and C.F. Zorumski, Eds. Malden, M. A.: Blackwell Publishing, 2005, pp.195-220.

[7] R. Cardinal and E. Bullmore, *The diagnosis of psychosis.* New York, N. Y.: Cambridge University Press, 2011.

[8] O. Freudenreich, "Differential diagnosis of psychotic symptoms: Medical "mimics," *Psychiatric Times*, vol. 27, no. 12, pp. 56-61, 2010.

[9] J. Kulkarni, and P. Power, "Initial treatment of first-episode psychosis," in *The recognition and management of early psychosis: A preventive approach,* P.D. McGorry and H.D. Jackson, Eds., Cambridge: Cambridge University Press, 1999, pp.184-205.

[10] D.V. Jeste, J. A. Gladsjo, L. A. Lindamer, and J. P. Lacro, "Medical comorbidity in schizophrenia," *Schizophrenia Bulletin,* vol. 22, no. 3, pp. 413-430, 1996.

[11] D.D. Miller and S. K. Schultz, "Differential diagnosis of schizophrenia," in Schizophrenia: A new guide for clinicians, *J.G. Csernansky*, Ed. New York, N. Y.: Marcel Dekker, 2002, pp.53-68.

[12] S.H. Fatemi, "Schizophrenia," in *The medical basis of psychiatry*, 2nd Ed., S. H. Fatemi and P. J. Clayton, Eds., New York, N. Y.: Humana Press, 2008, pp.403-417.

[13] C. Caton, S. Samet, and D. S. Hasin, "When acute-stage psychosis and substance use co-occur: Differentiating substance-induced and primary psychotic disorders," *Journal of Psychiatric Practice,* vol.6, pp. 256-266, 2000.

[14] Center for Substance Abuse Treatment, Assessment and treatment of patients with coexisting mental illness and alcohol and other drug abuse. Rockville, M. D.: Substance Abuse and Mental Health Services Administration, US, 1994.

[15] P. Schwartz and M. Weathers, "The psychotic patient," in *Clinical manual of emergency psychiatry,* M. B. Riba and D. Ravindranath, Eds. Arlington, V. A.: American Psychiatric Publishing, Inc, 2010, pp.115-140.

[16] W.T. Carpenter and R. W. Buchanan, "Schizophrenia," *The New England Journal of Medicine,* vol. 330, no. 10, pp.681-690, 1994.

[17] R.N. Rosenthal and C. R. Miner, "Differential diagnosis of substance induced psychosis and schizophrenia in patients with substance use disorders," *Schizophrenia Bulletin,* vol. 23, no. 2, pp. 187-193, 1997.

[18] B.B. Sheitman, H. Lee, R. Strauss, and J. A. Liebman, "The evaluation and treatment of first-episode psychosis," *Schizophrenia Bulletin,*vol. 23, no. 4, pp. 653-661, 1997.

[19] E. Albon, A. Tsourapas, E. Frew, C. Davenport, F. Oyebode, S. Bayliss, T. Arvanitis, and C. Meads, "Structural neuroimaging in psychosis: a systematic review and economic evaluation," *Health Technology Assessment,* vol. 12, no. 18, pp.1-184, 2008.

[20] D.R. Combs and K. T. Mueser, "Schizophrenia," in *Adult psychopathology and diagnosis*, 5th Ed., M. Hersen, S. Turner, and D. Beidel, Eds. New York, N. Y.: John Wiley Press, 2007, pp.234-285.

[21] P. Byrne, "Managing the acute psychotic episode," *British Medical Journal,* vol. 334, no. 7595, pp.686-692, 2007.

[22] D.P. Moore, *Textbook of clinical neuropsychiatry*, 2nd Ed. London: Hodder Arnold, 2001.

[23] J.L. Levenson, "Psychiatric issues in endocrinology," *Primary Psychiatry,* vol. 13, no. 4, pp. 27-30, 2006.

[24] M. Bauer and P. C. Whybrow, "Thyroid hormone, brain, and behavior," in *Hormones, Brain and Behavior*, 5th Ed., D.W. Pfaff, A. P. Arnold, A. M. Etgen, S. E. Fahrbach, and R. T. Rubin, Eds. San Diego, C. A.: Academic Press, 2002, pp.239-264.

[25] J.G. Hanly, G. McCurdy, L. Fougere, J-A. Douglas, and K. Thompson, "Neuropsychiatric events in systemic lupus erythematosus: Attribution and clinical significance," *The Journal of Rheumatology,* vol. 31, pp. 2156-2162, 2004.

[26] A.J. Mitchell, Neuropsychiatry and behavioural neurology explained. Edinburgh, W. B.: Saunders, 2004.

[27] J. Payer, T. Petrovic, L. Baqi, L. Lisy, and P. Langer, "Hashimoto's encephalopathy and rare cases of hyperthyroidism," *Endocrine Regulations,* vol. 43, no. 4, pp. 169-178, 2009.

[28] S. Reading and J. Little, "Psychosis secondary to infections," in *The spectrum of psychotic disorders: Neurobiology, etiology, and pathogenesis,* D. Fujii and I. Ahmed, Eds. Cambridge, U. K.: Cambridge University Press, 2007, pp. 316-336.

[29] B. Elliott, and J .S. Shorvon, "Delusions, illusions and hallucinations in epilepsy: 1.Elementary phenomena," *Epilepsy Research,* vol. 85, no. 2-3, pp. 162-171, 2009.

[30] P.S. Sachdev, "Schizophrenia-like psychosis and epilepsy," in *The spectrum of psychotic disorders: Neurobiology, etiology, and pathogenesis,* D. Fujii and I. Ahmed, Eds. Cambridge, U. K.: Cambridge University Press, 2007, pp. 262-284.

[31] W. A. M. Swinkels, J. Kuyk, R. vanDyck, and Ph. Spinoven, "Psychiatric comorbidity in epilepsy," *Epilepsy and Behavior,* vol. 7, pp. 37-50, 2005.

[32] J.L. Cummings, and B. L. Miller, "Visual hallucinations: Clinical occurrence and use in differential diagnosis," *Western Journal of Medicine,* vol. 146, pp. 46-51, 1987.

[33] T. Dolenc and T. Rummans, "Psychosis in patients with brain tumors," in *The spectrum of psychotic disorders: Neurobiology, etiology, and pathogenesis,* D. Fujii and I. Ahmed, Eds. Cambridge, U. K.: Cambridge University Press, 2007, pp. 302-315.

[34] M. Hopwood and L-M. Lim, "Brain tumors," in *Secondary schizophrenia,* P.S. Sachdev and M.S. Keshavan, Eds. Cambridge, UK: Cambridge University Press, 2010, pp.263-272.

[35] P.S. Sachdev, "Schizophrenia-like psychosis and traumatic brain injury," in *Secondary schizophrenia,* P.S. Sachdev and M.S. Keshavan, Eds. Cambridge, UK: Cambridge University Press, 2010, pp.186-196.

[36] C. Corcoran, and D. Malaspina, "Traumatic brain injury as a risk factor for schizophrenia," *Current Psychiatry Reviews,* vol. 3, no. 1, pp. 25-32, 2007.

[37] D. Fujii, and I. Ahmed, "Characteristics of psychotic disorder due to traumatic brain injury: An analysis of case studies in the literature," *The Journal of Neuropsychiatry and Clinical Neurosciences,* vol. 14, pp. 130-140, 2002.

[38] D. Fujii, I. Ahmed, and E. Hishinuma, "A neuropsychological comparison of psychotic disorder following traumatic brain injury, traumatic brain injury without psychotic disorder, and schizophrenia," *Journal of Neuropsychiatry and Clinical Neuroscience,* vol. 16, pp. 306-314, 2004.

[39] P.I. Rosebush, R. Anglin, and M. Mazurek, "Psychosis associated with leukodystrophies," in *Secondary schizophrenia,* P.S. Sachdev and M. S. Keshavan, Eds. Cambridge, UK: Cambridge University Press, 2010, pp.241-256.

[40] A. Feinstein, "Demyelinating disease and psychosis," in *Secondary schizophrenia,* P. S. Sachdev and M. S. Keshavan, Eds. Cambridge, UK: Cambridge University Press, 2010, pp.273-278.

[41] M. Walterfang and D. Velakoulis, "Storage disorders and psychosis," in *Secondary schizophrenia,* P. S. Sachdev and M. S. Keshavan, Eds. Cambridge, UK: Cambridge University Press, 2010, pp.214-228.

[42] E.C. Lauterbach and L. Lester-Burns, "Wilson's disease," in *Secondary schizophrenia,* P.S. Sachdev and M.S. Keshavan, Eds. Cambridge, UK: Cambridge University Press, 2010, pp.337-347.

[43] H.A. Ring, and J. Serra-Mestres, "Neuropsychiatry of the basal ganglia," *Journal of Neurology, Neurosurgery and Psychiatry,* vol. 72, pp. 12-21, 2002.

[44] K. Burns and H. Brodaty, "Fahr's disease and psychosis," in *Secondary schizophrenia,* P.S. Sachdev and M.S. Keshavan, Eds. Cambridge, UK: Cambridge University Press, 2010, pp.358-368.

[45] L. Marsh, "Psychosis in Parkinson's disease," *Primary Psychiatry,* vol. 12, no. 7, pp. 56-62, 2005.

[46] B. Ravina, K. Marder, H.H. Fernandez, J.H. Friedman, W. McDonald, D. Murphy, D. Aarsland, D. Babcock, J. Cummings, J. Endincott, S. Factor, W. Galpern, A. Lees, L. Marsh, M. Stacy, K. Gwinn-Hardy, V. Voon, and C. Goetz, "Diagnostic criteria for psychosis in Parkinson's disease: Reports of an NINDS, NIMH work group," *Movement Disorders,*vol. 22, no. 8, pp. 1061-1068, 2007.

[47] D. Weintraub and H.I. Hurtig, "Presentation and management of psychosis in Parkinson's disease and dementia with Lewy bodies," *American Journal of Psychiatry,*vol. 164, no. 10, pp. 1491-1498, 2007.

[48] E.S. Molho and S.A. Factor, "Psychosis," in *Parkinson's disease and nonmotor dysfunction,* R.F. Pfeiffer and I. Bodis-Wollner, Eds. Totowa, N.J.: Humana Press, 2005, pp.49-74.

[49] T.R. Kosten, and D.M. Ziedonis, "Substance abuse and schizophrenia," *Schizophrenia Bulletin,*vol. 23, no. 2, pp. 181-186, 1997.

[50] J. Thirthalli, V. Benegal, and B.N. Gangadhar, "Substance-induced psychosis: An overview," in *Secondary schizophrenia,* P.S. Sachdev and M.S. Keshavan, Eds. Cambridge, UK: Cambridge University Press, 2010, pp.112-126.

[51] Hausmann, and W.W. Fleischhacker, "Differential diagnosis of depressed mood in patients with schizophrenia: a diagnostic algorithm based on a review," *Acta Psychiatrica Scandinavica,* vol. 106, no. 2, pp. 83-96, 2002.

[52] G.A. Juhnke, Substance abuse assessment and diagnosis: A comprehensive guide for counselors and helping professionals. New York, N.Y.: Brunner-Routledge, 2002.

[53] J. Thirthalli and V. Benegal, "Psychosis among substance users," *Current Opinion in Psychiatry,* vol. 19, pp. 239-245, 2006.

[54] C. Brems and M.E. Johnson, "Clinical implications of the co-occurrence of substance use and other psychiatric disorders," *Professional Psychology: Research and Practice,*vol. 28, no. 5, pp. 437-447, 1997.

[55] M. Farrell, A. Boys, P. Bebbington, T. Brugha, J. Coid, R. Jenkins, G. Lewis, H. Meltzer, J. Marsden, N. Singleton, and C. Taylor, "Psychosis and drug dependence: results from a national survey of prisoners," *British Journal of Psychiatry,*vol. 181, pp. 393-398, 2002.

[56] M.H. Leamon, T.M. Wright, and H. Myrick, "Substance-related disorders," in *The American psychiatric publishing textbook of psychiatry,* R.E. Hales, S.C. Yudofsky, and G.O. Gabbard, Eds. Arlington, VA: American Psychiatric Publishing, Inc., 2008, pp. 365-406.

[57] C.E. Lewis, "Impact of substance abuse and dependence on patients with schizophrenia," in *Schizophrenia: A new guide for clinicians,* J.G. Csernansky, Ed. New York, N.Y.: Marcel Dekker, 2002, pp.267-284.

[58] L.M. Caton, R.E. Drake, D.S. Hasin, B. Dominguez, P.E. Shrout, S. Samet, and B. Schanzer, "Differences between early-phase psychotic disorders with concurrent substance abuse and substance-induced psychoses," *Archives of General Psychiatry,* vol. 62, no. 2, pp. 137-145, 2005.

[59] S.I. Cohen, "Overdiagnosis of schizophrenia: Role of alcohol and drug misuse," *The Lancet,* vol. 346, pp. 1541-1542, 1995.

[60] P.F. Buckley, B.J. Miller, D.S. Lehrer, and D.J. Castle, "Psychiatric comorbidities and schizophrenia," *Schizophrenia Bulletin,*vol. 35, no. 2, pp. 383-402, 2009.

[61] DeJong, R. Giel, C.J. Sboff, and D. Wiersma, "Relationships between symptomatology and social disability," *Social Psychiatry,*vol. 21, pp.200-205, 1986.

[62] B.J. Rounsaville, "DSM-V research agenda: Substance abuse/psychosis comorbidity," *Schizophrenia Bulletin,* vol. 23, no. 4, pp. 947-952, 2007.

[63] Munro, Delusional disorder: paranoia and related illnesses. Cambridge, UK: Cambridge University Press, 1999.

[64] J.R. Sands and M. Harrow, "Depression during the longitudinal course of schizophrenia," *Schizophrenia Bulletin,*vol. 25, no. 1, pp.157-171, 1999.

[65] C. Mulholland and S. Cooper, "The symptom of depression in schizophrenia and its management," *Advances in Psychiatric Treatment,* vol. 6, pp. 169-177, 2000.

[66] S.G. Siris, "Depression in schizophrenia: Perspective in the era of "atypical" antipsychotic agents," *American Journal of Psychiatry,* vol. 157, pp. 1379-1389, 2000.

[67] H. S. Akiskal, "Mood disturbances," in *The medical basis of psychiatry,* S.H. Fatemi and P.J. Clayton, Eds., New York, N.Y.: Humana Press, 2008, pp. 403-417.

[68] M.A. Escamilla, "Diagnosis and treatment of mood disorders that co-occur with schizophrenia," *Psychiatric Services,* vol. 52, no. 7, pp.911-919, 2001.

[69] C.M. Swartz and E. Shorter, *Psychotic depression.* New York, N.Y.: Cambridge University Press, 2007.

[70] E. Ivleva, G. Thaker, and C.A. Tamminga, "Comparing genes and phenomenology in the major psychoses: Schizophrenia and bipolar 1 disorder," *Schizophrenia Bulletin,* vol. 34, no. 4, pp. 734-742, 2008.

[71] A. Marneros, "The schizoaffective phenomenon: the state of the art," *Acta Psychiatrica Scandinavica,*vol. 108, suppl. 418, pp. 29-33, 2003.

[72] E. Cheniaux, J. Landeira-Fernandez, L. Lessa Telles, J.L. Lessa, A. Dias, T. Duncan, and M. Versiani, "Does schizoaffective disorder really exist? A systematic review of the studies that compared schizoaffective disorder with schizophrenia or mood disorders," *Journal of Affective Disorders,* vol. 106, no. 3, pp. 209-217, 2008.

[73] W. Coryell, "Schizoaffective and schizophreniform disorders," in *The medical basis of psychiatry*, 2nd Ed., S.H. Fatemi and P.J. Clayton, Eds., New York, N.Y.: Humana Press, 2008, pp.109-124.

[74] V. Kusumakar, D.J. Bond, and L.N. Yatham, "Diagnosis and treatment of mania and hypomania," in *Bipolar disorder : A clinician's guide to treatment management*, 2nd ed., L.N. Yatham and V. Kusumakar, Eds. New York, N.Y.: Routledge, 2009, pp. 1-19.

[75] R.T. Dolan-Sewell, R.F. Krueger, and M.T. Shea, "Co-occurrence with syndrome disorders," in *Handbook of personality disorders,* W.J. Livesley, Ed. New York, N.Y.: Guilford, 2001, pp.84-106.

[76] A.E. Skodol, "Manifestations, clinical diagnosis, and comorbidity," in *The American psychiatric publishing textbook of personality disorders,* J.M. Oldham, A.E. Skodol, and D.S. Bender, Eds. Washington, DC: American Psychiatric Publishing, 2005, pp.57-88.

[77] E.F. Coccaro and L.J. Siever, "Neurobiology," in *The American psychiatric publishing textbook of personality disorders,* J.M. Oldham, A.E. Skodol, and D.S. Bender, Eds. Washington, DC: American Psychiatric Publishing, 2005, pp.155-170.

[78] M.S. Keshavan, H.S. Duggal, G. Veergandham, N.M. McLaughlin, D.M. Montrose, G.L. Haas, and N.R. Schooler, "Personality dimensions in first-episode psychoses," *American Journal of Psychiatry,* vol. 162, pp. 102-109, 2005.

[79] L. Sperry, *Handbook of diagnosis and treatment of DSM-IV-TR personality disorders*, 2nd Ed., New York, N.Y.: Brunner-Routledge, 2003.

[80] E.F. Walker and S. Gale, "Neurodevelopmental processes in schizophrenia and schizotypal personality disorder," in *Schizotypal personality,* A. Raine, T. Lencz, and S.A. Mednick, Eds., New York, N. Y.: Cambridge University Press, 1995, pp. 56-78.

[81] L. J. Siever and K.L. Davis, "The pathophysiology of the schizophrenic disorders: Perspectives from the spectrum," *American Journal of Psychiatry,* pp.398-413.

[82] E.L. Merrin, "Delusional and other psychotic disorders," in *Review of general psychiatry,* 5th Ed., H.H. Goldman, Ed. McGraw Hill, 2000, pp. 251-263.

[83] S. Heckers, "Is schizoaffective disorder a useful diagnosis?" *Current Psychiatry Reports,* vol. 11, no. 4, pp. 332-337, 2009.

[84] Marneros, and F. Pillman, Acute and transient psychoses. Cambridge, UK: Cambridge University press, 2004.

In: Psychosis: Causes, Diagnosis and Treatment
Editor: Xenia Anastassiou-Hadjicharalambous
ISBN: 978-1-62081-516-8


*Chapter 2*

# PAEDIATRIC PSYCHOSIS: DIAGNOSIS, DEVELOPMENTAL TRAJECTORIES, CAUSES AND TREATMENT

***Xenia Anastassiou-Hadjicharalambous[1]*** *
***and Cecilia Essau[2]***

[1]Psychology Program, University of Nicosia, Nicosia, Cyprus
[2]Centre for Applied Research and Assessment in Child and Adolescent Wellbeing (CARACAW), School of Human and Life Sciences, Roehampton University, London, UK

## ABSTRACT

The term Psychosis refers to an abnormal condition of the mind that is characterized by disruptions in thinking and is accompanied by delusions and hallucinations. The purpose of the current chapter is to review the up to date state of empirical literature on Pediatric Psychosis as well as identify areas for future direction of research on an understudied disorder that is cumbersome to diagnose, differentiate and treat. The chapter begins with a brief overview of the diagnostic and associated features of the disorder and the factors implicated in making the diagnosis elusive and at times inaccurate. It continues with the differential diagnoses that are often implicated in the misdiagnosis of psychotic symptomatology. The next section covers the sparse epidemiological data on the prevalence followed by the factors implicated in the aetiology of the disorder. The developmental considerations of the disorder are covered next. The final section reports on the evidence-based status of the treatment approaches for Paediatric Psychosis and identifies future directions of research.

* E-mail: *hadjicharalambous.x@unic.ac.cy.*

# INTRODUCTION

Paediatric Psychosis (deriving from the Greek ψυχή "psyche", for soul or mind and -οσις "-osis", for abnormal condition) is a clinical condition characterized by disrupted thinking and accompanied by delusions[1] and hallucinations[2]. The child has no insight into the pathological nature of the hallucinations [1].

Historically, the definition of Psychosis in children has been surrounded by vagueness, confusion and debate primarily because of the developmentally appropriate role of imagination in the typically developing child. Paediatric Psychosis was originally conceptualized as part of the spectrum of the Pervasive Developmental Disorders. Gradually, by 1980 some consensus was reached that the essential features of Psychosis are essentially the same across age. In the most recent revision of Diagnostic and Statistical Manual of Mental Disorders, 4th edition, Text Revision (DSM-IV-TR) [1], the symptomatology of Paediatric Psychosis does not differ from the symptomatology of adult psychosis. This symptomatology includes disorganized or disturbed thought form and thought content, disorganized speech, disorganized or catatonic behaviour, flat affect, poverty of speech and lack of goal directed behaviour[1].

# CLINICAL FEATURES, DIAGNOSIS AND ASSESSMENT

The diagnosis of paediatric Psychotic Disorders remains an unresolved ongoing debate. In contrast to the diagnosis of adult Psychotic Disorders which is relatively reliable since their symptomatology and phenomenology are well established, in children and particularly the younger ones the diagnosis is elusive. The developmentally appropriate intrusions of fantasy for the young children along with the developing cognitive abilities make the diagnosis difficult to make and often inaccurate.

## Clinical Features of Psychotic Disorders

The term "psychotic" describes a clinical condition that is characterized by inability to evaluate the accuracy of one's thoughts and perceptions. Paediatric Psychotic Disorders in line with the adulthood onset Psychotic Disorders are characterized by the so called positive and negative symptoms. Positive symptoms are present in the psychotic patient and non-present in the non- patient. Negative symptoms describe normal functions that are present in the non- patient but absent in the psychotic patient. A psychotic symptom or clusters of symptoms are connected to a specific Psychotic Disorder as defined by a certain number of symptoms occurring over a specific duration of time with evident impairment. Delusions (false beliefs) and prominent hallucinations (erroneous perceptions) are usually considered as the basis of diagnosis of Psychotic Disorders [1].

---

[1] Illusions are false beliefs that typically involve a misinterpretation of perceptions or experiences.

[2] hallucinations may occur in any sensory modality (i.e. auditory, visual etc). Auditory hallucinations are the most common and they are experienced as voices that are perceived as distinct from the individual's own thoughts.

The DSM includes a section of specific Psychotic Disorders that are characterised by psychotic symptoms as prominent aspect of their presentation [1]. This section includes Schizophrenia, Schziphreniform Disorder, Delusional Disorder, Shared Psychotic Disorder, Substance Induced Psychotic Disorder, Brief Psychotic Disorder, Scizopaffective Disorder, Psychotic Disorder due to a General Medical Condition, and Psychotic Disorder Not Otherwise Spedified [1].

The Childhood-Onset Schizophrenia is characterized by the positive symptoms of gross disturbance of thought process or thought content, whereas delusions most possibly appear (or become apparent) with increasing age [2]. Negative symptoms in the schizophrenic child include flat affect, and paucity of speech and thought [3]. Younger children with Childhood-Onset Schizophrenia are reported to have fewer delusions and catatonic symptoms, but they exhibit hallucinations, disordered thought process and flattened affect [4]. For diagnostic purposes symptoms have to be present for a significant amount of time during one month with some characteristics of the disorder persisting for over 6 months [1]. This duration criteria is particularly important in the diagnosis of schizophrenia in childhood given the transient delusional or hallucinatory characteristics that the children could potentially present [5]. Further for diagnostic purposes the psychotic symptoms need to be accompanied by social dysfunction and should not be attributable to another disorder or a general medical condition [1]. For those children that they have previously been diagnosed with a Pervasive Developmental Disorder the additional diagnosis of Schizophrenia is given when delusions and/or hallucinations are present for one month [1].

The Schizophreniform Disorder is characterised by features that are identical to Schizophrenia apart from the Duration criterion. The Duration criterion for the diagnosis of the Schizophreniform Disorder is determined by the presence of psychotic symptomatology for a period of less than 6 months and more than 2 weeks (including prodromal, active and residual phases) [5].

Duration criterion is also the one that determines the diagnosis of Brief Psychotic Disorder which is characterised by the presence of psychotic features for more than a day and less than a month [1]. But given the transient delusional or hallucinatory characteristics that the children could potentially present [5] this disorder is considered of little importance for consideration in childhood diagnosis.

Of little clinical importance for consideration in childhood diagnosis are also considered the Delusional Disorder which is characterized by at least 1 month of non-bizarre delusions without other characteristics of Schizophrenia, the Shared Psychotic Disorder which is presented by delusions that are influenced by another individual who has longer-term delusions of similar content and the Substance-induced Psychotic Disorder which is considered to be the physiological consequent of a medical condition [5].

The Schizoaffective Disorder is characterized by positive and negative symptoms as well as symptoms of a Major Depressive Episode, a Manic Episode, or a Mixed Episode [1]. These clusters of symptoms and their interaction often make the diagnosis cumbersome. Particularly in the initial stages of Schizoaffective Disorder in children psychotic symptoms may be overshadowed by the presence of mood symptoms [2]. According to the DSM-IV the phase of the illness with psychotic symptoms only must last at least 2 weeks to distinguish Schizoaffective Disorder from a Mood Disorder with psychotic features. During these 2 weeks mood symptoms may be present but they are non-prominent. Often it is troublesome to make a decision of where to draw the line of non-prominent mood symptoms. Repeated observations and a combination of a set of multiple sources of information are necessary for a precise diagnosis [1].

The Psychotic Disorder Not Otherwise Specified is utilised to encompass characterized psychotic symptomatology for which there is not adequate information that would allow diagnosis of another Psychotic Disorder, for which there is contradictory information or do not meet full criteria for a specific psychotic disorder [1]. Despite that the Psychotic Disorder Not Otherwise Specified is included in the DSM its validity has been questioned and the reliable diagnosis of psychosis during childhood at present remains cumbersome.

The reliable diagnosis of Psychotic Disorders is further confounded by the fact that apart from the specific Psychotic Disorders that are included in the DSM section of Psychotic Disorders (on the basis of having psychotic symptoms as prominent aspect of their presentation) there is a series of other disorders that may present with psychotic symptoms as associated features [1] (e.g., Major Depressive Disorder with Psychotic Features, Bipolar Disorder with Psychotic Features, Substance-Induced Delirium. These Disorders do not have psychosis as their prominent feature, but, they may often be present with psychotic symptoms as associate features and in effect confound the diagnosis.

## Differential Diagnoses

Misdiagnosis of Paediatric Psychosis is common. For example an acute onset manic episode could be erroneously diagnosed as Schizophrenia, as hallucinations and delusions may be evident (usually mood congruent). Psychotic symptomatology in youngsters need to be differentiated against anticipatory anxiety related to Anxiety Disorders, to obsessions related to Obsessive-Compulsive Disorder, rumination related to Depression, perseverative thoughts related to Developmental Disorders, disorganized behaviour related to Attention-Deficit/Hyperactivity Disorder (ADHD), disorganised speech related to Communication Disorders [1]. Additionally, language and cognitive deficits related to mental retardation may erroneously be perceived as indicative of Psychosis in non-psychotic children [2]. Nonspecific symptoms, such as anxiety, distractibility, and irritability, may precede a psychotic symptom and confound the diagnosis. Furhemore temporal lobe epilepsy despite being quite elusive in its detection needs to be considered in differential diagnosis of Psychotic Disorders [6].

In adolescence, psychotic symptomatology could be associated with, or be secondary to a variety of other disorders such as epilepsy, substance abuse, mood disorders [7, 8] For instance affective psychosis (related to mood disorders), dissociative psychosis (i.e. related to Post Traumatic Stress Disorder – PTSD, or Dissociative Identity Disorder) or psychosis that is secondary to substance abuse is commonly seen in clinical practice [6] and can create diagnostic confusion. In effect, quite often in clinical practice the differential diagnosis of Psychotic Disorders is hard to be anticipated. For example the differentiation between Psychotic Disorders and Bipolar I Disorder (especially in adolescence is particularly cumbersome since these disorders may share a series of presenting symptoms such as grandiose and persecutory delusions, agitation, irritability and catatonic symptoms [1]. In such cases, features that discriminate between psychotic disorders and Bipolar I need to be considered. For instance, in contrast to Bipolar I Disorder, the Psychotic Disorders are characterised by periods of psychotic symptoms that occur in the absence of prominent mood symptoms [1]. On the other hand, manic and depressive symptoms could be present in Schizophrenia, Delusional Disorder and Psychotic Disorder Not Otherwishe Specified but they are rarely adequate (in terms of duration and pervasiveness) for diagnosis of a Manic or a Major Depressive Episode [1]. Apart from the accompanying prominent symptoms other parameters, such as appearance and developmental course of the displayed symptomatology, as well as family history can assist in the differential diagnosis.

## Associated Features

There is scarce empirical evidence that address plausible associated features of Paediatric Psychotic Disorders. Several empirical investigations have linked Paediatric Schizophrenia with gross and fine motor delays, hypotonia, poor coordination, sensory integration difficulties, and significant delays and dysfunctions in language development [9] that designate developmental abnormalities in language processes. Schizophrenic youngsters further display symptoms that are typically linked with Pervasive Developmental Disorders. These symptoms include stereotypic behaviour, such as hand flapping, preservative smelling and touching [2]. Further, children with Childhood-Onset Schizophrenia have shown clinical features that are associated with Attention Deficit Hyperactivity Disorder such as attention problems, distractibility, and other dysfunctions of executive functioning [10]. Further, children with Childhood-Onset Schizophrenia show diminished scores on IQ tests relative to the typically developing children [11]. However, neurocognitive studies reveal that these lower IQ scores may primarily be reflective of neurocognitive deficits [12].Youngsters with Paediatric Schizophrenia have shown neurobiological abnormalities such as reduced volume of the brain (frontal, temporal-limbic, thalamus, cerebellum), altered neuronal connections, enlarged ventricles, reduced brain activity, lower reaction of autonomic nervous system and neurotransmitter dysfunction (dopamine, serotonin, GABA, glutamate) [13].

Socioemotional deficits and characteristics of impaired communication such as withdrawal, isolation ineptness, moodiness, flat affect and absence of social interest have also been documented in schizophrenic samples of children [14].

While the few empirical studies that investigated associated features of paediatric psychoses focused on Schizophrenia there is scarce data that documented developmental delays and cognitive deficits (e.g. attention, learning, abstraction) in children with other psychotic disorders such as in Psychotic Disorder Not Otherwise Specified [15]. These data might be suggestive of the unidimentionality of the Psychotic Spectrum Disorders. However, the scarcity of the empirical evidence does not allow conclusions to be drawn with confidence.

Further the most empirical evidence derives from cross-sectional designs and in effect inferences of causality cannot be assumed. The development of the associated features of Psychotic Spectrum Disorders need to be studied from the very initial stages of the child's development and require explicit longitudinal validation.

## Assessment

Prior to diagnosis of psychosis, a comprehensive neurological examination is obligatory due to the fact that medical and neurological conditions could potentially mimic Psychotic Spectrum disorders.

Upon completion of medical and neurological examination, diagnosis of psychosis is based on multifaceted assessment encompassing a structured diagnostic interview such as the Schedule for Affective Disorders for School-Aged children (K-SADS) [16]. The structured diagnostic interview is further supplemented by a series of other assessments encompassing historical information, cognitive, psychological, behavioural and syndrome-specific assessments.

Turning first to historical information this includes information on pregnancy complications, developmental milestones, age of onset and course of symptomatology, and family history (including physical and mental health of extended family). Beyond historical information cognitive assessment includes IQ testing which has been considered a vital element of cognitive evaluation. IQ scores are expected to drop following onset of schizophrenia [17]. Empirical evidence has indeed shown negative correlation between IQ scores and schizophrenic symptomatology. For instance the FIQ (Full Scale IQ), VIQ (Comprehension and Knowledge of Verbal Concepts, and FFD (Freedom from Distractibility – i.e. later renamed as working memory in the WAIS -III) scales of WISC-III (Wechsler Intelligence Scale for Children – Third Edition), have been found to be negatively correlated with the number of loose associations [18]. Further IQ scores have been reported to be negatively correlated with negative symptoms [19]. Correlational data however need to be interpreted with caution since they allow no inferences of causality links.

Beyond intellectual deficits children with psychosis show deficits in adaptive functioning in areas such as social interaction, self-care and communication. The administration of an adaptive behaviour scale such as the Vineland Adaptive Scale (VABS) [20] or the Adaptive Behaviour Evaluation Scale (ABES) [21] provides useful information with respect to the specific adaptive skill deficit that would need to be addressed in the intervention plan.

Projective testing provides the clinician vital information about thought and perceptual processes and determine the nature of the thought disorder that potentially affects the psychotic child. The most commonly used projective test for evaluation of the nature of thought processes of psychotic children is the Thematic Apperception Test [22] and the Rorschach Test [23]. Incoherent, disorganized responses to projective testing are indicative of a thought disorder. Psychotic diagnosis however should not be ruled out on the basis of projective testing in isolation [24]. Some psychotic children are able to sustain an organized presentation during testing (especially if they are not stressed by the testing conditions) while others present with fluctuation of the degree of thought disorder depending whether they have a psychotic episode during testing. When they are not in a psychotic episode they are likely to give appropriate responses while when during a psychotic episode they will give a substantial number of awkward responses (e.g. combination of inappropriate images into a single whole – i.e. snake with 6 legs) that are assumed to reflect a breakdown in the thinking process [24]

The Kiddie Formal Thought Disorder Rating Scale [25] is an observer-rating scale of four types of thought disorder derived from DSM: illogical thinking, loose association, incoherence, and poverty of content of speech. It is administered by playing the Kiddie Formal Thought Disorder Story Game [25] with the child and then coding the child's answers to the game. The Kiddie Formal Thought Disorder Story Game has three parts: In the first part, the child listens to an audiotaped story and then s/he is required to repeat the story and answer questions that are based on the story. In the second part, the child is asked to create a story based on one of four topics. The third part is the same with the first part. The child's responses are videotaped for later scoring [26].The child's responses to the three parts of the story game are coded into the four thought disorder categories on the basis of operational definitions and illustrations for each category. A total score is derived by summing the category scores. Interrater reliability for the K-FTDS is considered satisfactory [26]. Illogical thinking, loose association, and total scores have been reported to discriminate between psychotic and non-psychotic samples [25]. Clinically, the K-FTDS is of limited utility because of its time-consuming coding procedure.

With respect to behavioural assessment, the Thought problems, Somatic Complains, and Withdrawal subscales of the Achenbach Child Behaviour Checklist CBCL) [27] the Teachers Report Forms (TRF) [28] and the Youth Self Reports [27] are likely to be elevated in the psychotic child and youth. The elevation of these subscales items however are not a sole characteristic of psychotic spectrum disorders but they are likely to be reflective of other psychiatric diagnoses as well and consequently caution should be exercised since no diagnostic specificity to psychoses applies to these elevated subscales. Further, none of the Achenbach scales addresses psychotic symptomatology.

A further behavioural assessment commonly used in the assessment of the psychotic child is the Behaviour Assessment System for Children (BASC) [29]. The BASC Atypicality Subscale includes items taping hallucinations, loss of control and loss of touch with reality. These items are consistent with the positive symptoms of Schizophrenia. Nonetheless, the BASC Atypicality Subscale also includes items that are reflective of other disorders such as Pervasive Developmental Disorders. Consequently, elevated scores on the BASC Atypicality Subscale should not be considers as indicator of only psychotic symptoms but also as indicative of other unusual behaviours as well. The BASC Withdrawal, Leadership and Social Skills Subscales consist of items indicative of the negative symptoms of schizophrenia as well as with items indicative of the social maladjustment characteristic of the disorder.

The Child Symptom Inventory - 4 (CSI-4) [30, 31] and the Adolescent Symptom Inventory (ASI-4)- [32, 33] parent and teacher report) include subsets of items that are intended to tap schizophrenic symptomatology as reflected in DSM-IV. The CSI-4 also includes subscales for depressive symptomatology, Pervasive Developmental Disorders, as well as anxiety symptomatology. The ASI-4 includes subscales for Depressive Disorders, Anxiety Disorders, Schizoid Personality Bipolar Disorder and Substance Abuse. Given the broad coverage of alternative symptomatology that is corresponsive to DSM symptomatology is particularly useful in determining alternative diagnosis or comorbit features to be probed in the structures interview.

The Personality Inventory for Youth (PIY) [34] provides useful insight into the youngsters' self reported symptomatology. On the PIY youngsters with Psychotic Spectrum Disorders show elevated Reality Distortion Subscale, Illusions and Hallucinations Subscale. The Social Withdrawal and Social Skills Deficits Scales provide information about social functioning and negative symptoms of Schizophrenia. More specifically the Isolation Subscale of the Social Withdrawal Scale indicates symptoms that are characteristic of withdrawal and isolation when the youngster displays negative symptoms of Psychosis.

Despite the variety of instruments that are available to the clinician for the multifaceted assessment of psychotic symptomatology the diagnosis of Paediatric Psychosis remains cumbersome, given that they are intertwined with the child's cognitive and socioemotional development. For instance the assessment of thought disorder is confounded by the young child's language skills. Additionally reported hallucinations are not always indicative of psychosis. Non-psychotic children report seeing ghosts or hearing voices [35, 36, 37]. These hallucinations do not designate symptomatology of psychosis.

While diagnosis of psychosis is young children is particularly troublesome it gets less problematic in adolescents whose thinking process gradually with age becomes more adult-like. Although even in adolescents reported hallucinations have not always shown to be indicative of fully-blown psychosis [38, 36] Consequently, the assessment and diagnostic findings of psychosis in children and adolescents should be treated with particular caution.

## EPIDEMIOLOGY

The epidemiology of Paediatric Psychotic Spectrum Disorders is still unclear. Sparse epidemiological data suggest that Paediatric Psychosis is rare. These epidemiological data provide estimates of paediatric Schizophrenia to be no more than 1% [39]. Schizophrenia with onset during middle to late adolescence is reported to be in the range of 0.5 to 1.5% [1]. Other reports provide even lower prevalence by suggesting that Schizophrenia in general population is around 1%. Among this 1% of individuals who develop Schizophrenia only 1% have age of onset prior to age 10 and another 4% have onset prior to age 15 [39]. In this variance on prevalence estimates, factors such as age, gender, race, ethnicity, assessment instruments, methods of combination of data between parent reports and child reports, as well as the employed diagnostic criteria and time could potentiality be implicated. With respect to age several investigations for instance report that Psychosis is diagnosed during adolescence rather than earlier [39]. This finding however does not necessarily mean that prevalence is higher in adolescence. It might be that many children with Psychosis are not referred until the disorder shows more adult-like features, or deteriorates. Further, as discussed above the developmentally appropriate fantasies in children makes the diagnosis in childhood elusive.

As far as gender is concerned, most empirical investigations report male-to-female ratio averaging 1.5-2:1. With respect to ethnic origin effects, certain population groups, for instance second generation African carrebians living in UK have been reported to have a far higher incidence [1]. However, the data are mixed and they may reflect biases deriving on overreliance on hospital records and they may not reflect community based samples. Further, birth cohort studies showed several geographical and historical variations in prevalence. For instance, higher risk has been reported in lower socioeconomic classes and in urban-born individuals versus rural-born individuals [40]. Also, lower prevalence has been reported for later-born versus earlier born birth cohorts [1]. Again most of these data sets concern Schizophrenia rather than the wider spectrum of Psychotic Disorders. The prevalence of this wider spectrum of Psychotic Disorders is even more difficult to be determined given the rarity of the diagnosis of these disorders and the diagnostic confusion with which they are characterised. For instance, the Psychotic Disorder Not Otherwise Specified in children is hard to determine, due to the vagueness of the term and the surrounded controversy over its validity.

As far as diagnostic criteria and time is concerned, it seems that prevalence rates are differentiated slightly with time as well as with the refinements in the diagnostic criteria. It seems that across time, prevalence rates will be more clearly set as our knowledge about childhood onset psychosis increases, as well as diagnostic criteria become more sensitive to the children's unique developmental characteristics. Further, it is possible that prevalence rates of Psychotic Spectrum Disorders are confounded by the diagnostic confusion that results in misdiagnosis of Psychosis.

A notable point in relation to prevalence rates and future direction of research is that the data primarily derive from Caucasian and African-American children. Further investigations are needed to look into prevalence rates across other cultures and factors implicated in the possible variance in prevalence rates across these cultures. Beyond cultural effects, developmental epidemiological studies are needed to determine prevalence patterns, as well as factors implicated in prevalence across developmental stages.

## AETIOLOGY

The current understanding about the aetiology of Paediatric Psychotic Disorders is limited and it primarily derives from adult schizophrenic samples with only a few studies focusing on child and adolescent samples. The preponderance of evidence is suggestive of no single cause of Psychosis. Most evidence indicates that Paediatric Psychosis is a Neurodevelopment Disorder that evolves from an underpinning genetic vulnerability, a prenatal insult to the developing brain, and stressful life events.

Turning first to the role of genetic vulnerability, its role has long been documented by empirical investigations. Empirical studies have reported increased prevalence of Schizophrenia and Psychotic Spectrum Disorders in first degree relatives of schizophrenic children. Systematic reviews of genetic research provide estimates of concordance rates of Schizophrenia to be two and a half to three times higher in identical twins than in dizygotic twins [41, 42]. Importantly, adoption studies provide further support to the genetic basis of the disorder. These studies documented that adopted children who develop Psychosis have increased number of biological (but not adoptive) relatives who develop the disorder. Also, there is evidence that affected children who were born by a psychotic mother but were adopted as babies are at the same risk level as the infants who were born and raised by a psychotic mother [43, 44]. In general, the risk of Schizophrenia has been reported to increase dramatically from 1 percent in individuals without family history of the illness, to 10 percent in individuals who have a first degree relative who is psychotic, to 50 percent in psychotic identical twins. In addition, children with first degree relatives that are affected are reported to have higher risk for earlier onset of the disorder [41, 42]. Further it has been documented that the risk for development of the disorder increases with the number of affected relatives. In other words, the more the affected relatives the higher the risk for the development of the disorder [41, 42]. In addition, it has been documented that even when relatives of affected individuals did not themselves develop the disorder they still had increased risk for other mental health problems such as mood disorders [45]. This finding provides support to the postulation that the increased risk documented in families of affected individuals might not be best accounted by a genetic transmission of psychoses, but, rather a more general model of risk of undifferentiated transmission of psychopathology might be implicated.

Apart from the well established genetic vulnerability, several investigations [46], but not all [47], have documented complications during pregnancy and delivery in adult samples with psychotic disorders. The combination of genetic predisposition and evidence of acquired damage has provided corroborative support to a neurodevelopmental theory with early Central Nervous System (CNS) abnormalities that contribute to an increased vulnerability to schizophrenia later in life. Prenatal insults may include viral infections, such as maternal influenza in the second trimester [48, 49], lack of oxygen at birth, starvation, and untreated blood type incompatibility. An augmentation in minor dysmorphic features has been considered as suggestive of prenatal-onset problems. An augmentation in hypoxia-associated complications was reported to increase the odds of developing earlier-onset Schizophrenia. Unlike most adult-onset patients, children who become psychotic prior to puberty show conspicuous evidence of progressively abnormal brain development. However, these findings need to be interpreted with caution, since they may be suggestive of increased risk for development of Psychosis, but, by no means can be considered as establishing causality.

Beyond genetic predisposition and prenatal insults to the developing brain, psychosocial stressors and dysfunctional family processes have been implicated in the development and deterioration of psychotic symptoms. For instance, family interaction characterised by dysfunctional thinking and attention, as well as, disturbed relationships has been linked to Schizophrenia [1]. Also, other extraordinary family stressors and their effect on the timing of onset or outburst of the illness in the genetically vulnerable individual is a domain of research that warrants further attention by empirical investigations.

To conclude, despite the empirical findings that established that Paediatric Psychoses are underpinned by genetic vulnerability, a prenatal insult to the developing brain, and stressful life events the interaction of these factors and the possibly differentiated patterns across the development of the child are yet to be determined. For instance, it is plausible that the genetic vulnerability could be diferentiately expressed depending on the timing of the stressful events coupled with each vulnerable's child unique temperamental characteristics. Future investigations need to address closely the complex interplay of numerous genetic and environmental factors implicated in the development of psychosis and the plausible differentiated interplay of these factors in the genesis and the development of psychosis.

## Developmental Trajectories and Prognosis

Psychosis in children is very seldom diagnosed before the age of 7. As discussed above the developmentally appropriate fantasy lives of young children would not allow diagnosis at earlier age. While Psychosis in young adults typically begins as an acute psychotic episode, in children and especially pre-adolescents in most of the cases it emerges progressively with only a few of the reported incidences to be showing abrupt onset. For instance in a study investigating the onset of the Disorder in children and adolescents aged 7-17 in most of the cases (60-78%) onset was insidious with gradual increase of the symptomatology. In only a small percentage the onset was acute [50]. Preliminary data on gender effects have documented a more insidious onset in boys relative to girls [51], but, this preliminary finding requires further investigation.

Empirical investigations have documented a variety of psychological symptoms of various disorders prior to providing adequate criteria for diagnosis of psychosis. Hyperactivity, agitation and marked mood changes have been reported to be commonly displayed prior to displaying symptomatology of psychosis [52]. Additionally, onset of the Paediatric Psychosis has been documented to be often preceded by developmental disturbances, such as lags in motor and speech/language development, school problems and "odd" personality [15, 7, 53]. The observation of these features as preceding to the onset of Psychosis has given rise to the question whether these characteristics can justifiably be interpreted as precursors of early manifestations of the disorder[13], and in effect allowing diagnosis of early onset Psychosis to become more likely during school age.

As it would be expected the developmental level of the affected child affects his/her psychotic experiences [54]. Young children's hallucinations typically include monsters, toys and animals and they are uncomplicated. Similarly, their delusions when they first make their appearance are simple (e.g. the monster will kill me), but, they gradually become more complex and systematic and as it would be expected they are intertwined with the child's cognitive and socioemotional development [55]. Adolescent onset Psychosis in comparison to Paediatric Onset Psychosis has relatively less insidious onset and as it would be expected it presents more adult like features of the disorder. For example, dilutions of Psychotic adolescents are relatively more systematized and more complex relative to Psychotic children's delusions [56].

Most empirical reports on the prognosis of child- and adolescent-onset Psychosis reveal a variable clinical course [57] most likely based on the severity and nature of the symptoms and the potential stressors in the youngster's life conditions. For most Psychotic children, Psychosis persists through lifetime. Most Psychotic youngsters will enter adulthood and their clinical condition will be characterized by exacerbations and remissions [58]. Among those youngsters whose condition persists into adulthood some will show a stable symptomatology, while others will show progressive deterioration with the expression of symptoms often fluctuating with the levels of stress experienced by the individual. Full recovery is extremely rare. 42-years follow up of cases that had age of onset by 14 years of age, 50% had a continuous severe course, 25 % had partial recovery, and 25 % were characterised as having recovered [59]. The 25 % that was characterized as having recovered is not low. Nonetheless, these findings should be interpreted with caution since often Psychotic individuals may not any more meet criteria for diagnosis of Psychosis, but, nonetheless their symptomatology is differentiately expressed as another form of psychopathology that warrants further investigation.

With respect to mortality, scarce data suggest relatively high premature mortality rates in individuals with child- and adolescent-onset Psychosis. Factors such as undetected medical conditions, suicide and other violent events have been considered to be implicated in the premature death of Psychotic individuals [60, 61]. Comorbit clinical conditions such as Depression could also be implicated in the link of Psychosis to premature death.

However, despite the fact in the most of the cases the prognosis of Psychosis can best be characterized as moderate and full recovery is extremely rare, there are a series of factors that are predictive of a better prognosis. These factors include associated mood disturbance, absence of structural brain abnormalities, and normal neurological functioning, treatment with antipsychotic soon after onset [1]. If significant time elapses between onset and treatment the potential consequences are worse, impacting the emotional, occupational, and social functioning of the individual in the long-term. Yet, the empirical data on the possible effect of resilience factors are still minimal. Future investigations need to examine risk and resilience factors and their potential interaction.

Further research also is needed to examine the plausible interactive factors implicated in spontaneous remission. More generally future prospective longitudinal studies are necessary for determining diverse developmental trajectories and factors implicated in these diverse trajectories.

## TREATMENT

To date, there is still minimal empirical data reporting on the efficacy of pharmaco therapy and psychosocial treatments specific to paediatric psychoses. Early diagnosis of paediatric psychoses is of crucial importance for the treatment outcome of the disorder. A complete multifaceted evaluation (described above) is necessary for the development of a comprehensive individual treatment plan to address individual difficulties.

Treatment strategies are typically intended to address the psychotic symptomatology, but, at the same time to address plausible comorbid conditions and psychosocial stressors. If there is corroborative evidence that delusions or hallucinations are the direct physiological consequence of a general medical condition, then, the very first step is to deal with these conditions. For example, treating a partial complex seizure disorder, managing a metabolic imbalance, or treating an underlying infection. In the cases when there is no evidence of a medical condition linked to psychotic symptomatology, then, the next step is to evaluate whether the psychotic features are secondary to another psychiatric diagnosis such as Depression or Mania. If the psychotic symptomatology is secondary to Depression for example, then, the child will be prescribed with antidepressant (e.g. selective serotonergic reuptake inhibitors such as flouxetine, paroxetine, sertraline, fluvoxamine, clomipramine) often accompanied by the use of antipsychotic medications.

Standard antipsychotic drugs appear to be effective for many psychotic youngsters. The atypical drug Clozapine has been found helpful for at least half of those youngsters who do not respond to other medication. In few cases, psychotic symptoms show substantial remission. However, despite the significant treatment outcomes of antipsychotic drugs children may be more susceptible than adults to the toxic effects of this medication. For instance, about one third of psychotic youngsters that are prescribed with Clozapine discontinue its' use it because of its' side effects and the serious risks that Clozapine carries. These risks include seizures and serious blood abnormalities, and therefore, it should solitarily be used only in cases that do not respond to other medications [15]. Newer antipsychotic drugs that may be safer and just as effective are now being under investigation.

While psychopharmacological treatment has been acknowledged as a promising treatment modality, findings reporting on the efficacy of this treatment must still be considered preliminary. Most data derive from clinical trials with older adolescents or adult samples. In fact, few randomised psychopharmacological studies have reported on the efficacy of psychopharmacological treatment approaches on Childhood Psychoses and most data derive from adult samples. In effect, rigorous studies on treatment outcome of pharmacological interventions are crucially needed.

While pharmacological intervention can be of value [39], since the developmental consequences of not controlling psychotic symptoms at an early age can be detrimental, it does not negate the need for psychosocial interventions. In brief, these interventions typically include family psychoeducational approaches that encompass psychoeducation of the child and the parent about psychoses, enhancing strategies for coping with the psychiatric condition, training in family communication, training in problem-solving and the provision of supportive psychotherapy during the recovery phase of the acute illness, and practical guidance of behaviour [15]. Ongoing supportive psychosocial treatment helps patients deal more effectively with psychosocial stressors. Clinicians also work with the parents with the schools and other social agencies to make sure that psychotic youngsters will continue their education while their individual needs will be addressed.

The most commonly used psychosocial treatment for psychotic children is the behavioural approach which focuses on the youngsters' observable behaviours, rather than on thoughts and perceptual processes. Behavioural treatment for Paediatric Psychosis appears to be promising [62]. It typically encompasses environmental structures, contingency management, and adaptive skill interventions [24]. Skill interventions are intended to improve the child's basic social, self-care, and organizational skills.

The Environmental Structure Interventions are intended to encourage internal structure of thought processes by increasing external structure which is expected to provide the child with a positive model of structure. Environmental Structure is achieved by organizing the child's living environment by increasing the predictability, organization, and scheduling of the child's daily life. Organization is reviewed and restored every day in ordered to maintain a well structured environment for the child on every day basis. The Environmental Structure also encompasses the child's daily schedule which is kept as predictable and active as possible. Social, mental, and physical activity is encouraged, and withdrawal is discouraged. The well structured environment and the predictability of the child's everyday activities are expected to reduce stress levels that would potentially evoke a psychotic episode.

The Contingency Management interventions are intended to decrease the frequency and severity of psychotic symptomatology. This intervention is based on the assumption that psychotic behaviour, like any other behaviour, can be reduced by altering the contingencies that sustain the behaviour. A series of behavioural techniques are utilized within the framework of contingency management. At the first step, the psychotic behaviours are operationally defined. Next, the antecedents and consequences of the behaviour are identified by the therapist with the assistance of the parents and the child. For a more accurate identification of the antecedents and consequences, the parent keeps record of antecedents and consequences for a period of time (usually 2 weeks). The frequency of the occurrences of the behaviour is also recorded in order to determine the severity of the displayed symptomatology and to have a baseline for reviewing treatment outcome. The Identification of the Antecedents and Consequences is followed by the Differential Reinforcement of Other Behaviour. In this step, the non-occurrence of the psychotic behaviour (differential reinforcement of other behaviour) and the occurrence of behaviours that are incompatible with the target behaviour (differential reinforcement of incompatible behaviour) are reinforced. Reinforcement is provided on a fixed-interval schedule, in which the psychotic child is rewarded if the behaviour does not occur for a certain period of time (depending on the initial frequency of the behaviour, this time period may range from 5 minutes to a day). In addition to the Differential Reinforcement of Other Behaviour, the technique of active ignoring of the target psychotic behaviour is also utilized. Finally, the technique of Antecedents' Management is used. For instance, a youngster who displays schizophrenic behaviours after loud arguments of the parents the antecedent management would be to address marital conflict. If this compilation of contingency management interventions work the intervention continues with newly targeted schizophrenic behaviours such as showing inappropriate affect, reported hallucinations, random babbling. For those behaviours that treatment has worked the intervals between reinforcement are increased and the amount of reinforcement is reduced. If the intervention does not work it is modified. For instance, reinforces may be modified to improve their effectiveness.

In most of the cases these behavioural interventions are further complemented by Adaptive Skills Interventions. The Adaptive Skills Interventions are intended to tap social, organization, and self-care deficits that often characterise children with psychosis. Upon identifying the specific adaptive skills deficit (e.g. eye contact, showing appropriate affect, apprehending the communication of others, keeping a clean working/living space, and keeping appropriate hygiene) with the utilisation of an adaptive scale – see section on this chapter on assessment) clear goals and expectations for social interaction and self-care, are set on the basis of each child's individualized deficits. Once adaptive skills deficits are identified goals reflecting the deficits are set. Once goals are set, modelling, rehearsal, and education are used to practice and demonstrate goal behaviour during therapeutic sessions, and the psychotic child is expected to record and evaluate progress toward the goal. The child's caregivers and professionals from the school setting (i.e. primary teacher) are also involved in the Adaptive Skills Intervention, by helping out in the process of s of identifying and achieving goal behaviours and rewarding the child when goal behaviours are achieved, utilising Contingency Management Techniques, such as those overviewed above.

A major part of Adaptive Skills package is the Social Skills Training which is often implemented in a group format so the child will have the opportunity to practice newly acquired social skills with peers. Depending on the level of deficits of psychotic children social skills programs are adjusted to tap the identified deficits. For instance, the social skills intervention for children that display a substantial degree of social skills deficits would target development of skills for appropriate eye contact, smiling, physical space, content of conversation, voice volume and inflection, acknowledgments, conversational openers, compliments, requests. For psychotic children that display relatively less deficits comparatively more advance social skills would be targeted. For instance, reading social cues, giving and receiving compliments, expressing oneself nonverbally, starting and ending a conversation, asking questions and answering questions when asked, expressing emotions and apprehending what others are thinking and feeling and developing empathy, joining a group conversation, disagreeing with others, setting limits on others and resisting peer pressure, and persuading others. The process of social skills training sessions which are typically group based include initial explanation of the skill followed by practice techniques such as modelling, role play, rehearsal and feedback from the therapists and the other group members. Once the newly acquired skill is achieved in the therapeutic setting, the next step is to be applied in the psychotic child's home environment and school setting with the reinforcement of the caregivers and teachers for the best possible learning outcome of the newly acquired skill.

While this combination of behavioural techniques have been reported to decrease psychotic symptomatology in certain samples of children with psychosis, behaviour techniques only indirectly address the cognitive characteristics of psychosis. Given that many children with Psychosis have been reported to have no control over their behaviour during a psychotic episode and in effect diminished ability to purposefully respond to a reinforcement schedule the utility of behaviour techniques for this subset of psychotic children has been questioned. Nonetheless, behavioural techniques can be of value in between psychotic episodes. Also, behaviour techniques when used in suitable timing in combination with pharmacotherapy can result in encouragement of appropriate behaviours. Behavioural therapy can also be useful when used in combination with pharmacotherapy at the timing when the medication reduces the negative symptoms.

Apart from the behaviour techniques family therapy has been utilized for the treatment of Psychotic Disorders. This approach addresses the child's psychotic symptomatology within the family system. In certain situations the child's symptomatology may serve the psychological needs of another family member. For instance, a mother who has the need to care for a highly depended child. In such a case the psychotic child serves the needs of the mother and therefore preserves the family system. In such cases the therapist would try to modify this system so the child's symptoms will no longer be needed to preserve the integrity of the system [24]. Family therapy is particularly useful when family conflict characterizes the family. Family conflict plays a detrimental role in exacerbating psychotic symptomatology. Family conflict results in significant distress within a vulnerable child, which in turn results in disorganization of thought and bizarre behaviour. In effect, family therapy attempts to modify the family system, so that it does not make things worse for the psychotic child. Of course, family therapy cannot be used in isolation for the treatment of the psychotic child, since it can address the family processes that are implicated in exacerbation of the symptoms of the psychotic child, but, it cannot treat the symptomatology of psychosis. It can nonetheless be utilized for addressing environmental factors that reduce the ability of the family to implement interventions such as medication compliance and behavioural therapy.

Apart from the behavioural and family interventions a much less common but yet sometimes used intervention for psychotic children is the play therapy. In the course of play therapy the therapists facilitates the psychotic child to play in unstructured, accepting therapy situation [63, 64]. This accepting therapy situation is considered to facilitate the child's growth and a self acceptance. Play therapy is based on the rationale that the psychotic children do not accept their selves as worthwhile, valuable persons. Play therapy is intended to allow psychotic children play in a nondirective, accepting atmosphere, is considered to provide the chance to them to explore themselves and to have their sense of self validated by the therapist. Play therapy is considered beneficial for psychotic children who have been neglected, rejected, or traumatized. However, the efficacy of play therapy for addressing the chore symptomatology of psychosis has not established.

Not rarely, none of the above treatment approaches works, either when used in isolation, or in when used in combination with others, especially for psychotic children with serious psychotic symptoms. In such cases, the level of adaptive functioning of the psychotic child is evaluated, and if their symptomatology has renter the non-manageable or dangerous, impatient hospitalization is considered. In the course of Inpatient treatment, most often a combination of medication intense behaviour therapy and family therapy (described above) are integrated in an intense therapeutic plan that aims to prevent the worsening of the displayed symptomatology, to stabilize the patient's condition and eventually result into producing lasting change in the child's behavior once s/he returns home. The effectiveness of the impatient treatment has provided promising results with respect to the stabilization of the child's condition, but evaluation of the long-term effectiveness of this integrative impatient intervention is yet to be determined.

Overall, despite the treatment approaches that are typically generated to address psychotic symptoms (either directly or indirectly by encouraging behaviour that is inconsistent with psychotic symptomatology) in children to date there is a crucial need for individualised treatment approaches that will be adjusted to each child's difficulties while developmental considerations will not be ignored. Further, methodologically rigorous controlled treatment studies that will evaluate the efficacy of each component of a treatment program, as well as, the long-term outcome of the treatment approaches are necessary.

Finally, of further potential concern is our lack of knowledge on treatment outcome among ethnic minorities. Several studies reported a less favourable attitude toward treatment for mental health problems in ethnic minorities [65, 66]. For instance, ethnic minority parents have been documented to be less favourable towards pharmacological intervention relative to Caucasian parents [67]. Ethnic differences in the perception and utilization of mental health treatments seems to be the outcome of several factors, such as the possible stigma attached to mental health treatment among ethnic minorities [68], the fear of possible institutionalization [69], and the lack of culturally sensitive treatment approaches [70]. Given that ethnic minorities are typically underrepresented in clinical trials future investigations need to evaluate the degree to which the factors involved in treatment outcome differentially affect ethnic minorities as well as other diverse populations.

## CONCLUSION

Although once a neglected disorder, Paediatric Psychosis has in the past two and a half decades received increased attention by empirical investigations. Nonetheless, despite the increase in the empirical investigations, still little is known about the interplay of the factors implicated in the aetiology, developmental course of the disorder, as well as, on empirically validated methods of treatment. Further, most studies report data on Caucasian and African American children, with very few studies reporting data from diverse cultures, as well as, addressing whether Psychosis is differentially presented across cultures, and determine whether cultural factors are implicated in the aetiology, developmental course, prognosis and treatment outcome of the disorder.

## REFERENCES

[1] American Psychiatric Association. *Diagnostic and Statistical Manual of Mental Disorders*, 4th ed, Text Revision. Washington, DC: American Psychiatric Association (2000).

[2] H. Courvoisie, M. Labellarte and M. Riddle Psychosis in Children: diagnosis and treatment. *Dialogues in Clinical Neuroscience* 3 (2), 79-98, (2001).
[3] American Academy of Child and Adolescent Psychiatry. Practice parameters for the assessment and treatment of children and adolescents with schizophrenia. *J. Am. Acad. Child. Adolesc. Psychiatry* 36 (suppl.), 177S-193S (1997).
[4] C. Eggers, D. Bunk, G. Volberg, B. Ropcke. The ESSEN study of childhood-onset schizophrenia: selected results. *Eur. Child Adolesc. Psychiatry* 8 (suppl. 1) 122-128. (1999).
[5] L. J. Rapoport and D. R. Ismond. DSM-IV Training Guide for Diagnosis of Childhood Disorders, Brunner-Routledge, New York Hove (1996).
[6] M. D. Claudio Cepeda. The Psychiatric Interview of Children and Adolescents, American Psychiatric Press, Washington, DC London, England (2000).
[7] J. McClellan, D. Breiger, C. McCurry and S. A. Hlastala. Premorbid functioning in early-onset psychotic disorders. *Journal of the American Academy of Child and Adolescent Psychiatry*, 42, 666-672 (2003).
[8] L. R. Ulloa. Psychosis in a pediatric mood and anxiety disorders clinic: Phenomenology and correlates. *Journal of the American Academy of Child and Adolescent Psychiatry*, 39, 337-345 (2000).
[9] J. Alaghband-Rad, K. McKenna, C. T. Gordon, et al. Childhood-onset schizophrenia: the severity of premorbid course. *J. Am. Acad. Child Adolesc. Psychiatry*,34, 1273-1283 (1995).
[10] I. Elman, M. Sigler, J. Kronenberg, et al. Characteristics of patients with schizophrenia successive to childhood attention hyperactivity disorder (ADHD). *Isr. J. Psychiatry*.35, 280-286 (1998).
[11] A. T. Russell. The clinical presentation of childhood-onset schizophrenia. *Schizophr. Bull.* 20, 631-646 (1994).
[12] M. R. Basso, H. A. Nasrallah, S. C. Olson, R. A. Bornstein. Cognitive deficits distinguish patients with adolescent - and adult-onset schizophrenia. *Neu-ropsychiatry Neuropsychol. Behav. Neurol.* 10, 107-112 (1997).
[13] J. R. Asarnow, and R. F. Asarnow, Childhood Onset Schziphrenia. In E. J. Mash and R. A. Barkley (Eds) *Child Psychopathology*. New York. Guilford Press (2003).
[14] S. Kumra, E. Wiggs, J. Bedwell, et al. Neuropsychological deficits in pediatric patients with childhood-onset schizophrenia and psychotic disorder not otherwise specified. *Schizophr. Res.* 42, 135-144 (2000).
[15] J. R. Asarnow, M. C. Thomson and E. P. McGratth Annotation: Childhood-onset schizophrenia: Clinical and treatment issues. *Journal of Child Psychology and Psychiatry*, 45, 180-194 (2004).
[16] P. J. Ambrosini. Historical development and present status of the Schedule for Affective Disorders and Schizophrenia for School-Age Children (K-SADS). *Journal of the American Academy of Child and Adolescent Psychiatry*, 39, 48-58. (2000).
[17] B. Fish, Antecedents of an acute schizophrenic break. *Journal of the American Academy of Child Psychiatry*, 25, 595-600. (1986).
[18] R. Caplan, J. G. Foy, R. F. Asarnow and T. Sherman, Information processing deficits of schizophrenic children with formal thought disorder. *Psychiatry Research*, 31, 169-177 (1990).

[19] B. A. Bettes, and E. Walker. Positive and negative symptoms in psychotic and other psychiatrically disturbed children. *Journal of Child Psychology and Psychiatry*, 28, 555-568 (1987).
[20] S. S. Sparrow, D. A. Balla and D. V. Cicchetti. Vineland Adaptive Behavior Scales. Circle Pines, M. N.: American Guidance Service (1984).
[21] S. B. McCarney, The Adaptive Behavior Evaluation Scale Home Version Technical Manual-Revised. Columbia, M. O.: Hawthorne Educational Services (1995).
[22] H. A. Murray. Thematic Apperception Test manual. Cambridge, M. A.: Harvard University Press (1943).
[23] J. E. Exner. The Rorschach: *A Comprehensive System* Volume 1: Basic Foundations (2nd ed). New York: Wiley. (1986).
[24] W. G. Kronenberger and R. G. Meyer. *The Cchild Clinician's Handbook*, Allyn and Bacon, Boston (second edition) (2001).
[25] R. Caplan, D. Guthrie, B. Fish, P. E. Tanguay and G. David-Lando, The Kiddie Formal Thought Disorder Scale (K-FTDS): Clinical assessment, reliability, and validity. *Journal of the American Academy of Child Psychiatry*, 28, 408-416. (1989).
[26] R. Caplan, S. Perdue, P. E. Tanguay and B. Fish, Formal thought disorder in childhood onset schizophrenia and schizotypal personality disorder. *Journal of Child Psychology and Psychiatry*, 31, 1103-1114 (1990b).
[27] T. M. Achenbach. Manual for the Child Behaviour Checklist/1-18 and 1991 Profile. Burlington, V. T.: University of Vermont Department of Psychiatry (1991).
[28] T. M. Achenbach. Manual for the Teacher's Report form and 1991 Profile. Burlington, V. T.: University of Vermont Department of Psychiatry. (1991b)
[29] C. R. Reynolds and R. W. Kamphaus. Behavior Assessment System for Children manual. Circle Pines, M. N.: American Guidance Service (1992).
[30] K. D. Gadow and. J. Sprafkin. Child Symptom Inventory-4 norms manual. Stony Brook, N. Y.: Checkmate plus, Ltd (1997).
[31] K. D. Gadow and J. Sprafkin. Child Symptom Inventory-4 screening manual. Stony Brook, N. Y.: Checkmate Plus, Ltd (1998).
[32] K. D. Gadow and J. Sprafkin. Child Symptom Inventory-4 screening manual. Stony Brook, N. Y.: Checkmate Plus, Ltd. (1997).
[33] K. D. Gadow and J. Sprafkin. Adolescent Symptom Inventory-4 norms manual. Stony Brook, N. Y.: Checkmate Plus, Ltd. (1998).
[34] D. Lachar and C. P. Gruber. Personality Inventory for Youth (P. I. Y.) manual. Los Angeles: Western Psychological Services (1995).
[35] R. McGee, S. William and. R. Poulton. Hallucinations in nonpsychotic children. *Journal of the American Academy of Child and Adolescent Psychiatry*, 39, 12-13 (2000).
[36] P. Mertin and S. Hartwing. Auditory hallucinations in nonpsychotic children: Diagnostic considerations. *Child and Adolescent Mental Health*, 9, 9-14 (2004).
[37] B. Vickers and E. Garralda. Hallucinations in nonpsychotic children. *Journal of the Academy of Child and Adolescent Psychiatry*, 39, 1073 (2000).
[38] H. Altman, M. Collins and. P. Mundy. Subclinical hallucinations and delusions in nonpsychotic adolescents. *Journal of Child Psychology and Psychiatry*, 38, 413-420 (1997).

[39] J. M. McClellan, Early onset schizophrenia. In B. J. Sadock and V. A., Sadock (Eds.) *Comprehensive Textbook of Psychiatry* (vol II) Philadelphia: Lippincott Williams and Wilkins (2005).

[40] A. S. Brown, M. Bresnahan, and E. S. Susser. Schizophrenia: environmental epidemiology. In B. J. Sadock and V. A. Sadock (Eds), *Comprehensive textbook of psychiatry.* Vol. 1. Philadelphia: Lippincott Williams and Wilkins (2005).

[41] I. I. Gottesman, Schizophrenia genesis: The origins of madness. New York: W. H. Freeman (1991).

[42] I. I. Gottesman, Blind men and elephants: Genetic and other perspectives on schizophrenia. I. L. L. Hall (ed), *Genetics and mental illness: Evolving issues from research and society*, (pp. 51-77) New York: Plenum. (1996).

[43] S. S. Kety. Schizophrenic illness in the families of schizophrenic adoptees: Findings from the Danish national sample. *Schizophrenia Bulletin*, 14, 217-222 (1988).

[44] S. S. Kety, Wender, P. H., Jacobsen, B., Ingraarm, L. J. Jasson, L. Faber, B. and D. K. Kinnery, Mental illness in the biological and adoptive relatives of schizophrenic adoptees: Replication of the Copenhagen Study in the rest of Denmark. *Archives of General Psychiatry,* 51, 442-455 (1994).

[45] E. K. Spencer and M. Campbell. Schizophrenic children: Diagnosis, phenomenology, and pharmacotherapy. *Schizophrenia Bulletin,* 20, 713-726. (1994).

[46] F. Gunther-Genta, P. Bovet and P. Hohlfeld. Obstetric complications and schizophrenia: A case-controlled study. *British Journal of Psychiatry,* 164, 165-170 (1994).

[47] W. H. Green, M. Pandron-Gaylo, A. S. Hardesty and M. Bassiri. Schizophrenia with childhood onset: A phenomenological study of 38 cases. *Journal of the American Academy of Child and Adolescent Psychiatry*, 31, 968-976 (1992).

[48] S. A. Mednick, R. A. Machon, M. O. Huttunen and D. Bonnett,. Fetal viral nfection and adult schizophrenia. *Archives of General Psychiatry*, 45, 189–192 (1988).

[49] P. Wright, N. Takei, L. Rifkin and R. M. Murray. Maternal influenza, obstetric complications, and schizophrenia. *American Journal of Psychiatry*, 152, 1714-1720 (1995).

[50] J. S. Werry, J. M. McClellan, L. K. Andrews, and M. Ham. Clinical features and outcome of child and adolescent schizophrenia. *Schizophrenia Bulletin,* 20, 619-630 (1994).

[51] J. Alaghband-Rad, S. D. Hamburger, J. N. Giedd, J. A. Frazier, and J. L. Rapoport. Childhood-onset schizophrenia: Biological markers in relation to clinical characteristics. *American Journal of Psychiatry*, 154, 64-68. (1997).

[52] J. M. McClellan and J. S. Werry, Schizophrenia. *Pediatric Psychopharmacology*, 15, 131-148 (1992).

[53] R. Nicolson, J. L. Rapoport. Childhood-onset schizophrenia: What can it teach us? In J. L. Rapoport (Ed) *Childhood onset of "adult" psychopathology*. Washington, DC: American Psychiatric Press. (2000).

[54] A. T. Russell, L. Bott, and C. Sammons. The phenomenology of schizophrenia occurring in childhood. *Journal of the American Academy of Child and Adolescent Psychiatry*, 28, 399-407 (1989).

[55] F. R. Volkmar, Childhood and adolescent psychosis: A review of the past 10 years. *Journal of the American Academy of Child and Adolescent Psychiatry*, 35, 843-851. (1996).

[56] F. R. Volkmar, D. Becker, R. A. King and T. H. McGlashan. Psychotic processes. In D. Cicchetti and D. J. Cohen (Eds), *Developmental psychopathology*. New York: John Wiley (1995).

[57] C. Eggers, D. Bunk and D. Krause. Schizophrenia with onset before the age of eleven: Clinical characteristics of onset and course. *Journal of Autism and Developmental Disorders*, 30, 29-38 (2000).

[58] C. Hollis, Adult outcomes of child – and adolescent-onset schizophrenia: Diagnostic stability and predictive validity. *American Journal of Psychiatry* 157, 1652-1659 (2000).

[59] C. Eggers, D. Bunk, The long-term course of childhood-onset schizophrenia: A 42-year follow up. *Schizophrenia Bulletin*, 23, 105-117 (1997).

[60] C. Hollis, Schizophrenia and allied disorders. In M. Rutter and E. Taylor (Eds.), *Child and adolescent psychiatry*. Oxford, UK: Blackwell Publishing (2002).

[61] H. Y. Meltzer, L. Alphs, A. I. Green, C. Altamura, R. Anand, A. Bertoldi, et al. Clozapine treatment for suicidality in schizophrenia. *Archives of General Psychiatry*, 60, 82-91 (2003).

[62] D. L. Evans, E. B. Foa, R. E. Gur, H. Hendin, C. P. O'. Brien, M. E. P. Seligman and B.T. (Eds). Treating and preventing adolescent mental health disorders. What we know and what we don't know: A research agenda for the mental health of our youth. New York: Oxford University Press (2005).

[63] V. M. Axline, Play therapy. New York: Ballantine (1969).

[64] D. M. Gelfand, W. R. Jenson and C. J. Drew. *Understanding child behavior disorders* (2nd ed.). New York: Harcourt Brace Jovanovich College Publishers (1988).

[65] A. E Kazdin. Acceptability of alternative treatments for child deviant behavior. *Journal of Applied Behavioral Analysis,* 13 (2), 259–273. (1980).

[66] K. J. Tarnowski, L. K. Rasnake, J. A. Mulisk and P. A. Kelly. Acceptability of behavioral treatments for self-injurious behavior. *American Journal of Mental Retardation,* 93(5), 575-580 (1989).

[67] D. A. Chavira, M. B. Stein, K. Bailey and M. T. Stein. Parental opinions regarding treatment for social anxiety disorder in youth. *Journal of Developmental and Behavioral Pediatrics,* 24(5), 315–322 (2003).

[68] K. M. Lin, T. S. Inui, A. M. Kleinman and W. M. Womach. Sociocultural determinants of the help-seeking behavior of patients with mental illness. *Journal of Nervous and Mental Disease,* 170 (2), 78–85 (1982).

[69] D. T. Takeuchi, K. T. Bui and L. Kim. The referral of minority adolescents to community mental health centers. *Journal of Health and Social Behavior,* 34(2), 153–164 (1993).

[70] P. B. Pederson. The multicultural context of mental health. In: T. B. Smith (Ed.), Practicing multiculturalism: affirming diversity in counseling and psychology. US: Pearson Education, Inc. (2004).

In: Psychosis: Causes, Diagnosis and Treatment
Editor: Xenia Anastassiou-Hadjicharalambous
ISBN: 978-1-62081-516-8


*Chapter 3*

# EARLY NEURODEVELOPMENT AND PSYCHOSIS RISK: ROLE OF NEUROHORMONES AND BIOLOGICAL SEX IN MODULATING GENETIC, PRENATAL AND SENSORY PROCESSING FACTORS IN BRAIN DEVELOPMENT

***Deborah J. Walder,*[1,2,3,*] *Luz Ospina,*[1,3] *Maureen Daly,*[2,3] *Marta Statucka*[2,3] *and Eva Raparia*[1]**

[1]Brooklyn College of The City University of New York, US
[2]Queens College of The City University of New York, US
[3]The Graduate Center of The City University of New York, US

## ABSTRACT

Schizophrenia is a psychiatric disorder largely believed to have neurodevelopmental origins with complex polygenic influences (including gene-environment interactions) that modify illness expression, as captured by the diathesis-stress model. It is now well known that the scope of these influences that render individuals vulnerable is broad and not necessarily illness specific, though many are believed to play a role in psychosis risk. Adverse pre-/peri-/post- natal events (e.g., prenatal maternal stress, teratogen exposure, obstetric complications) and genetic factors (e.g., candidate/susceptibility and modifier genes; epigenetics) represent two exemplary risk domains given they exert effects (though not exclusively) during early development (including impacting brain development). Relatively new to this field of study is consideration of sexual dimorphisms and the modulating role of one's biological sex and neurohormones (e.g., byproducts of the hypothalamic-pituitary-adrenal (HPA) and hypothalamic-pituitary-gonadal (HPG) axes; namely, cortisol and gonadal hormones) across the developmental trajectory in setting the stage for – and later potentiating (or buffering) - underlying vulnerability towards illness manifestation. This holds potential for better understanding etiology of, and risk for, psychosis from a diathesis-stress perspective. This chapter

[*]E-mail: dwalder@brooklyn.cuny.edu

focuses on select *early* neurodevelopmental risk factors for psychosis, particularly 1) evidence of genetic influences (from linkage to association studies, candidate susceptibility and modifier genes, and epigenetics), 2) pre-/peri- natal risk factors presumed to impact brain development and evidenced to occur in higher rates than normal in psychosis risk (with consideration of gene by environment interactions), and 3) sensory processing/early information-processing deficits (including sensorimotor gating) as an example of a vulnerability indicator; all of which are discussed with respect to hormonal influences and sexual differentiation. While an in-depth discussion of later developmental maturational processes (e.g., during adolescence) is beyond the scope of this paper, we briefly discuss this important developmental period in understanding psychosis risk and respective clinical implications. Throughout the paper, findings (and putative risk factors) are contextualized (and discussed) with respect to sex differences, the potential modulating role of neurohormones, and synergistic effects towards bolstering current theoretical models of psychosis proneness.

## I. Introduction

Schizophrenia is a debilitating psychiatric disorder largely believed to have neurodevelopmental origins [1], [2], with manifestation of prominent clinical features (e.g., hallucinations, delusions, behavioral deficits, bizarre/disorganized behavior) typically during late adolescence and early adulthood. With the implementation of contemporary study designs (e.g., genetic/family high-risk paradigms; prospective, longitudinal tracking of prodromal youth) and the advent of modern technological advances (e.g., neuroimaging, molecular genetics), the field has gained an increased appreciation of the role of early neuro-developmental susceptibility (or precursor) factors and how they interact with the environment towards yielding emergent cognitive, behavioral and clinical signs (and neurobiological correlates of) psychosis. These efforts reflect contemporary etiological models of psychotic disorders that emphasize complex polygenic influences (including gene-environment interactions) that modify illness expression, as captured by the diathesis-stress model. One iteration of this model, Walker and Diforio's [3] neural diathesis-stress model, highlights the import of the potentiating effects of neurohormonal mechanisms (e.g., hypothalamic-pituitary-adrenal (HPA) axis) on neurotransmitter systems (e.g., dopaminergic functioning) in the precipitation of psychosis.

Recent decades have yielded an increase in research elucidating early neuro-developmental mechanisms and their phenotypic expressions in psychotic spectrum disorders, which shed light on etiology and serve as bio-indicators of illness risk. In the context of stress-diathesis models and well-established sex differences (in prevalence, premorbid functioning, age at onset and course of illness) in psychotic disorders (for review see [4], [5]), newly emergent research has focused on the role of biological sex and neurohormones (e.g., byproducts of the hypothalamic-pituitary-gonadal (HPG) and HPA axes) as potential modulators of illness manifestation. These influences on latent vulnerability may exert their impact at various points through development and illness trajectory, with critical (or at least more sensitive) windows noted prenatally and during adolescence, both periods marked by neuromaturation.

It is now well known that the scope of genetic and other early neurodevelopmental and environmental factors that render individuals vulnerable to illness is broad. Moreover, these vulnerability factors are not necessarily illness specific, though many are believed to play a role in psychosis risk. Various susceptibility and modifier genes, for example, have been implicated in a range of psychiatric disorders including psychosis (see [6]). Likewise, prenatal (during pregnancy), perinatal (around delivery) and early postnatal factors such as fetal malnutrition, teratogen exposure, obstetric complications and maternal stress, and later environmental influences such as adverse stressful life events have been demonstrated to occur more frequently in psychosis [7], depression [8] and autism [9].

Adverse prenatal events and genetic factors represent two exemplary risk domains given they exert effects (though not exclusively) during early development and interact with other influences such as neurohormonal milieus. Until recently, the 'organizational' effects of gonadal hormones – such as sexual differentiation of brain structure – were of primary interest. More recent discoveries, however, point to the role of prenatal stress (and associated adrenal hormone exposure) in brain development and long-term behavioral outcome [10], [11]. This is predominantly evidenced by experimental findings in the animal literature (e.g., [12]), though there is some recent corroborative evidence in the human literature; notably, an association of prenatal maternal stress exposure with dermatoglyphic abnormalities in offspring (e.g., [13]; see [14]). The epigenome is sensitive to environmental influences not only prenatally, but also during neonatal development, puberty and old age (see [15]). This is a reminder that while early neurodevelopment warrants heed in consideration of causal factors in mental (and physical/neurological) health, a lifespan perspective need also be considered.

An interest in gonadal hormones in psychosis risk arose initially from evidence of sex differences in psychosis (e.g., age at onset; see [16]). The notion that prenatal gonadal hormones influence sexually differentiated clinical, cognitive, behavioral and morpholologic traits (and general CNS organization) associated with psychosis vulnerability have arisen from several converging lines of investigation. Recent examples in our work include evidence of sex differences in aspects of neurocognition (e.g., [17]) and neuroanatomic substrates of these sex differences (e.g., [18]) in schizophrenia, sex differences in neurocognition as an indicator of risk for conversion to psychosis [19], and indirect evidence of disruptions in the prenatal gonadal hormone milieu in risk for psychosis [20]. With consideration of Meehl's [21] notion that psychopathology falls along a continuum, we recently investigated the modulating role of menstrual cycle status (an indirect index of the natural gonadal hormone milieu) and one's biological sex on cortisol secretion and psychiatric symptoms in a non-clinical sample of young adults [22]. Findings were interpreted with respect to the complex (proposed dose response) interplay of gonadal and adrenal hormone systems and one's biological sex in modulating non-clinical psychiatric symptoms. Newer on scene is evidence that glucocorticoids can alter brain development, with some sex-specific effects and implications for psychosis risk. To date, several morphologic (e.g., dermatoglyphics), cognitive (e.g., neuropsychological), behavioral (e.g., neuromotor) and neurohormonal (e.g., cortisol) abnormalities marked by sexual differentiation have been identified in psychosis risk, many of which are believed to reflect disruptions in prenatal development. There remain, however, several cognitive and behavioral deficits that may represent putative indicators of psychosis risk that are not as clearly linked with prenatal influences. One example is sensory processing deficits, particularly in auditory, visual and (more recently) olfactory domains. These deficits, evidenced in both patients and high-risk populations, have been largely understood in terms of dysfunctional transmission at N-methyl-D-aspartate (NMDA)-type glutamate receptors [23]. Another emerging area of interest is that of sensorimotor gating deficits in schizophrenia. Less well understood, however, are somatosensory and gustatory processing deficits. Given the relative dearth of research examining these factors in psychosis risk, it is not surprising that consideration of the role of genetics and prenatal events (as well as neurohormones and sex effects) on the integrity of these systems is not well understood. We begin this chapter with a review of genetic influences on psychosis risk, including evolving methodological approaches (from linkage to association studies), candidate susceptibility and modifier genes, and epigenetics (which may lead to alterations in phenotypic expression without altering DNA sequence, and may be heritable). We then turn to a review of pre- and peri- natal factors presumed to impact brain development and evidenced to occur in higher rates than normal in psychosis risk, with consideration of gene by environment interactions. We then briefly review the domain of sensory processing deficits in psychosis, as an example of an indicator of vulnerability. Integrity of some domains of sensory processing have been linked to the prenatal environment [24], [25], and well documented as sexually differentiated in the general population (see [26] for review). Deficits in sensory processing and sensorimotor gating/early information-processing in psychosis, however, have only limitedly been discussed with respect to hormonal influences and sexual differentiation (for meta-analysis, see [27]), and genetic factors (e.g., [28], [29]). While an in-depth discussion of later maturational processes (e.g., during adolescence) is beyond the scope of this paper, we briefly discuss this important developmental period in understanding psychosis risk and respective clinical implications. Importantly, throughout each section we contextualize findings (and discuss putative risk factors) with respect to sex differences, the potential modulating role of neurohormones, and synergistic effects towards bolstering current theoretical models of psychosis proneness.

## II. Genetic Factors: Candidate/Susceptibility Genes and Modifier Genes/Epigenetics

*Primary Genetic Risk Factors/Candidate Genes.* It is widely believed that schizophrenia (as with many disorders of mental health) involves a substantial genetic component, though identifying the specific role of genes has proven difficult. From a behavioral genetics perspective, family and twin studies have revealed that risk to siblings of an affected individual is approximately 10 times greater than in the general population, and heritability is 80% or more [30], [31]. Even though heritability is high, concordance in monozygotic (MZ) twins is 41-65% [30]. This phenotypic discordance implicates a role of environmental factors, including suboptimal to severely adverse events occurring as early as prenatal and early postnatal development. Moreover, family studies suggest that simple major gene effects are unlikely. Predominant contemporary genetic hypotheses ascribe to a polygenic model, whereby several common alleles of small to moderate effects and possibly a few rare alleles with larger effects [32], [33] are believed to serve as susceptibility markers. In addition to susceptibility/candidate genes, modifer genes have more recently been suggested to influence clinical/phenotypic expression of illness independent of liability. Together, these findings collectively support the widely accepted notion that multiple genetic factors (whether candidate or modifer genes) act in concert (bidirectionally) with the environment, through development, towards manifestation of psychiatric illness, including psychosis. There remains debate as to the complex nature and direction of these relationships. Discussion of the multifaceted, interactive gene-environment processes that underlie risk for psychosis remains beyond the scope of this chapter, though a comprehensive overview of this literature can be found elsewhere (see [34]). Here we review some of the more prominent candidate and modifier genes linked with psychosis risk and the role of epigenetics.

*Linkage studies.* A number of approaches have been utilized to seek genes for schizophrenia. Work in psychiatric genetics began with linkage studies, which assessed the tendency of certain loci to be inherited together. Early linkage studies were based upon a small number of families with a high number of affected individuals and have progressively used larger numbers of individuals [35], [36]; although many candidate genes have been reported, findings have not been consistently replicated [37]. However, a recent meta-analysis of 32 linkage studies reported a number of significant linkages than would be expected by chance, particularly on chromosomes 2q and 5q [38]. These and similar regions may be involved in conferring weak or moderate effects for the disorder; advanced DNA sequencing methods are required to confirm and define their role in the etiology of schizophrenia. Positional candidate gene studies, which prioritize genes in putative linkage regions, have been more successful in discovering promising susceptibility genes in multiple genetic studies [39]. The most highly implicated genes in positional candidate studies are: Neuroligin 1 *(NRG1), Dysbindin (DTNBP1), D Amino Acid Oxidase Activator (DAOA)*, and *DISC1. NRG1* was identified as a candidate gene via fine-mapping of a locus on chromosome 8 [40] and has been subsequently linked with schizophrenia. *NRG1* encodes many mRNA species and proteins which influence cell-cell signaling, axon guidance, synaptogenesis, glial differentiation, myelination and neurotransmission [41]; however, the mechanisms by which altered *NRG1* function might lead to schizophrenia are unclear. *DTNBP1* was first identified as a gene associated with schizophrenia through linkage on the chromosome 6p [42], and has been replicated in subsequent studies. The function of *DTNBP1* is not well understood, although findings report that *DTNBP1* influences glutamate neurotransmission [43] and reduced levels of *DTNBP1* expression have been found in schizophrenic brains [44]. Chromosome 13, which includes the *DAOA* gene, has strong linkage regions to schizophrenia; replication and a meta-analysis study have supported this finding [45]. *DAOA* activates D amino acid oxidase, which is a coagonist at NMDA glutamate receptors. Therefore, there is plausibility for both *DTNBP1*and *DAOA* to be candidate genes based on the glutamate hypothesis for schizophrenia. Finally, *DISC1* on chromosome 1 has been implicated in schizophrenia, bipolar disorder and other major mental illnesses [46]. Although its molecular mechanism is unknown, *DISC1* is thought to be involved in brain development and adult neuronal functioning such as neuronal migration and maturation, synaptic transmission and plasticity.

*Association studies.* The limited power of linkage studies to identify genes of modest effect led to the recent development of association studies. Genetic association studies are based on the assumption that common diseases are a result of the contribution of many, small-effect genes and that susceptibility alleles will be shared by a significant proportion of common variants with small effect sizes. The recent creation of a genome-wide map of 3.1 million single nucleotide polymorphisms (SNPs) spanning the entire genome has allowed researchers to conduct genome-wide association studies (GWAS) of large clinical and non-clinical samples [47]. GWAS combines the qualities of association (power to detect small effects) with that of linkage studies (no requirement for specific knowledge of pathogenesis). One GWAS study based on pooled DNA sampling, where DNA from multiple cases is mixed together, has reported a significant association to the *REELIN* gene which is believed to encode a protein involved in neuronal positioning and neuronal development [48]; further replication is needed to confirm this particular finding. GWAS based on individual genotyping have implicated genes such as *colony stimulating factor 2 receptor alpha* (*CSF2RA*) which is thought to regulate granulocytes and macrophages, and *short stature homeobox isoform b* (*SHOX*) which is a transcription factor whose involvement is still unknown [49]. Interestingly, another GWAS based on individual genotyping for schizophrenia revealed a significant result for the *zinc finger protein 804A* gene (*ZNF804A*) only when the phenotype was expanded to include bipolar disorder [50]. Therefore, *ZNF804A* is very likely a susceptibility locus for schizophrenia and bipolar disorder, two disorders that share similar clinical symptomatology.

*Copy number variants (CNVs).* The same technology that allows for GWAS also permits the detection of CNVs. CNVs are stretches of genomic deletions and duplications ranging from 1 kb to several Mb that can vary between individuals; thus, they are likely to have larger phenotypic effects than SNPs. One of the most consistent findings is the role of chromosome 22q11; a deletion of chromosome 22q11 increases the risk for schizophrenia approximately 25-fold [51]. Recently, there has been compelling evidence that additional CNVs contribute to the etiology of schizophrenia. For example, major recurrent CNVs associated with schizophrenia are 1q21 deletions [52], and 15q13 deletions [53]. With regards to individual CNVs implicating specific genes, [54] identified a rare deletion affecting part of gene *NRXN1*, which has been previously implicated in autism and mental retardation [55]. They also observed a *de novo* duplication of *amyloid beta A4 precursor protein-binding* (APBA2), a protein which interacts with *NRXN1*. Together, *NRXN1*and APBA2 is believed to play a role in synaptic development and function. Also, preliminary results appear to implicate the *CNTNAP2* gene, which codes for the *contactin-associated protein-like 2*, a cell adhesion protein. Although researchers are still uncertain to what extent CNVs contribute to the disorder, CNV analysis has the potential to identify novel pathogenic mechanisms and provide insight into a broader neuropsychiatric spectrum for schizophrenia.

*Epigenetics.* As discussed above, twin studies do not reveal a 100% concordance rate for schizophrenia; rather, if one twin has schizophrenia, the other has approximately a 50% risk for developing the disorder [56]. This suggests environmental effects also likely contribute to the pathophysiology of schizophrenia. One method in which the environment may render an individual susceptible to developing the disorder is through environmental influence on epigenetic mechanisms. Epigenetics is the study of heritable, but reversible changes in gene expression that occurs without any changes in the genomic DNA sequence [57]. These changes arise primarily through alterations in DNA methylation and chromatin structure, which contribute to the regulation of gene activity in the central nervous system. DNA methylation is characterized by the direct, covalent modification of DNA, where at least three encoded enzymes known as DNA methyltransferases (DNMTs) catalyze the addition of a -CH3 group to cytosine residues at the 5-position of the pyrimidine ring [58]. DNA methylation has been implicated in a number of developmental processes such as genomic imprinting and cellular differentiation [59] as well as neurodevelopmental disorders such as Fragile X mental retardation [60]. Although epigenetic processes play a crucial role in normal cellular differentiation during embryogenesis, recent studies reveal that epigenetic alternation of DNA can also occur during the life span due to environmental influences or stochastic changes [57], and even hormonal stimulation [61]. Therefore, it is reasonable to hypothesize that epigenetic effects can contribute to the etiology of schizophrenia.

Growing evidence for DNA methylation in schizophrenia mainly involves candidate genes associated with neurotransmitter function. For example, *REELIN*, which is expressed primarily by GABAergic interneurons that regulate neighboring glutamatergic neurons, and *GAD1*, which aids in the synthesis of GABA from glutamate, are down-regulated in individuals with schizophrenia [61]. Down-regulation of either of these genes through epigenetic mechanisms can certainly disrupt GABAergic neurotransmission, and altered GABA activity appears responsible for at least some of the clinical features of schizophrenia [62]. Indeed, research has shown that both *DNMT1* mRNA and protein levels are significantly increased in the cortex of individuals with schizophrenia, and these increases parallel deficits in both *REELIN* and *GAD1* [63]. Altered function of serotonin has also been implicated in the increased susceptibility of a number of psychiatric disorders, including schizophrenia [64]. Variation of the gene encoding the 5-HT2A receptor (*HTR2A*) has been associated with schizophrenia in a number of studies. In one study, the methylation of the *HTR2A* C102 allele was found to correlate with *DNMT1* expression levels; furthermore, methylation of the promoter correlated with *HTR2A* expression levels [65]. However, this result has not been consistently replicated; further testing is necessary to elucidate the effects of epigenetic variation and imprinting of *HTR2A* in schizophrenia.

Dysfunction of the limbic pathway and associated dopamine release is thought to heavily influence the pathophysiology of schizophrenia; therefore, understanding the regulation of dopamine levels by focusing on Catecholamine-*O*-Methyltransferase (*COMT)* is one approach for understanding the etiology of schizophrenia. *COMT* is located on chromosome 22q11, an area previously implicated with schizophrenia [51] and is responsible for the metabolism of dopamine in the dorsolateral prefrontal cortex. DNA methylation analyses of *COMT* have been conducted in postmortem brains, and have revealed that methylation of the membrane-bound *COMT* gene promoter was reduced approximately 50% in patients with schizophrenia [66].

*Brain-derived neurotrophic factor* (*BDNF*) is another gene known to play a role in aberrant cognition and mental disorders [67]. Postmortem reports have demonstrated decreased levels of *BDNF* protein and mRNA levels in the prefrontal cortex and hippocampus of schizophrenia patients [68]. Furthermore, one study revealed modest evidence for a correlation between DNA methylation in the *BDNF* gene and a neighboring SNP that has been previously associated with psychosis [69].

Psychosis and other positive symptoms of schizophrenia have also been associated with low activity of *dopamine beta hydroxylase (DβH)* [70], though not consistently [71]. Located in human serum, DβH is a key enzyme that catalyzes the conversion of dopamine to norepinephrine. One early study suggested that individuals with schizophrenia (particularly paranoid subtype) appear to have lower serum DβH concentration than controls [70]. Early linkage studies discovered that the major gene controlling serum DβH activity is linked to ABO on human chromosome 9q34 [72]. Cubells and colleagues [73] demonstrated that the DβH genotype is a major quantitative trait locus for plasma DβH activity, and that it also influences DβH levels in cerebrospinal fluid (CSF). In turn, low plasma or CSF levels of DβH protein have been shown to be associated with greater vulnerability to positive psychotic symptoms in a range of psychiatric disorders [70], [74]. They [74] subsequently demonstrated that genetic variant at DβH associated with low DβH activity ('Del-a' haplotype) is also associated with cocaine-induced paranoia. Similarly, [75] provided evidence suggesting the Del-a haplotype is associated with greater psychiatric symptoms among schizophrenia patients suggesting that, although not causal, the DβH gene may modify psychotic symptoms and illness severity. Cubells and colleagues [76] investigated this possibility through linkage analysis of schizophrenia patients and their relatives; results yielded the first direct evidence for linkage between DβH and plasma DβH activity. This line of research opens the door to novel avenues of investigation exploring modifier genes of psychosis.

Overall, data suggest that DNA methylation may be a viable epigenetic mechanism that contributes to the development of schizophrenia. In particular, some of the genes currently hypothesized to play a role in psychosis via DNA methylation include *REELIN*, *HTR2A*, *COMT*, and *BDNF*. Exciting newly emergent research also suggests a role of DβH in modulating psychotic symptoms. Further research in this area of epigenetics hold promise for elucidating etiological pathways to schizophrenia.

*Sex differences and hormone regulation of genetic risk.*_To date, the genetic basis of observed sex differences in schizophrenia in areas such as premorbid functioning, phenotypic characteristics and course of illness is not well understood. Sex-specific effects of particular genes in psychosis are one possible contender. Neurohormonal influences on early central nervous system development constitute a second viable prospect under increasing investigation.

*Sex differences in genetic risk for psychosis.*_Some sex-specific associations in schizophrenia have been reported for a number of genes such as *COMT* [77] whereby one SNP distributed in the *COMT* gene, rs165599, demonstrated a highly significant effect in affected women compared to men. More evidence for female-specific findings includes polymorphisms of the *nogo* gene, which is a myelin-associated protein associated with neurite growth and regeneration in schizophrenia [78], as well as the *SPEC2*, *PDZ-GEF2* and *ACSL6* genes, which are purported to be involved in signal transduction and enzymatic processes [79].

However, the results of these studies have not been corroborated or replicated in subsequent analyses. More recently, [48] conducted a GWAS for schizophrenia in an Ashkanazi Jewish population using DNA pooling and discovered a female-specific SNP, rs7341475, which is part of the *REELIN* gene; therefore, this common variant of *REELIN* may confer a sex-specific risk for schizophrenia in women.

A recent meta-analysis confirms [48] results implicating *REELIN* as the strongest evidence for genetically-linked sex differences in schizophrenia [80]. Other evidence of sexually differentiated genetic risk for schizophrenia is limited, warranting further investigation. For example, a couple of studies detail a trend towards sex differences. Specifically, greater levels of serotonin mRNA were expressed in peripheral leukocyte among (primarily male) schizophrenia patients compared to healthy controls; within-sex comparisons yielded elevations in mRNA expression in male patients versus decreases in mRNA expression among female patients compared to their healthy counterparts [81].

Moreover, a polymorphism of the DRD3 gene was linked with worse premorbid social functioning and earlier age of onset among women (but not men) with schizophrenia [82].

*The modulating role of genetic factors and neurohormones.* Interestingly, new lines of investigation are pointing to a role of genes (e.g., *COMT*) in modulating neurohormone activity (e.g., HPA byproduct) believed to play a role in potentiating psychosis [83] and, in turn, a role of neurohormones (e.g., cortisol, estrogen) yielded by the HPA and hypothalamic-pituitary-gonadal (HPG) axes in modulating neurotransmitter (e.g., dopamine) activity [84] and vulnerability for psychosis [85], [86].

Interest in the HPA axis arises from neurodevelopmental models of schizophrenia positing a potentiating role of cortisol (a byproduct of the HPA axis, which is known to play a key role in the mammalian biological stress response) on the dopaminergic system towards triggering and exacerbating psychotic symptom expression (see [3]). There is relatively recent evidence of longitudinal, developmental increases in cortisol over time among psychiatric at-risk youth [83] and adolescents with schizotypal personality disorder (SPD; [85]) and an association of cortisol with psychotic-like symptoms among SPD adolescents [85], suggesting postpubertal HPA maturation that moderates psychiatric symptom expression [85].

Moreover, youth at-risk who subsequently developed psychosis showed significantly higher cortisol over time compared to youth who did not convert [86]. Given genetic factors account for approximately 50% of cortisol secretion variability [87], it is reasonable to deduce that genes converge with other genetic and environmental factors [88] towards yielding individual differences in HPA activity and risk for psychiatric illness. In support of this possibility, Walder and colleagues [83] demonstrated differential cortisol levels for *COMT Met* homozygotes (compared with Val carriers) suggesting that *COMT* modulates longitudinal changes in cortisol during adolescence. Genes appear to be implicated in modulating neurohormone secretion, particularly during developmentally sensitive periods (e.g., adolescence) associated with neuromaturation and increased risk for psychosis.

A comprehensive review of the wide range of possible environmental contributors is beyond the scope of this chapter. The next section therefore focuses on the earliest environments encountered in the developmental process; namely, the pre-/peri natal environments, and how influences during this developmental window interface with genetic factors towards psychosis risk.

## III. Pre-/Peri- Natal Factors: Gene-Environment Interactions

Numerous pre- and peri- natal events are believed to alter neurodevelopment, increasing risk for schizophrenia spectrum disorders (SSD) during adolescence and young adulthood. These disruptions range from adverse events experienced by the mother during pregnancy (e.g., prenatal maternal stress) that negatively impact the health and psychological well-being of the mother, to obstetric complications (OCs) during pregnancy and around birth (e.g., preeclampsia, viral exposure, malnutrition). In line with the diathesis-stress model, such pre- and peri- natal disruptions have not only been linked with schizophrenia [89], [90]; (see [91] for review) and in a sex-dependent manner [92], [93]; (see [5] for review), but also may serve as one type of stressor interacting with genes towards precipitation of psychosis. One example of this is a study demonstrating genes involved in neurovascular function (e.g., AKT1,

BDNF, DTNBP1, GRM3) may interact with obstetric complications in psychosis risk [94]; a more extensive discussion of this follows below.

*Seasonality of birth and prenatal viral exposure.* One of the first environmental etiological risk factors for schizophrenia reported in the literature is the so-called seasonality of birth effect [95]. Most studies have consistently observed an excess of winter-spring births in individuals with schizophrenia (see [96] for review). Although a number of factors have been proposed to account for this seasonality effect including meteorological variables, maternal hormones, sperm quality, nutrition and external toxins, one of the most extensively studied factors is prenatal exposure to viral infection [97]. Seminal work by Mednick and colleagues [98] first examined a Finnish birth cohort and showed that individuals exposed to the 1957 type A2 influenza epidemic in Helsinki during their second trimester of fetal development were at elevated risk for being diagnosed with schizophrenia in adulthood. Subsequent research examining different cohorts narrowed the critical risk period further. Machon et al. [99] found that individuals who were exposed to the 1969 Hong Kong influenza epidemic during week 23 of the $6^{th}$ month of gestation had elevated scores on an index of schizotypal personality characteristics – a proposed indicator of genetic vulnerability for developing SSD. Exposure to other infections including a wide variety of respiratory infection [100], rubella [101], and poliovirus infection [102] during the first and second trimesters have been associated with significantly increased risk of SSD. More recently, Mortensen et al. [103] showed that elevated levels of maternal herpes simplex virus 2 (HSV-2) antibodies were associated with increased risk in the Danish National Birth Cohort.

Several researchers are currently using animal models in an attempt to better understand the brain pathology that results from prenatal viral exposure, which might increase vulnerability for SSD. In a mouse model, maternal exposure to influenza (H1N1) virus resulted in upregulation of serotonin ($5HT_2A$) receptors and downregulation of glutamate ($mGlu_2$) receptors in the frontal cortex of the offspring [104]. In a monkey model, one year old offspring of mothers who had been infected with influenza (H3N2) virus in the early third trimester showed reduced cortical gray matter especially in the cingulate and parietal areas and a reduction in parietal white matter [105]. These neurochemical and neuroanatomical changes are similar to pathology observed in patients with schizophrenia.

Though extensively studied, the association between viral exposure and schizophrenia risk remains controversial for a number of reasons. First, not all research has found evidence of elevated risk in exposed individuals [106]. Secondly, most viruses do not cross the placental barrier and therefore direct viral exposure of the fetus is not a viable explanation for the elevated risk observed. Thus, researchers have suggested that the deleterious effects of prenatal viral exposure may be due to maternal antiviral responses such as the release of pro-inflammatory cytokines. From assays in archived prenatal sera, Ellman et al. [107] determined that exposure to cytokine interleukin-8 (IL-8) was associated with increases in ventricular cerebrospinal fluid and decreases in left entorhinal cortex volume and right posterior cingulate volume, all areas consistently implicated in schizophrenia research. Boksa [108] provides a review of behavioral, structural, and functional changes in rodent models exposed to prenatal immune activation including the potential role of immunogens, cytokines, prostaglandins, and oxidative stress on neurodevelopment.

*Prenatal maternal malnutrition.* Another extensively studied prenatal risk factor for SSD is maternal malnutrition. This body of research was sparked by another cohort study led by Susser and colleagues [90], [109]. These studies showed that both men and women conceived during the 1944-1945 Dutch Hunger Winter and born to severely malnourished mothers were at a twofold increased risk for later developing schizophrenia. Similar results have been reported in cohorts of individuals exposed to the 1959-1961 famine in China [110], [111]. Nutritional deficiencies implicated include folate, essential fatty acids, retinodis, vitamin D, and iron (see [112] for review). In a Finnish birth cohort, failure to take vitamin D supplements during the first year of life was associated with increased risk only in males [113]. Vitamin D in rat models has been associated with structural and functional changes in the brain including altered dopaminergic function (see [114] for review). As is the case with prenatal viral exposure, the underlying mechanisms that may lead to these brain changes are unclear. Some research, however, has shown that malnourished pregnant rats show increased levels of pro-inflammatory cytokines similar to those seen during viral infection and this might help explain the deleterious effects on offspring [115].

*Prenatal maternal stress.* In addition to viral exposure and maternal malnutrition which can have obvious physiological implications for the developing fetal nervous system, prenatal maternal stress has also been implicated as an important etiological factor that may alter fetal brain development. Maternal stressors experienced during pregnancy that have been examined include bereavement [116-118], military invasion/war [119], [120], and natural disasters such as floods [121], earthquakes [122], and tornados [123]. Stress exposure results in activation of the HPA axis and increased glucocorticoid release.

Some researchers have suggested that exposure to these environmental stressors during prenatal development particularly affects regions of the brain responsible for negative feedback of the HPA axis such as the hippocampus (see [124] for review), and thus may lead to dysregulation of the system and hypersensitivity to stress [3]. In a mouse model, offspring of mothers exposed to a stressor showed a transient period of abnormal growth of brain cells during postweaning and in adolescence, followed by dramatic dendritic atrophy in the same area during adulthood [125]. Notably, the affected region (cerebellar vermis) has considerable connections with brain regions involved in HPA axis regulation. Interestingly, offspring of rats exposed to the glucocorticoid receptor agonist dexamethasone during gestation demonstrate behavioral deficits (e.g., decreased social play, blunted startle reflex, increased prepulse inhibition (PPI) of startle, reduced amphetamine-induced motor activity) characteristic of SSD [126].

*Obstetric complications (OCs).* Beyond maternal environmental stressors, substantive research has supported a link between complications during pregnancy and elevated risk for SSD. These complications include preeclampsia [92], bleeding during pregnancy [92], [93], [127], diabetes mellitus during pregnancy (see [128] for review), rhesus incompatibility [129] and maternal-fetal genotype incompatibility [130], low birth weight [131-134], and complications during delivery including asphyxia [135], uterine atony [93], and emergency Cesarean section [136], [137] (see [91], [138] for review). Though these OCs are diverse, some researchers have proposed that the underlying mechanism for all pre- and peri- natal complications associated with later SSD is fetal hypoxia [139]. Using individuals from the National Collaborative Perinatal Project, Cannon and colleagues [140] reported that individuals that experience three or more hypoxia-related OCs were five times more likely to develop schizophrenia than individuals with no history of hypoxia-related OCs.

*Gene-environment interactions.* Although the association between SSD and OCs appears strong, a history of OCs is associated with increased risk for a number of psychiatric disorders including autism [141-143], attention deficit hyperactivity disorder (ADHD) [144-146], anorexia nervosa and bulimia nervosa [147], [148], and mood disorders [127], [149]. This lack of diagnostic specificity seems to suggest that complications during prenatal development and birth may increase one's vulnerability to psychopathology in general, and the clinical expression of this vulnerability will depend on later gene-environment interactions [150], [151]. For instance, Jablensky and colleagues [152] reported that women with schizophrenia were more likely to experience placental abruption, to give birth to low birth-weight babies, and to have babies with cardiovascular congenital anomalies and that these complications were more likely to occur after psychiatric diagnosis had been made. It therefore appears that risk of OCs is significantly higher in babies that already carry genetic vulnerability for SSD and that an interaction between these two factors may determine the clinical expression of this vulnerability.

Studies investigating the interaction between putative schizophrenia vulnerability genes and winter birth have yielded mixed results. Narita et al. [153] found an excess of winter births in patients with schizophrenia with HLA-DR1 genotype, though Tochigi et al. [154] failed to replicate these findings. Chotai et al. [155] found polymorphisms of 5-HTTLPR and DRD4 to be associated with season of birth in female schizophrenia patients only, whereas Muntjewerff et al. [156] found neither winter birth, MTHFR 677TT genotype, nor their interaction was associated with increased schizophrenia risk.

Given that hypoxia-related OCs have been linked with schizophrenia risk, one study examined the rate at which several candidate genes for schizophrenia are also known to be sensitive to hypoxia regulation and/or may be related to vascular expression [157]. Results indicated that over 50% of the identified schizophrenia vulnerability genes (e.g., AKT1, BDNF, COMT, NRG1, RELN, TNF among others) met these criteria, suggesting that genes linked with schizophrenia susceptibility may (in part) exert their influence via regulating hypoxia during development and modulating cerebrovascular function [157].

There is recent evidence that hypoxia-related OCs may interact with some schizophrenia candidate genes. In the first study to empirically test for interaction between genetic risk factors and OCs, Nicodemus et al. [94] reported that several genes involved in vascular function in the brain or regulated by hypoxia – specifically AKT1, BDNF, DTNBP1, and GRM3 – interacted with a history of serious OCs toward increased risk for schizophrenia. Abazyan et al. [158] observed an interaction between mutant human disrupted-in-schizophrenia 1 (mhDISC1) gene and exposure to an immunostimulant (polyinosinic: polycytidylic acid) in a mouse model which produced behavioral abnormalities such as elevated anxiety, depression-like responses, altered sociability, and attenuated reactivity to stress. This interaction also yielded neurobiological abnormalities that resemble those seen in mood disorders and SSD including decreased HPA reactivity, decreased serotonin neurotransmission in the hippocampus, reduced enlargement of lateral ventricles, reduced amygdala and periaqueductal gray matter volumes, and reduced density of hippocampus dendritic spines.

The field's identification of schizophrenia vulnerability and modifier genes (and their interactions) continues to expand. This, together with an evolving appreciation of diverse pre-/peri- natal factors and their complex interplay with polygenic factors brings us closer to understanding their underlying mechanisms of action that contribute to psychosis risk. Future investigations of both the independent effects of, and interactions among, these important etiological factors is clearly warranted.

*Sex differences, hormonal influences and prenatal insults affect early brain development.* In line with conceptualizations of schizophrenia as having neurodevelopmental origins, one factor believed to influence fetal central nervous system development is gonadal hormones. Disruptions in the prenatal gonadal hormone milieu have been implicated in a variety of conditions such as immune dysfunction and autism [159], and more recently in risk for psychosis, as evidenced by disrupted sex differences in a distal indicator of prenatal gonadal hormone; namely digit ratio [20]. Complementary to this literature, there is substantive data supporting a strong association of OCs with a range of neurobiological and behavioral deficits in schizophrenia, more so among males than females; including neuropsychological functioning [160], neurological soft signs [161], and behavior [162]. As outlined by Walder et al. [20], findings of sexual dimorphisms in behavioral sequelae of prenatal insult are consistent with research suggesting the male fetus (compared to the female fetus) may be more susceptible to prenatal gonadal hormone disruptions, adverse pre- and peri- natal events [93] which in turn may contribute to schizophrenia [135], [163], [164] and be sexually differentiated [5], neurodevelopomental abnormalities [165], and neonatal mortality [166]. Sex differences are noted in obstetric complication rates in schizophrenia (males>females) [167], [168] though not uniformly (see [5] for review). Moreover, compared to girls, boys born small for gestational age or exposed to pre-eclampsia or asphyxia at birth are also at increased risk for schizophrenia [93].

Taken together, the aforementioned lines of investigation point to the potential role of one's biological sex, prenatal gonadal hormones and other neurohormonal systems and their byproducts in modulating effects of prenatal events/insults (such as obstetric complications) on brain development and psychosis risk. More focused research on these possibilities, together with consideration of genetic influences, lie imminently on the horizon within this field of study with exciting potential for better understanding the neurobiological and environmental basis (including underlying mechanisms) of psychosis risk.

## IV. Sensory Processing (and Sensorimotor Gating) Deficits as Putative Indicators of Risk for Psychosis

Sensory processing deficits have been implicated in an etiological model of schizophrenia involving dysfunctional transmission at N-methyl-D-aspartate (NMDA)-type glutamate receptors [23]. These deficits in schizophrenia patients and individuals at high-risk have been well characterized in auditory, visual, and (increasingly) olfactory domains, whereas somatosensory and gustatory processing deficits are less well understood. Peripherally relevant to primary sensory processing deficits are impairments in sensory gating in schizophrenia. This section outlines sensory processing and sensory gating functions - as putative indicators of psychosis proneness - across the schizophrenia spectrum, with later consideration of sex differences and the modulating role of gonadal hormones.

*Auditory processing and psychosis risk.* Sensory processing deficits in schizophrenia have been most widely explored in the auditory domain, and are associated with poorer functioning over the course of the illness [169]. For example, schizophrenia patients demonstrate tone matching [170] and speech perception deficits [171] relative to controls.

Neurophysiological evidence using electroencephalography (EEG) and magnetoencephalography (MEG) corroborate behavioral findings in that schizophrenia patients exhibit auditory processing abnormalities in initial sensory registration, prediction and temporal integration in paired speech stimulus to noise paradigms, mismatch negativity (MMN) response component, and early N1/P1 response components (for a review see [172]).

Two principal neurophysiological measures in understanding the pathophyisology of auditory processing deficits in schizophrenia are P300 and MMN. The P300 component is conceptualized as an index of context updating and/or stimulus categorization of higher cognitive processing. Schizophrenia patients exhibit reduced P300 amplitude related to reduced superior temoporal gyrus (STG) volume ([173]; for a review see [174]). Schizophrenia patients tend to exhibit prominent STG gray matter reductions [175], [176] and decreased volumes of pyramidal neurons in layer 3 of primary and secondary auditory cortices suggestive of feed-forward auditory processing deficits [177].

The MMN component can be elicited independent of attention with various stimuli (e.g., auditory, visual, somatosensory), and across developmental and clinical populations. The MMN response component is dependent on NMDA-type glutamate receptor functioning [178], and has been implicated in the pathophysiology of schizophrenia [170]. Schizophrenia patients consistently exhibit attenuated auditory MMN (aMMN; [179]) responses, and the neural generators of this component have been well-characterized, primarily localized to the STG [180]. Diminished aMMN in schizophrenia patients is associated with greater illness severity and cognitive deficits [181], and greater functional decline [169].

The electrophysiological auditory steady state response (ASSR) is a measure of the integrity of synchronous oscillatory brain activity in response to temporally-linked stimuli, and is modified by attention (see [182] for a review). Consistent with the aforementioned neurophysiological findings with respect to P300 and MMN, ASSR deficits are associated with decreased bilateral activity in the STG. Inhibitory GABAergic interneurons and interactions with glutamatergic mechanisms (specifically via NMDA-type receptors) are thought to modulate gamma oscillations and may underlie ASSR disruptions in schizophrenia [182], though the neural mechanisms are still not fully understood.

*Auditory processing and genetics in psychosis.* Genetic findings in relation to neurophysiological components (e.g., P300, MMN) assist in the identification of the underlying pathophysiology of auditory processing deficits in schizophrenia [174]. For example, reduced NoGo-P300 differences indicative of deficits in response inhibition and monitoring associated with anterior cingulate functioning have been associated with dysbindin gene polymorphisms that modulate the glutamatergic neurotransmitter system and have been linked to schizophrenia [183].

Findings are mixed regarding associations between decreased MMN amplitude and genetic risk for schizophrenia [184-186]. MMN has been linked with catechol-O-methyltransferase (COMT) gene variants, a key enzyme in dopamine degradation [187]. Increased dopamine degradation in prefrontal regions reduces inhibitory GABAergic projections to subcortical regions (e.g., basal ganglia), which in turn results in increases in tyrosine-hydroxylase mRNA and unregulated increases in subcortical dopamine release. This cascade is associated with poorer prefrontal executive functioning, loose associations and positive symptoms of schizophrenia (see [174] for a review).

With regard to ASSR, it remains unclear whether gamma frequency range (30-50Hz) deficits in this component represent a risk marker versus indicator of sensitivity to psychosis expression [182]. There is some evidence of ASSR gamma frequency deficits in schizophrenia patients [188] and first-degree relatives but not medicated schizophrenia patients [189] or individuals with schizotypal personality disorder [182, 190]. This pattern of findings is suggestive of ASSR as a genetic biomarker of risk for schizophrenia, though perhaps not an indicator of clinical high risk [182]. More research examining the link between steady state response and genetic risk is indicated.

*Visual processing.* Schizophrenia patients exhibit visual processing deficits in motion and form perception, low spatial frequency and location discrimination, perceptual organization, and backward masking performance that are modulated by distinguishable neural mechanisms (see [23] for a review). The visual system is characterized by two pathways: magnocellular (M) and parvocellular (P), which project to the dorsal (i.e., parieto-occipital) and ventral streams (i.e., temporo-occipital), respectively. Neurons of the M pathway have large cell bodies and rapidly respond to low-contrast, low spatial resolution stimuli, and motion, but not color or fine-details. Conversely, neurons of the P pathway have smaller cell bodies and respond relatively slowly to fine details, high-resolution stimuli, and color, but not low contrast stimuli. Visual processing can be understood in terms of gain control (i.e., adaptation and optimization of responses to visual stimuli) and integration (i.e., coordinated neural responses via co-activation that subsequently guide behavior; [191]). Gain control is directly influenced by NMDA-type glutamate receptor functioning as demonstrated by decreases in stimulus response amplitude and lateral inhibition following administration of NMDA antagonists, and may be more closely associated with the M than P pathway, yet both are involved. The response of M neurons sharply increases with increases in luminance contrast, but then plateau at approximately 16%, whereas P neurons begin to respond at a luminance contrast of approximately 10%, and increase linearly. Schizophrenia patients exhibit decreases in gain control as evidenced in motion perception, contrast sensitivity, and lateral inhibition paradigms (see [191] for a review). Opposite to healthy controls, schizophrenia patients demonstrate greater susceptibility to an illusion that is typically endorsed more frequently with decreasing contrast, but demonstrated less susceptibility to visual illusions that become more prominent with increasing contrast, indicating deficits in contrast sensitivity [192]. Kantrowitz and colleagues [192] suggest the differential pattern of susceptibility to visual illusions in schizophrenia patients relative to controls is mediated by deficits in the M processing stream that may disrupt higher order cognitive-perceptual processing.

Disruptions of early visual processing mediated by the M pathway are implicated in facial emotion identification deficits commonly seen in schizophrenia patients [193]. Schizophrenia patients exhibit M-dependent contrast sensitivity deficits of emotional stimuli relative to controls, and deficits are associated with facial emotion identification (i.e., fear, anger, happiness, sadness, and neutral) and differentiation of facial emotion intensity [194]. Poorer emotion identification is associated with reduced steady state visual evoked potentials (ssVEP) specific to M-based, but not P-based, neural responses [194]. Among schizophrenia patients, poorer social cognition, as assessed via emotion perception, is a predictor of less social support, deficits in social competence, and poorer global functional outcome [195]. Similarly, visual steady state response (VSSR) paradigms suggest that schizophrenia patients exhibit decreased power in frontal and parietal regions in the alpha frequency range (9-12 Hz). Furthermore, the deficits tend to reflect disruptions in the M (e.g., luminance) pathway rather than the P (e.g., chromatic) pathway, and are consistent with reductions in gray matter thickness in the occipital cortex present at first-episode, as well as reduced white matter tract integrity of the optic radiations (see [182] for a review).

Visual integration deficits in schizophrenia patients 1) have been demonstrated in response to contrast, contour, form and motion stimulus paradigms; 2) are associated with disorganized symptom presentation [196] and poorer premorbid social functioning [197]; and, 3) are also thought to be modulated by NMDA-type glutamatergic activity (i.e., decreased lateral excitation signaling integration of relevant spatial features; [191], [198]). For example, schizophrenia patients tend to perform better than controls on tasks of contrast discrimination, indicating specific abnormalities of visual processing (i.e., deficits of orientation-specific surround suppression) in the primary visual cortex functioning, which is inconsistent with a generalized perceptual deficit hypothesis [199].

Early visual processing of the M pathway, integration, and selective visual attention may be modulated by aberrant hemispheric asymmetries among schizophrenia patients relative to controls [200]. Performance on a global-local task (i.e., a large letter made up of small letters, respectively) can assess a predominately right hemisphere response to global stimuli and a predominately left hemisphere response to local stimuli, as well as effects of shifting, priming and interference on task performance. Schizophrenia patients exhibit impaired shifting from global/low frequency to local/high frequency stimulus identification, but not vice versa, suggestive of disruptions in the shift from right hemisphere to left hemisphere engagement [200], possibly modulated by M system disruptions secondarily affecting P system functioning [201] rather than generalized errors. Also, local interference in global processing (i.e., longer reaction time) is consistent with global processing deficits implicating M pathway dysfunction.

*Olfaction.* Olfactory processing is mediated by frontal and temporolimbic regions, and deficits in identification, detection threshold sensitivity, and memory of odors have been proposed as biomarkers of risk for schizophrenia (for review see [202]). Odor molecules enervate receptors in the olfactory bulb and, via the lateral olfactory tract, enervate the primary olfactory cortex, which makes this system one of the most direct pathways from the external environment to the central nervous system. The primary olfactory cortex then sends projections to various structures (i.e., anterior olfactory nucleus, olfactory tubercle, piriform cortex, amygdala, entorhinal cortex) that project directly to the frontal cortex, and indirectly to the orbitofrontal cortex via the thalamus, the hypothalamus via the amygdala, and the hippocampus via entorhinal cortex [203].

*Olfaction and prenatal disruptions.* The olfactory system is thought to be functional late in fetal development, is susceptible to environmental perturbations (e.g., exposure to toxins) that disrupt typical development, and structures involved in olfaction have also been implicated in the pathophysiology of schizophrenia (for review see [202]). Thus, some suggest that insults that affect olfactory system development may also affect neurodevelopment more broadly, perhaps increasing risk for psychopathology [204]. This is the closest evidence (we are aware of to date) that links prenatal disruptions with olfactory deficits.

While the olfactory system is less well studied in schizophrenia, it holds particular promise given the unique feature that the olfactory epithelium cells regenerate approximately every 2 to 3 months. This trait provides an opportunity for the examination of neurodevelopmental changes involved in basic sensory processing of odors in live individuals. In fact, biopsies of olfactory epithelium cells of living schizophrenia patients are abnormal relative to controls [205]. Smell identification deficits (SID) are relatively specific to schizophrenia and the negative symptom dimension [206], and have been identified in young adults with psychotic disorders [207] and first-degree relatives of schizophrenia patients relative to controls (see [204] for a review), suggestive of a link between olfactory deficits and genetic risk for the illness. Moreover, behavioral findings have been corroborated by neuroanatomical and neurophysiological findings. Schizophrenia patients exhibit regional amplitude reductions of N1 (inferior frontotemporal) and P2 (medial parietal) olfactory event-related potentials (OERPs) relative to healthy controls [204], indicative of central processing deficits.

*Somatosensory processing.* Behavioral somatosensory measures permit non-invasive means to examine proprioception (e.g., weight discrimination), exteroceptive touch sensitivity (e.g., two-point discrimination), tactile spatial resolution (e.g., grating orientation), and complex cognitive somatosensory processing (e.g., graphesthesia). Basic elementary sensory processing (e.g., proprioception, tactile stimulation) begins in cutaneous and subcutaneous receptors, crosses the midline and ascends the medial lemniscal tract, enervating the ventroposterolateral thalamic nuclei and projecting to primary somatosensory cortex (SI); complex cognitive somatosensory processing (e.g., graphesthesia task) also occurs in the secondary somatosensory association cortex (SII; [208]). Thalamic nuclei also send projections to the supplementary motor area and superior parietal lobe.

Schizophrenia patients and first-degree relatives exhibit somatosensory deficits relative to controls, whereas first-degree relatives of bipolar patients do not, suggesting specificity to schizophrenia [209]. Among nonclinical undergraduate students, elevated two-point discrimination thresholds are related to greater levels of schizotypy [210]. Elementary sensory functions are disrupted in patients with SI lesions, but spared in patients with parietal lesions sparing SI (see [211] for a review). Electrophysiological research indicates that schizophrenia patients exhibit: 1) disruptions in sensorimotor and frontal-parietal-temporal networks in response to somatosensory stimuli [212], 2) abnormal somatosensory evoked potentials [213], and 3) reversed asymmetry and displaced somatosensory evoked field potentials [214]. The neural circuitry associated with somatosensory duration-processing sensitivity in response to vibrotactile stimuli can be assessed via the mismatch negativity (MMN) component of human event-related potentials [180]. However, little is known regarding somatosensory MMN (sMMN) among clinical populations. Two-point discrimination performance is associated with the N20 component generated by SI (areas 3b and 1; [215]); moreover, schizophrenia patients have exhibited high frequency oscillations with prolonged latency and higher amplitude in the low frequency range of N20 relative to controls, which may be indicative of decreased thalamic inhibition and related to positive symptoms [213].

While some suggest that somatosensory processing deficits (based on behavioral measures) among nonclinical [210] and genetic high risk [209], [216], [217] are independent of broad cognitive functioning, others propose "panmodal processing imprecision" as a primary etiological factor in schizophrenia [218], [219].

*Sex differences and neurohormonal effects in sensory processing and sensorimotor gating.* Overall, few studies of sensory processing deficits in schizophrenia examine sex differences. In the realm of olfactory function, sex differences - notably a female advantage (see [26] for review) - are well established in the general population. Few diagnosis-specific sex differences in odor identification, detection threshold sensitivity, discrimination, and memory have been demonstrated. It has been posited that this is likely due to the shortage of studies examining olfactory processing by sex in schizophrenia patients relative to controls

[27]. One study of schizophrenia patients found that male patients performed worse than female patients, male controls and female controls, whereas the latter three groups performed comparably, suggesting a differential sex effect in patients [220]. There is also evidence that male schizophrenia patients exhibited hedonic deficits in experiencing pleasant odors relative to female schizophrenia patients, suggesting that subjective odor judgments, associated with affect, may differ by sex [221]. By comparison, one recent large, retrospective study of young psychotic patients (in the early course of illness) found a normal pattern of sex differences in smell identification among patients [222]. These studies (albeit limited in number) suggest a potential relation of olfactory sex differences with illness duration (and possibly age); the lack of research in this area highlights the need for future investigation along these lines.

Interestingly, while there is a dearth of literature on sex differences in sensory processing in schizophrenia, there is an emerging body of literature pointing to sex differences and hormonal influences in sensorimotor gating and implications for psychosis (for review see [223]). As outlined by Kumari [223], sensorimotor gating generally refers to the process (or ability) to filter out (or gate) irrelevant or interfering information/stimuli within the environment. One operational index of sensorimotor gating is prepulse inhibition (PPI), or attenuation of the startle response. Impaired gating of stimulus interference (or PPI) was initially demonstrated in schizophrenia over three decades ago [224], lending support to the theory that this disorder involved early stage information processing deficits, which are believed to contribute to sensory overload [225] and play a role in psychotic symptoms [226].

PPI is of marked interest in the field – particularly as a potential endophenotypic marker of psychosis - given it is highly heritable [227], reduced across the schizophrenia spectrum [228], [229], and genetically mediated [223], [230]. Kumari [223] emphasizes that some genetic influences, however, appear to be specific to healthy men, whereas PPI in healthy women is speculated to vary as a function of the menstrual cycle. The author reviews the literature demonstrating that PPI is sexually dimorphic (though not prior to 8 years of age) and sensitive to menstrual cycle phase in healthy women – with more PPI during early follicular (when estrogen levels are low) relative to luteal phase (when estrogen and progesterone levels are high). PPI is additionally of interest in light of research suggesting that 1) second generation antipsychotics may attenuate PPI impairments in schizophrenia [231] and 2) progesterone may have antipsychotic-like effects, including PPI restoration, among healthy young women during the luteal menstrual phase [232].

## Conclusion

It is now well established that schizophrenia has neurodevelopmental origins, as evidenced (in part) by a wide range of neurobiological findings that link vulnerability factors and disruptions in early development with subsequent illness manifestation. As reviewed in this chapter, some prime influences include genetic factors (i.e., candidate/susceptibility genes, modifier genes, epigenetics) and pre-/peri- natal factors that impact brain development, as well as sensory processing/sensorimotor gating deficits that may serve as potential vulnerability indicators of psychosis risk. Associations across these influences and their interactions (e.g., gene-environment interactions) are increasingly being considered with respect to etiology of, and risk for, psychosis from a diathesis-stress perspective. Relatively new to this field of study is consideration of sexual dimorphisms and the modulating role of neurohormones in setting the stage for – and later potentiating - underlying vulnerability towards illness manifestation. Emerging awareness of the import of neurohormonal influences in psychosis risk and outcome, particularly during adolescence, as evidenced (in part) by longitudinal pubertal elevations in hormones that are exaggerated in psychosis risk (e.g., [85]; see [233]), sex differences [234], and menstrual cycle (natural fluctuations in gonadal hormone) effects on stress hormones and non-clinical psychiatric symptoms in young adulthood [22], brings to our attention the role of neuromaturational processes that extend beyond the earliest of neurodevelopmental periods. This is reinforced by evidence that the epigenome, for example, is sensitive to environmental influences beginning in the prenatal period, through puberty and into old age (see [15]). Though extensive discussion is beyond the scope of this chapter, elucidation of early developmental (e.g., genetic; pre-/peri- natal) influences, how these are modified by later developmental events - both environmental and neurobiological in nature (e.g., pubertal hormone surge) – and, importantly, their underlying neural mechanisms have important implications for early identification of at-risk youth and future development of means of prevention and early intervention across the psychotic spectrum.

## REFERENCES

[1] T. F. McNeil and E. Cantor-Graae, "Neuromotor markers of risk for schizophrenia.," *Australian and New Zealand journal of psychiatry*, vol. 34, pp. S86-90, Nov. 2000.

[2] E. F. Walker, T. Savoie, and D. Davis, "Neuromotor Precursors of Schizophrenia," *Schizophrenia bulletin*, vol. 20, no. 3, pp. 441-451, 1994.

[3] E. F. Walker and D. Diforio, "Schizophrenia: a neural diathesis-stress model.," *Psychological review*, vol. 104, no. 4, pp. 667-685, Oct. 1997.

[4] E. F. Walker, D. J. Walder, R. Lewine, and R. Loewy, "Sex differences in the origins and premorbid development of schizophrenia," in *Psychiatric illness in women: emerging treatments and research*, F. Lewis-Hall, T. S. Williams, J. A. Panetta, and J. H. Herrera, Eds. Washington, D.C.: American Psychiatric Publishing, 2002, pp. 193-214.

[5] J. M. Goldstein and D. J. Walder, "Sex differences in schizophrenia: the case for developmental origins," in *The early course of schizophrenia*, T. Sharma and P. Harvey, Eds. New York, NY: Oxford University Press, 2006, pp. 143-173.

[6] A. H. Fanous and K. S. Kendler, "Genetic heterogeneity, modifier genes, and quantitative phenotypes in psychiatric illness: searching for a framework.," *Molecular psychiatry*, vol. 10, no. 1, pp. 6-13, Jan. 2005.

[7] T. D. Cannon, I. M. Rosso, C. E. Bearden, L. E. Sanchez, and T. Hadley, "A prospective cohort study of neurodevelopmental processes in the genesis and epigenesis of schizophrenia.," *Development and psychopathology*, vol. 11, no. 3, pp. 467-85, Jan. 1999.

[8] J. Kaufman et al., "Social supports and serotonin transporter gene moderate depression in maltreated children.," *Proceedings of the National Academy of Sciences of the United States of America*, vol. 101, no. 49, pp. 17316-21, Dec. 2004.

[9] D. K. Kinney, A. M. Miller, D. J. Crowley, E. Huang, and E. Gerber, "Autism prevalence following prenatal exposure to hurricanes and tropical storms in Louisiana.," *Journal of autism and developmental disorders*, vol. 38, no. 3, pp. 481-8, Mar. 2008.

[10] M. Weinstock, "The long-term behavioural consequences of prenatal stress.," *Neuroscience and biobehavioral reviews*, vol. 32, no. 6, pp. 1073-86, Aug. 2008.

[11] M. Weinstock, "Sex-dependent changes induced by prenatal stress in cortical and hippocampal morphology and behaviour in rats: An update," *Stress*, vol. 14, no. 6, pp. 604-13, 2011.

[12] J. R. Seckl and M. J. Meaney, "Glucocorticoid programming," in *Biobehavioral stress response: protective and damaging effects*, B. Yehuda and R. McEwen, Eds. New York, NY: New York Academy of Sciences, 2004, pp. 63-84.

[13] S. King, A. Mancini-Marïe, A. Brunet, E. Walker, M. J. Meaney, and D. P. Laplante, "Prenatal maternal stress from a natural disaster predicts dermatoglyphic asymmetry in humans.," *Development and Psychopathology*, vol. 21, pp. 343-353, 2009.

[14] E. F. Walker, H. D. Trotman, J. Brasfied, M. Esterberg, and M. Larsen, "Stress hormones, genes and neuronal signaling in adolescence," in *The dynamic genome and mental health: The role of genes and environments in youth development*, K. S. Kendler, S. R. Jaffee, and D. Romer, Eds. New York, NY: Oxford University Press, 2011, pp. 388-408.

[15] D. C. Dolinoy, R. Das, J. R. Weidman, and R. L. Jirtle, "Metastable epialleles, imprinting, and the fetal origins of adult diseases.," *Pediatric research*, vol. 61, no. 5 Pt 2, p. 30R-37R, May. 2007.

[16] H. Hafner, "Gender differences in schizophrenia.," *Psychoneuroendocrinology*, vol. 28, pp. 17-54, 2003.

[17] D. J. Walder, L. J. Seidman, N. Cullen, J. Su, M. T. Tsuang, and J. M. Goldstein, "Sex differences in language dysfunction in schizophrenia," *American Journal of Psychiatry*, vol. 163, pp. 470-477, 2006.

[18] D. J. Walder, L. J. Seidman, N. Makris, M. T. Tsuang, D. N. Kennedy, and J. M. Goldstein, "Neuroanatomic substrates of sex differences in language dysfunction in schizophrenia: a pilot study.," *Schizophrenia research*, vol. 90, no. 1-3, pp. 295-301, Feb. 2007.

[19] D. J. Walder, V. Mittal, H. D. Trotman, a L. McMillan, and E. F. Walker, "Neurocognition and conversion to psychosis in adolescents at high-risk.," *Schizophrenia research*, vol. 101, no. 1-3, pp. 161-8, Apr. 2008.

[20] D. J. Walder, T. L. C. Andersson, A. L. McMillan, S. M. Breedlove, and E. F. Walker, "Sex differences in digit ratio (2D:4D) are disrupted in adolescents with schizotypal personality disorder: altered prenatal gonadal hormone levels as a risk factor.," *Schizophrenia research*, vol. 86, no. 1-3, pp. 118-22, Sep. 2006.

[21] P. E. Meehl, "Schizotaxia, schizotypy, schizophrenia.," *American Psychologist*, vol. 17, no. 12, pp. 827-838, 1962.

[22] D. J. Walder, M. Statucka, M. P. Daly, K. Axen, and M. Haber, "Biological sex and menstrual cycle phase modulation of cortisol levels and psychiatric symptoms in a non-clinical sample of young adults," *Psychiatry Research*, In Press.

[23] D. C. Javitt, "When doors of perception close: bottom-up models of disrupted cognition in schizophrenia.," *Annual review of clinical psychology*, vol. 5, pp. 249-75, Jan. 2009.

[24] R. T. Lacy, C. F. Mactutus, and S. B. Harrod, "Prenatal IV nicotine exposure produces a sex difference in sensorimotor gating of the auditory startle reflex in adult rats.," *International journal of developmental neuroscience*, vol. 29, no. 2, pp. 153-61, May. 2011.

[25] M. L. Schneider, C. F. Moore, and M. M. Adkins, "The effects of prenatal alcohol exposure on behavior: rodent and primate studies.," *Neuropsychology Review*, vol. 21, pp. 186-203, 2011.

[26] K. Good and L. Kopala, "Sex differences in olfactory function," in *Smell and the brain: window to the mind*, W. Brewer, D. Castle, and C. Pantelis, Eds. Cambridge, UK: Cambridge University Press, 2006, pp. 183-202.

[27] P. J. Moberg, R. Agrin, R. E. Gur, R. C. Gur, B. I. Turetsky, and R. L. Doty, "Olfactory dysfunction in schizophrenia: a qualitative and quantitative review.," *Neuropsychopharmacology*, vol. 21, no. 3, pp. 325-40, Sep. 1999.

[28] B. Quednow et al., "The schizophrenia risk allele C of the TCF4 rs9960767 polymorphism disrupts sensorimotor gating in schizophrenia spectrum and healthy volunteers," *Journal Neuroscience*, vol. 31, pp. 6684-6691, 2011.

[29] L. C. Kopala, K. P. Good, K. Morrison, A. S. Bassett, M. Alda, and W. G. Honer, "Impaired olfactory identification in relatives of patients with familial schizophrenia.," *American Journal Psychiatry*, vol. 158, pp. 1286-1290, 2001.

[30] A. G. Cardno and I. I. Gottesman, "Twin studies of schizophrenia: from bow-and-arrow concordances to star wars Mx and functional genomics," *American Journal of Medical Genetics*, vol. 97, no. 1, pp. 12-17, 2000.

[31] P. F. Sullivan, K. S. Kendler, and M. C. Neale, "Schizophrenia as a complex trait: evidence from a meta-analysis of twin studies," *Archives of General Psychiatry*, vol. 60, no. 12, pp. 1187-1192, Dec. 2003.

[32] I. I. Gottesman and J. Shields, "A polygenic theory of schizophrenia," *Proceedings of the National Academy of Sciences of the United States of America*, vol. 58, no. 1, pp. 199-205, Jul. 1967.

[33] W. Y. Wang, B. J. Barratt, D. G. Clayton, and J. A. Todd, "Genome-wide association studies: theoretical and practical concerns," *Nature reviews.Genetics*, vol. 6, no. 2, pp. 109-118, Feb. 2005.

[34] K. Kendler, S. Jaffee, and D. Romer, *The dynamic genome and mental health: The role of genes and environments in youth development.* New York, NY: Oxford University Press, 2011.

[35] N. M. Williams et al., "A systematic genomewide linkage study in 353 sib pairs with schizophrenia," *American Journal of Human Genetics*, vol. 73, no. 6, pp. 1355-1367, Dec. 2003.

[36] B. K. Suarez et al., "Genomewide linkage scan of 409 European-ancestry and African American families with schizophrenia: suggestive evidence of linkage at 8p23.3-p21.2 and 11p13.1-q14.1 in the combined sample," *American Journal of Human Genetics*, vol. 78, no. 2, pp. 315-333, Feb. 2006.

[37] M. J. Owen, N. Craddock, and M. C. O'Donovan, "Schizophrenia: genes at last?," *Trends in genetics*, vol. 21, no. 9, pp. 518-525, Sep. 2005.

[38] M. Y. Ng et al., "Meta-analysis of 32 genome-wide linkage studies of schizophrenia," *Molecular psychiatry*, vol. 14, no. 8, pp. 774-785, Aug. 2009.

[39] C. A. Ross, R. L. Margolis, S. A. Reading, M. Pletnikov, and J. T. Coyle, "Neurobiology of schizophrenia," *Neuron*, vol. 52, no. 1, pp.

[40] P. J. Harrison and A. J. Law, "Neuregulin 1 and schizophrenia: genetics, gene expression, and neurobiology," *Biological psychiatry*, vol. 60, no. 2, pp. 132-140, Jul. 2006.

[41] G. Corfas, K. Roy, and J. D. Buxbaum, "Neuregulin 1-erbB signaling and the molecular/cellular basis of schizophrenia," *Nature neuroscience*, vol. 7, no. 6, pp. 575-580, Jun. 2004.

[42] R. E. Straub et al., "Genetic variation in the 6p22.3 gene DTNBP1, the human ortholog of the mouse dysbindin gene, is associated with schizophrenia," *American Journal of Human Genetics*, vol. 71, no. 2, pp. 337-348, Aug. 2002.

[43] T. Numakawa et al., "Evidence of novel neuronal functions of dysbindin, a susceptibility gene for schizophrenia," *Human molecular genetics*, vol. 13, no. 21, pp. 2699-2708, Nov. 2004.

[44] N. J. Bray et al., "Haplotypes at the dystrobrevin binding protein 1 (DTNBP1) gene locus mediate risk for schizophrenia through reduced DTNBP1 expression," *Human molecular genetics*, vol. 14, no. 14, pp. 1947-1954, Jul. 2005.

[45] S. D. Detera-Wadleigh and F. J. McMahon, "G72/G30 in schizophrenia and bipolar disorder: review and meta-analysis," *Biological psychiatry*, vol. 60, no. 2, pp. 106-114, Jul. 2006.

[46] W. Hennah, P. Thomson, L. Peltonen, and D. Porteous, "Genes and schizophrenia: beyond schizophrenia: the role of DISC1 in major mental illness," *Schizophrenia bulletin*, vol. 32, no. 3, pp. 409-416, Jul. 2006.

[47] I. H. Consortium et al., "A second generation human haplotype map of over 3.1 million SNPs," *Nature*, vol. 449, no. 7164, pp. 851-861, Oct. 2007.

[48] S. Shifman et al., "Genome-wide association identifies a common variant in the reelin gene that increases the risk of schizophrenia only in women," *PLoS genetics*, vol. 4, no. 2, p. e28, Feb. 2008.

[49] T. Lencz et al., "Converging evidence for a pseudoautosomal cytokine receptor gene locus in schizophrenia," *Molecular psychiatry*, vol. 12, no. 6, pp. 572-580, Jun. 2007.

[50] M. C. O'Donovan et al., "Identification of loci associated with schizophrenia by genome-wide association and follow-up," *Nature genetics*, vol. 40, no. 9, pp. 1053-1055, Sep. 2008.

[51] K. C. Murphy, L. A. Jones, and M. J. Owen, "High rates of schizophrenia in adults with velo-cardio-facial syndrome," *Archives of General Psychiatry*, vol. 56, no. 10, pp. 940-945, Oct. 1999.

[52] H. C. Mefford et al., "Recurrent rearrangements of chromosome 1q21.1 and variable pediatric phenotypes," *The New England journal of medicine*, vol. 359, no. 16, pp. 1685-1699, Oct. 2008.

[53] A. J. Sharp et al., "A recurrent 15q13.3 microdeletion syndrome associated with mental retardation and seizures," *Nature genetics*, vol. 40, no. 3, pp. 322-328, Mar. 2008.

[54] G. Kirov et al., "Comparative genome hybridization suggests a role for NRXN1 and APBA2 in schizophrenia," *Human molecular genetics*, vol. 17, no. 3, pp. 458-465, Feb. 2008.

[55] A. G. P. Consortium et al., "Mapping autism risk loci using genetic linkage and chromosomal rearrangements," *Nature genetics*, vol. 39, no. 3, pp. 319-328, Mar. 2007.

[56] M. Tsuang, "Schizophrenia: genes and environment," *Biological psychiatry*, vol. 47, no. 3, pp. 210-220, Feb. 2000.
[57] R. Pidsley and J. Mill, "Epigenetic studies of psychosis: current findings, methodological approaches, and implications for postmortem research," *Biological psychiatry*, vol. 69, no. 2, pp. 146-156, Jan. 2011.
[58] A. Bird, "DNA methylation patterns and epigenetic memory," *Genes and development*, vol. 16, no. 1, pp. 6-21, Jan. 2002.
[59] P. K. Yang and M. I. Kuroda, "Noncoding RNAs and intranuclear positioning in monoallelic gene expression," *Cell*, vol. 128, no. 4, pp. 777-786, Feb. 2007.
[60] S. Das et al., "Methylation analysis of the fragile X syndrome by PCR," *Genetic testing*, vol. 1, no. 3, pp. 151-155, 1997.
[61] H. M. Abdolmaleky et al., "Methylomics in psychiatry: Modulation of gene-environment interactions may be through DNA methylation," *American journal of medical genetics. Part B (Neuropsychiatric genetics)*, vol. 127, no. 1, pp. 51-59, May. 2004.
[62] Z. J. Daskalakis, P. B. Fitzgerald, and B. K. Christensen, "The role of cortical inhibition in the pathophysiology and treatment of schizophrenia," *Brain Research Reviews*, vol. 56, no. 2, pp. 427-442, Dec. 2007.
[63] M. Veldic, A. Guidotti, E. Maloku, J. M. Davis, and E. Costa, "In psychosis, cortical interneurons overexpress DNA-methyltransferase 1," *Proceedings of the National Academy of Sciences of the United States of America*, vol. 102, no. 6, pp. 2152-2157, Feb. 2005.
[64] J. H. Gaddum and K. A. Hameed, "Drugs which antagonize 5-hydroxytryptamine," *British journal of pharmacology and chemotherapy*, vol. 9, no. 2, pp. 240-248, Jun. 1954.
[65] O. O. Polesskaya, C. Aston, and B. P. Sokolov, "Allele C-specific methylation of the 5-HT2A receptor gene: evidence for correlation with its expression and expression of DNA methylase DNMT1," *Journal of neuroscience research*, vol. 83, no. 3, pp. 362-373, Feb. 2006.
[66] H. M. Abdolmaleky et al., "Hypomethylation of MB-COMT promoter is a major risk factor for schizophrenia and bipolar disorder," *Human molecular genetics*, vol. 15, no. 21, pp. 3132-3145, Nov. 2006.
[67] F. Angelucci, S. Brene, and A. A. Mathe, "BDNF in schizophrenia, depression and corresponding animal models," *Molecular psychiatry*, vol. 10, no. 4, pp. 345-352, Apr. 2005.
[68] C. S. Weickert et al., "Reductions in neurotrophin receptor mRNAs in the prefrontal cortex of patients with schizophrenia," *Molecular psychiatry*, vol. 10, no. 7, pp. 637-650, Jul. 2005.
[69] J. Mill et al., "Epigenomic profiling reveals DNA-methylation changes associated with major psychosis," *American Journal of Human Genetics*, vol. 82, no. 3, pp. 696-711, Mar. 2008.
[70] K. Fujita et al., "Serum dopamine-beta-hydroxylase in schizophrenic patients," *Journal of neurochemistry*, vol. 30, no. 6, pp. 1569-1572, Jun. 1978.

[71] H. Y. Meltzer, H. W. Cho, B. J. Carroll, and P. Russo, "Serum dopamine-beta-hydroxylase activity in the affective psychoses and schizophrenia. Decreased activity in unipolar psychotically depressed patients," *Archives of General Psychiatry*, vol. 33, no. 5, pp. 585-591, May. 1976.

[72] A. F. Wilson, R. C. Elston, R. M. Siervogel, and L. D. Tran, "Linkage of a gene regulating dopamine-beta-hydroxylase activity and the ABO blood group locus," *American Journal of Human Genetics*, vol. 42, no. 1, pp. 160-166, Jan. 1988.

[73] J. F. Cubells et al., "Dopamine beta-hydroxylase: two polymorphisms in linkage disequilibrium at the structural gene DBH associate with biochemical phenotypic variation," *Human genetics*, vol. 102, no. 5, pp. 533-540, May. 1998.

[74] J. F. Cubells et al., "A haplotype at the DBH locus, associated with low plasma dopamine beta-hydroxylase activity, also associates with cocaine-induced paranoia," *Molecular psychiatry*, vol. 5, no. 1, pp. 56-63, Jan. 2000.

[75] K. Yamamoto et al., "Dopamine beta-hydroxylase (DBH) gene and schizophrenia phenotypic variability: a genetic association study," *American journal of medical genetics. Part B (Neuropsychiatric genetics)*, vol. 117, no. 1, pp. 33-38, Feb. 2003.

[76] J. F. Cubells et al., "Linkage analysis of plasma dopamine β-hydroxylase activity in families of patients with schizophrenia," *Human genetics*, vol. 130, no. 5, pp. 635-643, 2011.

[77] S. Shifman et al., "A highly significant association between a COMT haplotype and schizophrenia," *American Journal of Human Genetics*, vol. 71, no. 6, pp. 1296-1302, Dec. 2002.

[78] E. C. Tan, S. A. Chong, H. Wang, E. Chew-Ping Lim, and Y. Y. Teo, "Gender-specific association of insertion/deletion polymorphisms in the nogo gene and chronic schizophrenia," *Molecular brain research*, vol. 139, no. 2, pp. 212-216, Oct. 2005.

[79] X. Chen et al., "Haplotypes spanning SPEC2, PDZ-GEF2 and ACSL6 genes are associated with schizophrenia," *Human molecular genetics*, vol. 15, no. 22, pp. 3329-3342, Nov. 2006.

[80] R. Magi, C. M. Lindgren, and A. P. Morris, "Meta-analysis of sex-specific genome-wide association studies," *Genetic epidemiology*, vol. 34, no. 8, pp. 846-853, Dec. 2010.

[81] G. Wang et al., "Overexpression of serotonin receptor and transporter mRNA in blood leukocytes of antipsychotic-free and antipsychotic-naïve schizophrenic patients: Gender differences," *Schizophrenia Research*, vol. 121, no. 1-3, pp. 160-171, 2010.

[82] B. R. Godlewska, L. Olajossy-Hilkesberger, J. Limon, and J. Landowski, "Ser9Gly polymorphism of the DRD3 gene is associated with worse premorbid social functioning and an earlier age of onset in female but not male schizophrenic patients," *Psychiatry research*, vol. 177, no. 1-2, pp. 266-267, May. 2010.

[83] D. J. Walder, H. D. Trotman, J. F. Cubells, J. Brasfield, Y.-L. Tang, and E. F. Walker, "Catechol-O-methyltransferase modulation of cortisol secretion in psychiatrically at-risk and healthy adolescents.," *Psychiatric genetics*, vol. 20, no. 4, pp. 166-70, Aug. 2010.

[84] M. F. Dallman et al., "Chronic Stress-Induced Effects of Corticosterone on Brain: Direct and Indirect," *Annals of the New York Academy of Sciences*, vol. 1018, pp. 141-150, 2004.

[85] E. F. Walker, D. J. Walder, and F. Reynolds, "Developmental changes in cortisol secretion in normal and at-risk youth.," *Development and psychopathology*, vol. 13, no. 3, pp. 721-32, Jan. 2001.

[86] E. F. Walker, P. A. Brennan, M. Esterberg, J. Brasfield, B. Pearce, and M. T. Compton, "Longitudinal changes in cortisol secretion and conversion to psychosis in at-risk youth.," *Journal of Abnormal Psychology*, vol. 119, no. 2, pp. 401-8, 2010.

[87] P. Linkowski, A. Van Onderbergen, M. Kerkhofs, D. Bosson, J. Mendlewicz, and E. Van Cauter, "Twin study of the 24-h cortisol profile: evidence for genetic control of the human circadian clock," *American Journal of Physiology*, vol. 264, no. 2 Pt. 1, pp. 173-181, 1993.

[88] J. van Os, M. Hanssen, M. Bak, R. V. Bijl, and W. Vollebergh, "Do Urbanicity and Familial Liability Coparticipate in Causing Psychosis?," *American journal of psychiatry*, vol. 160, pp. 477-482, 2003.

[89] R. H. Yolken and E. F. Torrey, "Viruses, schizophrenia, and bipolar disorder.," *Clinical microbiology reviews*, vol. 8, no. 1, pp. 131-45, Jan. 1995.

[90] E. Susser et al., "Schizophrenia after prenatal famine. Further evidence.," *Archives of general psychiatry*, vol. 53, no. 1, pp. 25-31, Jan. 1996.

[91] M. Cannon, P. B. Jones, and R. M. Murray, "Obstetric Complications and Schizophrenia: Historical and Meta-Analytic Review," *American journal of psychiatry*, vol. 159, pp. 1080-1092, 2002.

[92] C. Dalman, P. Allebeck, J. Cullberg, C. Grunewald, and M. Koster, "Obstetric complications and risk of schizophrenia: a longitudinal study of a national birth cohort," *Archives of general psychiatry*, vol. 56, pp. 234-240, May. 1999.

[93] C. M. Hultman, P. Sparén, N. Takei, R. M. Murray, and S. Cnattingius, "Prenatal and perinatal risk factors for schizophrenia, affective psychosis, and reactive psychosis of early onset: case-control study.," *British Medical Journal*, vol. 318, no. 7181, pp. 421-6, Feb. 1999.

[94] K. K. Nicodemus et al., "Serious obstetric complications interact with hypoxia-regulated/vascular-expression genes to influence schizophrenia risk.," *Molecular psychiatry*, vol. 13, no. 9, pp. 873-7, Sep. 2008.

[95] M. Tramer, "Über die biologische Bedeutung des Geburtsmonates insbesondere für die Psychoseerkrankung. / The biological significance of the birth month, with special reference to psychosis.," *Schweizer Archiv für Neurologie und Psychiatrie*, vol. 24, pp. 17-24, 1929.

[96] E. F. Torrey, J. Miller, R. Rawlings, and R. H. Yolken, "Seasonality of births in schizophrenia and bipolar disorder: a review of the literature.," *Schizophrenia research*, vol. 28, no. 1, pp. 1-38, Nov. 1997.

[97] M. Tochigi, Y. Okazaki, N. Kato, and T. Sasaki, "What causes seasonality of birth in schizophrenia?," *Neuroscience Research*, vol. 48, no. 1, pp. 1-11, Jan. 2004.

[98] S. A. Mednick, R. A. Machon, M. O. Huttunen, and D. Bonett, "Adult Schizophrenia Following Prenatal Exposure to an Influenza Epidemic," *Archives of General Psychiatry*, vol. 45, no. 2, pp. 189-192, 1988.

[99] R. A. Machón et al., "Adult schizotypal personality characteristics and prenatal influenza in a Finnish birth cohort.," *Schizophrenia research*, vol. 54, no. 1-2, pp. 7-16, Mar. 2002.

[100] A. S. Brown et al., "Maternal exposure to respiratory infections and adult schizophrenia spectrum disorders: a prospective birth cohort study.," *Schizophrenia bulletin*, vol. 26, no. 2, pp. 287-95, Jan. 2000.
[101] A. S. Brown, P. Cohen, S. Greenwald, and E. Susser, "Nonaffective Psychosis After Prenatal Exposure to Rubella," *American Journal of Psychiatry*, vol. 157, no. 3, pp. 438-443, Mar. 2000.
[102] J. Suvisaari, J. Haukka, A. Tanskanen, T. Hovi, and J. Lönnqvist, "Association between prenatal exposure to poliovirus infection and adult schizophrenia.," *The American journal of psychiatry*, vol. 156, no. 7, pp. 1100-2, Jul. 1999.
[103] P. B. Mortensen et al., "A Danish National Birth Cohort study of maternal HSV-2 antibodies as a risk factor for schizophrenia in their offspring.," *Schizophrenia research*, vol. 122, no. 1-3, pp. 257-63, Sep. 2010.
[104] J. L. Moreno et al., "Maternal influenza viral infection causes schizophrenia-like alterations of 5-HT2A and mGlu2 receptors in the adult offspring.," *The Journal of neuroscience*, vol. 31, no. 5, pp. 1863-72, Feb. 2011.
[105] S. J. Short et al., "Maternal influenza infection during pregnancy impacts postnatal brain development in the rhesus monkey.," *Biological psychiatry*, vol. 67, no. 10, pp. 965-73, May. 2010.
[106] J. P. Selten, A. S. Brown, K. G. Moons, J. P. Slaets, E. S. Susser, and R. S. Kahn, "Prenatal exposure to the 1957 influenza pandemic and non-affective psychosis in The Netherlands.," *Schizophrenia research*, vol. 38, no. 2-3, pp. 85-91, Aug. 1999.
[107] L. M. Ellman et al., "Structural brain alterations in schizophrenia following fetal exposure to the inflammatory cytokine interleukin-8.," *Schizophrenia research*, vol. 121, no. 1-3, pp. 46-54, Aug. 2010.
[108] P. Boksa, "Effects of prenatal infection on brain development and behavior: a review of findings from animal models.," *Brain, behavior, and immunity*, vol. 24, no. 6, pp. 881-97, Aug. 2010.
[109] E. S. Susser and S. P. Lin, "Schizophrenia after prenatal exposure to the Dutch Hunger Winter of 1944-1945.," *Archives of general psychiatry*, vol. 49, no. 12, pp. 983-8, Dec. 1992.
[110] D. St Clair et al., "Rates of Adult Schizophrenia Following of 1959-1961," *Journal of the American Medical Association*, vol. 294, no. 5, pp. 557-562, 2005.
[111] M.-Q. Xu et al., "Prenatal malnutrition and adult schizophrenia: further evidence from the 1959-1961 Chinese famine.," *Schizophrenia bulletin*, vol. 35, no. 3, pp. 568-76, May. 2009.
[112] A. S. Brown and E. S. Susser, "Prenatal nutritional deficiency and risk of adult schizophrenia.," *Schizophrenia bulletin*, vol. 34, no. 6, pp. 1054-63, Nov. 2008.
[113] J. McGrath et al., "Vitamin D supplementation during the first year of life and risk of schizophrenia: a Finnish birth cohort study.," *Schizophrenia research*, vol. 67, no. 2-3, pp. 237-45, Apr. 2004.
[114] J. J. McGrath, T. H. Burne, F. Féron, A. Mackay-Sim, and D. W. Eyles, "Developmental vitamin D deficiency and risk of schizophrenia: a 10-year update.," *Schizophrenia bulletin*, vol. 36, no. 6, pp. 1073-8, Nov. 2010.
[115] Q. Shen et al., "The role of pro-inflammatory factors in mediating the effects on the fetus of prenatal undernutrition: implications for schizophrenia.," *Schizophrenia research*, vol. 99, no. 1-3, pp. 48-55, Feb. 2008.

[116] M. O. Huttunen and P. Niskanen, "Prenatal loss of father and psychiatric disorders.," *Archives of general psychiatry*, vol. 35, no. 4, pp. 429-31, Apr. 1978.

[117] C. Dalman, S. Wicks, and P. Allebeck, "Prenatal loss of father and subsequent psychosis: a national cohort study," in *The International Congress on Schizophrenia Research*, 2005.

[118] A. S. Khashan et al., "Higher risk of offspring schizophrenia following antenatal maternal exposure to severe adverse life events.," *Archives of general psychiatry*, vol. 65, no. 2, pp. 146-52, Feb. 2008.

[119] J. van Os and J. P. Selten, "Prenatal exposure to maternal stress and subsequent schizophrenia. The May 1940 invasion of The Netherlands," *The British Journal of Psychiatry*, vol. 172, no. 4, pp. 324-326, Apr. 1998.

[120] D. Malaspina et al., "Acute maternal stress in pregnancy and schizophrenia in offspring: a cohort prospective study.," *BMC psychiatry*, vol. 8, p. 71, Jan. 2008.

[121] J. P. Selten, Y. van der Graaf, R. van Duursen, C. C. Gispen-de Wied, and R. S. Kahn, "Psychotic illness after prenatal exposure to the 1953 Dutch Flood Disaster.," *Schizophrenia research*, vol. 35, no. 3, pp. 243-5, Feb. 1999.

[122] J. B. Watson, S. A. Mednick, M. Huttunen, and X. Wang, "Prenatal teratogens and the development of adult mental illness.," *Development and Psychopathology*, vol. 11, no. 3, pp. 457-466, 1999.

[123] D. K. Kinney, W. Hyman, C. Greetham, and S. Tramer, "Increased relative risk for schizophrenia and prenatal exposure to a severe tornado (abstract).," *Schizophrenia research*, vol. 36, no. 1-3, pp. 45-46, 1999.

[124] A. Charil, D. P. Laplante, C. Vaillancourt, and S. King, "Prenatal stress and brain development.," *Brain research reviews*, vol. 65, no. 1, pp. 56-79, Oct. 2010.

[125] R. Pascual, D. Ebner, R. Araneda, M. J. Urqueta, and C. Bustamante, "Maternal stress induces long-lasting Purkinje cell developmental impairments in mouse offspring.," *European journal of pediatrics*, vol. 169, no. 12, pp. 1517-22, Dec. 2010.

[126] K. Kleinhaus et al., "Effects of excessive glucocorticoid receptor stimulation during early gestation on psychomotor and social behavior in the rat.," *Developmental psychobiology*, vol. 52, no. 2, pp. 121-32, Mar. 2010.

[127] A. Sacker, D. J. Done, T. J. Crow, and J. Golding, "Antecedents of schizophrenia and affective illness. Obstetric complications," *The British Journal of Psychiatry*, vol. 166, no. 6, pp. 734-741, Jun. 1995.

[128] R. J. Van Lieshout and L. P. Voruganti, "Diabetes mellitus during pregnancy and increased risk of schizophrenia in offspring?: a review of the evidence and putative mechanisms," *Journal of Psychiatry and Neuroscience*, vol. 33, no. 5, pp. 395-404, 2008.

[129] J. M. Hollister, P. Laing, and S. A. Mednick, "Rhesus Incompatibility as a Risk Factor for Schizophrenia in Male Adults," *Archives of general psychiatry*, vol. 53, no. 1, pp. 19-24, 1996.

[130] C. G. S. Palmer et al., "RHD maternal-fetal genotype incompatibility increases schizophrenia susceptibility.," *American journal of human genetics*, vol. 71, no. 6, pp. 1312-9, Dec. 2002.

[131] E. A. Lane and G. W. Albee, "Comparative birth weights of schizophrenics and their siblings," *Journal of Psychology*, vol. 64, pp. 227-231, 1966.

[132] G. Wrede, S. A. Mednick, M. O. Huttunen, and C. G. Nilsson, "Pregnancy and delivery complications in the births of an unselected series of Finnish children with schizophrenic mothers.," *Acta Psychiatrica Scandinavica*, vol. 62, no. 4, pp. 369-381, 1980.

[133] L. Rifkin, S. Lewis, P. Jones, B. Toone, and R. Murray, "Low birth weight and schizophrenia," *The British Journal of Psychiatry*, vol. 165, no. 3, pp. 357-362, Sep. 1994.

[134] H. Kunugi, S. Nanko, and R. M. Murray, "Obstetric complications and schizophrenia: prenatal underdevelopment and subsequent neurodevelopmental impairment," *The British Journal of Psychiatry*, vol. 178, no. 40, p. s25-s29, Apr. 2001.

[135] C. Dalman, H. V. Thomas, A. S. David, J. Gentz, G. Lewis, and P. Allebeck, "Signs of asphyxia at birth and risk of schizophrenia: Population-based case-control study," *The British Journal of Psychiatry*, vol. 179, no. 5, pp. 403-408, Nov. 2001.

[136] R. E. Kendell, K. McInneny, E. Jusczak, and M. Bain, "Obstetric complications and schizophrenia: Two case-control studies based on structured obstetric records," *The British Journal of Psychiatry*, vol. 176, no. 6, pp. 516-522, Jun. 2000.

[137] M. Byrne et al., "Labour and delivery complications and schizophrenia: Case--control study using contemporaneous labour ward records," *The British Journal of Psychiatry*, vol. 176, no. 6, pp. 531-536, Jun. 2000.

[138] M. C. Clarke, M. Harley, and M. Cannon, "The role of obstetric events in schizophrenia.," *Schizophrenia bulletin*, vol. 32, no. 1, pp. 3-8, Jan. 2006.

[139] J. R. Geddes et al., "Schizophrenia and complications of pregnancy and labor: an individual patient data meta-analysis.," *Schizophrenia bulletin*, vol. 25, no. 3, pp. 413-23, Jan. 1999.

[140] T. D. Cannon, I. M. Rosso, J. M. Hollister, C. E. Bearden, L. E. Sanchez, and T. Hadley, "A prospective cohort study of genetic and perinatal influences in the etiology of schizophrenia.," *Schizophrenia bulletin*, vol. 26, no. 2, pp. 351-66, Jan. 2000.

[141] P. F. Bolton, M. Murphy, H. Macdonald, B. Whitlock, A. Pickles, and M. Rutter, "Obstetric complications in autism: consequences or causes of the condition?," *Journal of the American Academy of Child and Adolescent Psychiatry*, vol. 36, no. 2, pp. 272-81, Feb. 1997.

[142] L. Burd, R. Severud, J. Kerbeshian, and M. G. Klug, "Prenatal and perinatal risk factors for autism.," *Journal of Perinatal Medicine*, vol. 27, no. 6, pp. 441-450, 1999.

[143] N. Juul-dam, J. Townsend, and E. Courchesne, "Prenatal, perinatal, and neonatal factors in autism, pervasive developmental disorder-not otherwise specified, and the general population," *Pediatrics*, vol. 107, p. E63, 2001.

[144] S. Sprich-Buckminster, J. Biederman, S. Milberger, S. V. Faraone, and B. K. Lehman, "Are perinatal complications relevant to the manifestation of ADD? Issues of comorbidity and familiality.," *Journal of the American Academy of Child and Adolescent Psychiatry*, vol. 32, no. 5, pp. 1032-7, Sep. 1993.

[145] S. Deb, K. B. Prasad, H. Seth, and J. M. Eagles, "A comparison of obstetric and neonatal complications between children with autistic disorder and their siblings.," *Journal of intellectual disability research*, vol. 41 ( Pt 1), pp. 81-86, 1997.

[146] S. Milberger, J. Biederman, S. V. Faraone, J. Guite, and M. T. Tsuang, "Pregnancy, delivery and infancy complications and attention deficit hyperactivity disorder: issues of gene-environment interaction.," *Biological psychiatry*, vol. 41, no. 1, pp. 65-75, Jan. 1997.

[147] S. Cnattingius, C. M. Hultman, M. Dahl, and P. Sparén, "Very preterm birth, birth trauma, and the risk of anorexia nervosa among girls.," *Archives of general psychiatry*, vol. 56, no. 7, pp. 634-8, Jul. 1999.

[148] D. L. Foley, L. R. Thacker, S. H. Aggen, M. C. Neale, and K. S. Kendler, "Pregnancy and perinatal complications associated with risks for common psychiatric disorders in a population-based sample of female twins.," *American Journal of Medical Genetics*, vol. 105, no. 5, pp. 426-431, 2001.

[149] A. S. Brown, J. van Os, C. Driessens, H. W. Hoek, and E. S. Susser, "Further Evidence of Relation Between Prenatal Famine and Major Affective Disorder," *American Journal of Psychiatry*, vol. 157, no. 2, pp. 190-195, Feb. 2000.

[150] H. Verdoux and A.-L. Sutter, "Perinatal risk factors for schizophrenia: diagnostic specificity and relationships with maternal psychopathology.," *American journal of medical genetics*, vol. 114, no. 8, pp. 898-905, Dec. 2002.

[151] H. Verdoux, "Perinatal risk factors for schizophrenia: how specific are they?," *Current psychiatry reports*, vol. 6, no. 3, pp. 162-7, Jun. 2004.

[152] A. V. Jablensky, V. Morgan, S. R. Zubrick, C. Bower, and L.-anne Yellachich, "Pregnancy, delivery, and neonatal complications in a Population Cohort of Women With Schizophrenia and Major Affective Disorders," *American journal of psychiatry*, vol. 162, pp. 79-91, 2005.

[153] K. Narita et al., "Human leukocyte antigen and season of birth in Japanese patients with schizophrenia.," *The American journal of psychiatry*, vol. 157, no. 7, pp. 1173-5, Jul. 2000.

[154] M. Tochigi et al., "Human leukocyte antigen-A specificities and its relation with season of birth in Japanese patients with schizophrenia," *Neuroscience Letters*, vol. 329, no. 2, pp. 201-204, Aug. 2002.

[155] J. Chotai, A. Serretti, E. Lattuada, C. Lorenzi, and R. Lilli, "Gene-environment interaction in psychiatric disorders as indicated by season of birth variations in tryptophan hydroxylase (TPH), serotonin transporter (5-HTTLPR) and dopamine receptor (DRD4) gene polymorphisms.," *Psychiatry research*, vol. 119, no. 1-2, pp. 99-111, Jul. 2003.

[156] J.-W. Muntjewerff, R. a Ophoff, J. E. Buizer-Voskamp, E. Strengman, and M. den Heijer, "Effects of season of birth and a common MTHFR gene variant on the risk of schizophrenia.," *European neuropsychopharmacology*, vol. 21, no. 4, pp. 300-5, Apr. 2011.

[157] R. Schmidt-Kastner, J. van Os, H. W M Steinbusch, and C. Schmitz, "Gene regulation by hypoxia and the neurodevelopmental origin of schizophrenia.," *Schizophrenia research*, vol. 84, no. 2-3, pp. 253-71, Jun. 2006.

[158] B. Abazyan et al., "Prenatal interaction of mutant DISC1 and immune activation produces adult psychopathology.," *Biological psychiatry*, vol. 68, no. 12, pp. 1172-81, Dec. 2010.

[159] J. T. Manning, S. Baron-Cohen, S. Wheelwright, and G. Sanders, "The 2nd to 4th digit ratio and autism.," *Developmental medicine and child neurology*, vol. 43, no. 3, pp. 160-4, Mar. 2001.

[160] C. Casar, M. Artamendi, M. Gutiérrez, P. Gil, M. J. García, and M. J. Cuesta, "[Neuropsychological deficits, obstetric complications and premorbid adjustment in patients with the first psychotic episode].," *Actas luso-españolas de neurología, psiquiatría y ciencias afines*, vol. 25, no. 5, pp. 303-7.

[161] A. Lane et al., "Schizophrenia and neurological soft signs: gender differences in clinical correlates and antecedent factors.," *Psychiatry research*, vol. 64, no. 2, pp. 105-14, Sep. 1996.

[162] M. Hadders-Algra, H. J. Huisjes, and B. C. Touwen, "Perinatal risk factors and minor neurological dysfunction: significance for behaviour and school achievement at nine years.," *Developmental Medicine and Child Neurology*, vol. 30, no. 4, pp. 482-491, 1988.

[163] E. O'Callaghan et al., "Risk of schizophrenia in adults born after obstetric complications and their association with early onset of illness: a controlled study.," *British Medical Journal*, vol. 305, no. 6864, pp. 1256-9, Nov. 1992.

[164] I. M. Rosso, T. D. Cannon, T. Huttunen, M. O. Huttunen, J. Lönnqvist, and T. L. Gasperoni, "Obstetric risk factors for early-onset schizophrenia in a Finnish birth cohort.," *The American journal of psychiatry*, vol. 157, no. 5, pp. 801-7, May. 2000.

[165] A. Hoff and W. Kremen, "Sex differences in neurocognitive function in schizophrenia," in *Psychiatric illness in women: emerging treatments and research*, F. Lewis-Hall, T. S. Williams, J. A. Panetta, and J. H. Herrera, Eds. Washington, D.C.: American Psychiatric Publishing, 2002, pp. 215-238.

[166] M. J. Khoury, J. S. Marks, B. J. McCarthy, and S. M. Zaro, "Factors affecting the sex differential in neonatal mortality: the role of respiratory distress syndrome.," *American journal of obstetrics and gynecology*, vol. 151, no. 6, pp. 777-82, Mar. 1985.

[167] A. Foerster, S. W. Lewis, M. J. Owen, and R. M. Murray, "Low birth weight and a family history of schizophrenia predict poor premorbid functioning in psychosis," *Schizophrenia Research*, vol. 5, no. 1, pp. 13-20, Jul. 1991.

[168] H. Matsumoto, N. Takei, F. Saito, K. Kachi, and N. Mori, "The association between obstetric complications and childhood-onset schizophrenia: a replication study.," *Psychological Medicine*, vol. 31, no. 5, pp. 907-914, 2001.

[169] G. A. Light and D. L. Braff, "Stability of mismatch negativity deficits and their relationship to functional impairments in chronic schizophrenia.," *The American journal of psychiatry*, vol. 162, no. 9, pp. 1741-3, Sep. 2005.

[170] D. C. Javitt, A. Shelley, and W. Ritter, "Associated deficits in mismatch negativity generation and tone matching in schizophrenia.," *Clinical neurophysiology*, vol. 111, no. 10, pp. 1733-7, Oct. 2000.

[171] R. E. Hoffman, J. Rapaport, C. M. Mazure, and D. M. Quinlan, "Selective speech perception alterations in schizophrenic patients reporting hallucinated 'voices'," *American Journal of Psychiatry*, vol. 156, no. 3, pp. 393-399, 1999.

[172] R. A. Adcock et al., "When top-down meets bottom-up: auditory training enhances verbal memory in schizophrenia.," *Schizophrenia bulletin*, vol. 35, no. 6, pp. 1132-41, Nov. 2009.

[173] B. F. O'Donnell et al., "Identification of neural circuits underlying P300 abnormalities in schizophrenia," *Psychophysiology*, vol. 36, no. 3, pp. 388-398, Aug. 1999.
[174] S. Bender, M. Weisbrod, and F. Resch, "Which perspectives can endophenotypes and biological markers offer in the early recognition of schizophrenia?," *Journal of neural transmission*, vol. 114, no. 9, pp. 1199-215, Sep. 2007.
[175] M. E. Shenton, C. C. Dickey, M. Frumin, and R. W. McCarley, "A review of MRI findings in schizophrenia.," *Schizophrenia research*, vol. 49, no. 1-2, pp. 1-52, Apr. 2001.
[176] J. Sun, J. J. Maller, L. Guo, and P. B. Fitzgerald, "Superior temporal gyrus volume change in schizophrenia: a review on region of interest volumetric studies.," *Brain research reviews*, vol. 61, no. 1, pp. 14-32, Jun. 2009.
[177] R. A. Sweet, S. E. Bergen, Z. Sun, M. J. Marcsisin, A. R. Sampson, and D. a Lewis, "Anatomical evidence of impaired feedforward auditory processing in schizophrenia.," *Biological psychiatry*, vol. 61, no. 7, pp. 854-64, Apr. 2007.
[178] D. C. Javitt, M. Steinschneider, C. E. Schroeder, and J. C. Arezzo, "Role of cortical N-methyl-D-aspartate receptors in auditory sensory memory and mismatch negativity generation: implications for schizophrenia.," *Proceedings of the National Academy of Sciences of the United States of America*, vol. 93, no. 21, pp. 11962-7, Oct. 1996.
[179] M. I. Garrido, J. M. Kilner, K. E. Stephan, and K. J. Friston, "Clinical Neurophysiology The mismatch negativity: A review of underlying mechanisms," *Clinical Neurophysiology*, vol. 120, no. 3, pp. 453-463, 2009.
[180] J. S. Butler, S. Molholm, I. C. Fiebelkorn, M. R. Mercier, T. H. Schwartz, and J. J. Foxe, "Common or redundant neural circuits for duration processing across audition and touch.," *The Journal of neuroscience*, vol. 31, no. 9, pp. 3400-6, Mar. 2011.
[181] T. Baldeweg, A. Klugman, J. Gruzelier, and S. R. Hirsch, "Mismatch negativity potentials and cognitive impairment in schizophrenia," *Schizophrenia Research*, vol. 69, no. 2-3, pp. 203-217, Aug. 2004.
[182] C. A. Brenner et al., "Steady state responses: electrophysiological assessment of sensory function in schizophrenia.," *Schizophrenia bulletin*, vol. 35, no. 6, pp. 1065-77, Nov. 2009.
[183] A. J. Fallgatter et al., "DTNBP1 (dysbindin) gene variants modulate prefrontal brain function in healthy individuals.," *Neuropsychopharmacology*, vol. 31, no. 9, pp. 2002-10, Sep. 2006.
[184] F. Jessen et al., "Amplitude reduction of the mismatch negativity in first-degree relatives of patients with schizophrenia.," *Neuroscience letters*, vol. 309, no. 3, pp. 185-8, Aug. 2001.
[185] P. T. Michie, H. Innes-Brown, J. Todd, and A. V. Jablensky, "Duration mismatch negativity in biological relatives of patients with schizophrenia spectrum disorders.," *Biological psychiatry*, vol. 52, no. 7, pp. 749-58, Oct. 2002.
[186] E. Bramon, "Mismatch negativity in schizophrenia: a family study," *Schizophrenia Research*, vol. 67, no. 1, pp. 1-10, Mar. 2004.
[187] K. Baker, T. Baldeweg, S. Sivagnanasundaram, P. Scambler, and D. Skuse, "COMT Val108/158 Met modifies mismatch negativity and cognitive function in 22q11 deletion syndrome.," *Biological psychiatry*, vol. 58, no. 1, pp. 23-31, Jul. 2005.
[188] J. S. Kwon et al., "Gamma frequency-range abnormalities to auditory stimulation in schizophrenia.," *Archives of general psychiatry*, vol. 56, no. 11, pp. 1001-5, Nov. 1999.

[189] L. E. Hong et al., "Evoked gamma band synchronization and the liability for schizophrenia.," *Schizophrenia research*, vol. 70, no. 2-3, pp. 293-302, Oct. 2004.

[190] C. A. Brenner, O. Sporns, P. H. Lysaker, and B. F. O'Donnell, "EEG synchronization to modulated auditory tones in schizophrenia, schizoaffective disorder, and schizotypal personality disorder.," *The American journal of psychiatry*, vol. 160, no. 12, pp. 2238-40, Dec. 2003.

[191] P. D. Butler, S. M. Silverstein, and S. C. Dakin, "Visual perception and its impairment in schizophrenia.," *Biological psychiatry*, vol. 64, no. 1, pp. 40-7, Jul. 2008.

[192] J. T. Kantrowitz, P. D. Butler, I. Schecter, G. Silipo, and D. C. Javitt, "Seeing the world dimly: the impact of early visual deficits on visual experience in schizophrenia.," *Schizophrenia bulletin*, vol. 35, no. 6, pp. 1085-94, Dec. 2009.

[193] C. G. Kohler, J. B. Walker, E. a Martin, K. M. Healey, and P. J. Moberg, "Facial emotion perception in schizophrenia: a meta-analytic review.," *Schizophrenia bulletin*, vol. 36, no. 5, pp. 1009-19, Sep. 2010.

[194] P. D. Butler et al., "Sensory contributions to impaired emotion processing in schizophrenia.," *Schizophrenia bulletin*, vol. 35, no. 6, pp. 1095-107, Nov. 2009.

[195] J. Brekke, D. D. Kay, K. S. Lee, and M. F. Green, "Biosocial pathways to functional outcome in schizophrenia.," *Schizophrenia research*, vol. 80, no. 2-3, pp. 213-25, Dec. 2005.

[196] P. J. Uhlhaas, W. A. Phillips, and S. M. Silverstein, "The course and clinical correlates of dysfunctions in visual perceptual organization in schizophrenia during the remission of psychotic symptoms.," *Schizophrenia research*, vol. 75, no. 2-3, pp. 183-92, Jun. 2005.

[197] S. M. Silverstein, R. A. Knight, S. B. Schwarzkopf, L. L. West, L. M. Osborn, and D. Kamin, "Stimulus configuration and context effects in perceptual organization in schizophrenia," *Journal of abnormal psychology*, vol. 105, no. 3, pp. 410-420, 1996.

[198] W. A. Phillips and S. M. Silverstein, "Convergence of biological and psychological perspectives on cognitive coordination in schizophrenia.," *The Behavioral and brain sciences*, vol. 26, no. 1, pp. 65-82; discussion 82-137, Feb. 2003.

[199] J. H. Yoon et al., "Diminished orientation-specific surround suppression of visual processing in schizophrenia.," *Schizophrenia bulletin*, vol. 35, no. 6, pp. 1078-84, Nov. 2009.

[200] M. J. Coleman et al., "Schizophrenia patients show deficits in shifts of attention to different levels of global-local stimuli: evidence for magnocellular dysfunction.," *Schizophrenia bulletin*, vol. 35, no. 6, pp. 1108-16, Nov. 2009.

[201] P. D. Butler et al., "Subcortical visual dysfunction in schizophrenia drives secondary cortical impairments.," *Brain□: a journal of neurology*, vol. 130, no. 2, pp. 417-30, Feb. 2007.

[202] A. D. Nguyen, M. E. Shenton, and J. J. Levitt, "Olfactory Dysfunction in Schizophrenia: A Review of Neuroanatomy and Psychophysiological Measurements," *Harvard review of psychiatry*, vol. 18, no. 5, pp. 279–292, 2010.

[203] L. B. Buck, "Smell and taste: The chemical senses," in *Principles of Neural Science*, 4th ed., E. R. Kandel, J. H. Schwartz, and T. M. Jessell, Eds. New York: McGraw-Hill, 2000, pp. 625-647.

[204] B. I. Turetsky, C.-G. Hahn, K. Borgmann-Winter, and P. J. Moberg, "Scents and nonsense: olfactory dysfunction in schizophrenia.," *Schizophrenia bulletin*, vol. 35, no. 6, pp. 1117-31, Nov. 2009.

[205] F. Féron, C. Perry, M. H. Hirning, J. McGrath, and A. Mackay-Sim, "Altered adhesion, proliferation and death in neural cultures from adults with schizophrenia.," *Schizophrenia research*, vol. 40, no. 3, pp. 211-8, Dec. 1999.

[206] D. Malaspina and E. Coleman, "Olfaction and social drive in schizophrenia.," *Archives of general psychiatry*, vol. 60, no. 6, pp. 578-84, Jun. 2003.

[207] C. Corcoran et al., "Olfactory deficits, cognition and negative symptoms in early onset psychosis.," *Schizophrenia research*, vol. 80, no. 2-3, pp. 283-93, Dec. 2005.

[208] H. Blumenfeld, *Neuroanatomy Through Clinical Cases*. Sunderland: Sinauer Associates, Inc., 2002, p. 951.

[209] B. P. Chang and M. F. Lenzenweger, "Somatosensory processing and schizophrenia liability: proprioception, exteroceptive sensitivity, and graphesthesia performance in the biological relatives of schizophrenia patients.," *Journal of abnormal psychology*, vol. 114, no. 1, pp. 85-95, Feb. 2005.

[210] M. F. Lenzenweger, "Two-point discrimination thresholds and schizotypy: illuminating a somatosensory dysfunction.," *Schizophrenia research*, vol. 42, no. 2, pp. 111-24, Apr. 2000.

[211] R. M. Bauer and J. A. Demery, "Agnosia," in *Clinical Neuropsychology*, 4th ed., K. M. Heilman and E. Valenstein, Eds. New York: Oxford University Press, 2003, p. 716.

[212] M.-X. Huang et al., "Somatosensory system deficits in schizophrenia revealed by MEG during a median-nerve oddball task.," *Brain topography*, vol. 23, no. 1, pp. 82-104, Mar. 2010.

[213] C. Norra et al., "High-frequency somatosensory thalamocortical oscillations and psychopathology in schizophrenia.," *Neuropsychobiology*, vol. 49, no. 2, pp. 71-80, Jan. 2004.

[214] M. Reite, P. Teale, T. L. Benkers, and J. Carlson, "in Schizophrenia," *Psychiatry: Interpersonal and Biological Processes*, no. December, pp. 2148-2153, 2003.

[215] S. Knecht, E. Kunesch, and a Schnitzler, "Parallel and serial processing of haptic information in man: effects of parietal lesions on sensorimotor hand function.," *Neuropsychologia*, vol. 34, no. 7, pp. 669-87, Jul. 1996.

[216] B. P. Chang and M. F. Lenzenweger, "Somatosensory processing in the biological relatives of schizophrenia patients: A signal detection analysis of two-point discrimination.," *Journal of Abnormal Psychology*, vol. 110, no. 3, pp. 433-442, 2001.

[217] B. P. Chang and M. F. Lenzenweger, "Investigating graphesthesia task performance in the biological relatives of schizophrenia patients.," *Schizophrenia bulletin*, vol. 30, no. 2, pp. 327-34, Jan. 2004.

[218] D. C. Javitt, E. Liederman, A. Cienfuegos, and A. M. Shelley, "Panmodal processing imprecision as a basis for dysfunction of transient memory storage systems in schizophrenia.," *Schizophrenia bulletin*, vol. 25, no. 4, pp. 763-75, Jan. 1999.

[219] D. C. Javitt, "Sensory processing in schizophrenia: neither simple nor intact.," *Schizophrenia bulletin*, vol. 35, no. 6, pp. 1059-64, Nov. 2009.

[220] L. Kopala, C. Clark, and T. A. Hurwitz, "Sex differences in olfactory function in schizophrenia," *American Journal of Psychiatry*, vol. 146, no. 10, pp. 1320-1322, Oct. 1989.

[221] P. J. Moberg et al., "Impairment of Odor Hedonics in Men With Schizophrenia," *American Journal of Psychiatry*, vol. 160, no. 10, pp. 1784-9, Jan. 2003.

[222] K. P. Good, R. A. Leslie, J. McGlone, H. I. Milliken, and L. C. Kopala, "Sex differences in olfactory function in young patients with psychotic disorders.," *Schizophrenia research*, vol. 97, no. 1-3, pp. 97-102, Dec. 2007.

[223] V. Kumari, "Sex differences and hormonal influences in human sensorimotor gating: implications for schizophrenia.," *Current topics in behavioral neurosciences*, vol. 8, pp. 141-54, Jan. 2011.

[224] D. Braff, C. Stone, E. Callaway, M. Geyer, I. Glick, and L. Bali, "Prestimulus effects on human startle reflex in normals and schizophrenics.," *Psychophysiology*, vol. 15, no. 4, pp. 339-43, Jul. 1978.

[225] L. A. Gottschalk, J. L. Haer, and D. E. Bates, "Effect of sensory overload on psychological state. Changes in social alienation-personal disorganization and cognitive-intellectual impairment.," *Archives of general psychiatry*, vol. 27, no. 4, pp. 451-7, Oct. 1972.

[226] D. L. Braff and M. A. Geyer, "Sensorimotor gating and schizophrenia. Human and animal model studies.," *Archives of general psychiatry*, vol. 47, no. 2, pp. 181-8, Feb. 1990.

[227] W. Hasenkamp et al., "Heritability of acoustic startle magnitude, prepulse inhibition, and startle latency in schizophrenia and control families.," *Psychiatry research*, vol. 178, no. 2, pp. 236-43, Jul. 2010.

[228] V. Kumari, E. Antonova, and M. A. Geyer, "Prepulse inhibition and 'psychosis-proneness' in healthy individuals: an fMRI study.," *European psychiatry*, vol. 23, no. 4, pp. 274-80, Jul. 2008.

[229] K. S. Cadenhead, N. R. Swerdlow, K. M. Shafer, M. Diaz, and D. L. Braff, "Modulation of the startle response and startle laterality in relatives of schizophrenic patients and in subjects with schizotypal personality disorder: evidence of inhibitory deficits.," *The American journal of psychiatry*, vol. 157, no. 10, pp. 1660-8, Oct. 2000.

[230] N. Petrovsky et al., "Sensorimotor gating is associated with CHRNA3 polymorphisms in schizophrenia and healthy volunteers.," *Neuropsychopharmacology*, vol. 35, no. 7, pp. 1429-39, Jun. 2010.

[231] V. Kumari, E. Antonova, M. A. Geyer, D. Ffytche, S. C. R. Williams, and T. Sharma, "A fMRI investigation of startle gating deficits in schizophrenia patients treated with typical or atypical antipsychotics.," *The international journal of neuropsychopharmacology*, vol. 10, no. 4, pp. 463-77, Aug. 2007.

[232] V. Kumari et al., "Evidence for a role of progesterone in menstrual cycle-related variability in prepulse inhibition in healthy young women.," *Neuropsychopharmacology*, vol. 35, no. 4, pp. 929-37, Mar. 2010.

[233] E. Walker and D. J. Walder, "Neurohormonal aspects of the development of psychotic disorders," in *Neurodevelopmental mechanisms in psychopathology*, D. Cichetti and E. Walker, Eds. Boston, MA: Cambridge University Press, 2002, pp. 526-544.

[234] E. Walker, Z. Sabuwalla, A. Bollini, and D. Walder, "Gender and stress," in *Women's mental health: a life-cycle approach*, S. Roman and M. Seeman, Eds. New York, NY: Lippincott, Williams and Wilkins, 2005, pp. 35-47.

In: Psychosis: Causes, Diagnosis and Treatment
Editor: Xenia Anastassiou-Hadjicharalambous
ISBN: 978-1-62081-516-8


*Chapter 4*

# PSYCHOSES IN A CHILD AND ADOLESCENT PSYCHIATRIC POPULATION AND THEIR OUTCOME IN ADULTHOOD

*Ulf Engqvist*[*]

Ulf Engqvist, PhD, Senior lecturer in Social Work,
Department of Social Work, Mid-Sweden University,
Östersund, Sweden

## ABSTRACT

The purpose of this chapter is to give answers to a number of questions concerning a group of former child and adolescent psychiatric (CAP) patients diagnosed during childhood, adolescence or adulthood as suffering from schizophrenia, schizotypal disorder, delusional disorders and/or psychotic mood disorders.

At what age was the diagnosis made? Was this diagnosis later changed and, if so, in what manner? Were early signs of the disorder detectable prior to or at the time of admission to CAP care? Which CAP patients were later diagnosed as psychotic in general (adult) psychiatry (GenP) and how did this latter group differ from those who had already received a diagnosis before the age of 18 years? 1,400 CAP patients admitted 1975-1990 to inpatient or outpatient CAP care in Jämtland County, Sweden were followed until 2003. Jämtland County is located in the western part of middle Sweden at the border to Norway.

The status of the patients' mental health was monitored until 2003 using official registries and hospital records. A specific re-examination of CAP hospital records for those having a psychosis diagnosis either at CAP and or in GenP was performed in 2007.

The records were evaluated using the Comprehensive Assessment of At-Risk Mental States (CAARMS), in which any possible early signs of psychosis were noted. Sixty-two former CAP patients (4.4%;) received a psychosis diagnosis during the observation time, 48 of them within the diagnosis block of Schizophrenia, schizotypal and delusional disorders and 14 within the Psychotic mood disorders block.

[*] E-mail: ulf,engqvist@miun.se

Mean age at first onset was 21.4 years (SD 6.4). Behavioral changes, including social isolation, refusal to go to school, loneliness and odd behavior in general and positive symptoms were the initial signs and symptoms most frequently observed prior or upon admission to CAP care.

Psychotic disorders have been and continue to be relatively uncommon among patients admitted to CAP care in Sweden. Psychotic disorders in average have a debut during late adolescence and early adult-life. Disorders in the ICD category of Schizophrenia, schizotypal and delusional disorders are more common than those classified as Psychotic mood disorders.

However, individuals experiencing early onset of disorders categorized as Schizophrenia, schizotypal and delusional disorders may already exhibit typical symptoms upon admission to CAP care at the age of 13-17; whereas with late-onset disorders, it appears not be associated with any obvious signs or symptoms years before the disorder has developed fully.

## INTRODUCTION

In this chapter, the occurrence of psychoses in a CAP population in a smaller county council and province study area in Sweden is described. It also describes the outcome in adulthood for patients having psychoses in childhood and adolescence in terms of later GenP care and diagnoses, mortality and criminality.

Psychoses refer to the category of mental health problems that include schizophrenia, schizotypal disorder, delusional disorders and/or psychotic mood disorders. They are defined by ICD-10 chapter V, block F20-29 and block F30-F39.

## TWO PSYCHIATRIC SETTINGS WITHIN SWEDISH PSYCHIATRY

Psychiatry is one of the most large-scale caring sectors in our time. It is probably the most changeable and widely prejudice-loaded sector in the health care system in Sweden. The most rapidly growing, controversy-ridden, and attention-attracting area of history over the past generation has been the history of psychiatry [1].

Psychiatry is not at all a uniform concept. In Sweden, there are three psychiatric settings, GenP, forensic psychiatry and CAP working with adult patients, children and young people up to 18 years and mentally disordered offenders, respectively [2]. Without being a specialty, there are also units for geriatric psychiatry in some hospitals. Particularly, in the research work, delimitation of psychiatry is made with consideration to method and theoretical basis in, for example, dynamic psychiatry, social psychiatry and biological psychiatry [3].

Psychiatry has a history dating back to medieval times when the church organized the first care of the sick in Sweden and the healthcare facilities belonged to the monasteries. In the 18th century, the madhouses played a more important role. General hospitals for care of physical diseases were established but the mentally ill remained at the "madhouses" [4]. Around 1860, several large changes within psychiatry and psychiatric care in Sweden was effected. A new regulation was sanctioned and psychiatry became an established branch of learning at the medical seats of learning and more hospitals were built [5]. In 1851, the

Government laid the foundation for psychiatry as a medical specialty [6]. Construction of new mental hospitals after the turn of the century took off and grew in the following decades, until the 1960's as an expression of a general institutionalization trend. From 1900 to 1950, the number of beds at the mental hospitals increased from 4,600 to 25,000. In the beginning of the1960s, there were 31 free-standing mental hospitals in Sweden [7]. In 1967, when the county councils took over the responsibility for mental health services from the Government, the number of inpatient beds was approximately 36,000; most of them in mental hospitals.

On January 1, 1995, the Community Mental Health Care reform [8] came into effect; a reform that all political parties supported. The reform made clear the liability for the municipality to provide for occupation and housing so that the psychiatric disabled patients could adapt themselves to the society. They were now seen as mentally handicapped and placed under the same act as individuals with a bodily handicap, The Act on Support and Service (LSS) [9].

In 2001, only 5,565 beds for inpatient psychiatric care remained and in 2006, the number was 4,600 beds. An increasing population and decreasing number of beds has lead to more individuals out of society [10].

The national psychiatry coordinator (which was appointed as an investigator of psychiatry at the beginning of the 2000s) established that the Community Mental Health Care Reform from 1995 has implied an increased supply of housing and occupation in the municipalities and that the needs of the target group has been attended to in a better way than before. But the weak support in law for the reform, the lack of local political support and the lack of evidence-based methods for the community-based support caused obstacles that to a great extent, remains more than ten years later [9].

For a long time, children and young were not separated from adults in the psychiatric context. As a medical specialty, CAP is altogether a 20th century matter but intelligence defects and psychoses among children had been paid attention to through earlier centuries. They were treated together with adults in the "madhouses" [11].

Within pediatrics, it was observed early during the latter part of the 19th century that children could also show nervous and mental diseases. Sweden was the first country in the world to set up special chairs on child diseases. The first psychiatric guidance unit was established in Stockholm in 1914. School psychiatry was also a form of early child psychiatry. The child custody authority in Stockholm established the Child Guidance Clinics Centrals in the beginning of the 1930s.

Professorships in CAP were established from 1958 onwards. In November 1960, the mental healthcare was subsidized by the State. Ten independent CAP clinics were active in Sweden at that time. In 1971, all county councils have an organization with in- and outpatient services for CAP. The State subsidy regulation remained to the end of 1975 when the number of clinics was 30 [12-13].

Three years after the Community Mental Health Care reform in 1995, another governmental report on CAP was published. That report established, among other things, that psychiatric care for youths with severe psychological disturbances such as eating disorders, autism, schizophrenia, severe obsessive-compulsive disorders and depression with suicide risk did not seem to be working in a satisfactory manner. Many proposals were given in the report but few were realized [14-16].

During the 1990s, the inflow of admissions to CAP increased to a large extent. The waiting lists grow and it was not unusual with more than yearlong periods of waiting for care.

This caused debate in the media and in the authorities [14-17]. The history of GenP in Jämtland County follows the history for the rest of the country. Frösö Hospital, which was finished in 1912, was one of the largest mental hospitals built in Sweden at that time. As late as the start of the 1980s, there were more than 20 psychiatric wards with more than 1,000 inpatients. During the 1980s, the psychiatry was divided in sectors. At the start of the 1990s, psychiatry was transferred from Frösö hospital to Östersunds hospital and became a psychiatric unit integrated with the physical care. Today there are five wards and less than 100 beds.

As early as in 1944, Jämtland County Council came to a decision that child and youth care should be organized in the County and the activity started in August 1946 and was closed in the beginning of 1948 when the chief physician left his post. The work was conducted without a treatment ward but with the possibility to use three beds at the pediatric ward. Consulting hours existed at not less than nine different places in the County [18].

It took more than twenty years before CAP again was established in Jämtland. In September 1970, the activity started with one children's ward and one youth ward with seven beds each. The children's ward was transformed to a family ward in 1977 but that was closed one year later. From 1978 up to and until 1993, there was one ward with five beds. In the beginning, the care was characterized by traditional nursing- a successive change and development towards environment therapy and family therapy. In 1984, a treatment home was opened and it was closed ten years later.

The inpatient activities were replaced in the mid 1990s by an intensified systemic outpatient treatment at the same time as the treatment home and the ward were closed [18-19]. During the time for CAP care, this chapter comprises both outpatient and inpatient care at a ward and a treatment home that was active.

## Similarities and Differences between General Psychiatry and Child and Adolescent Psychiatry

There are many similarities between GenP and CAP. The two disciplines have operated in parallel during the last 100 years. Despite the similarities, there is a lack of significant and reliable information regarding, for instance, the relationship between psychiatric deviations and behavioral disturbances in childhood and psychiatric disorders and social adjustment problems and or criminality later in adulthood.

Information about the relationship between behavioral disturbances in childhood and criminality in later life has, however, developed further compared to information about psychological deviations during childhood and later psychiatric illness. There is also a virtual lack of information regarding possible early symptoms of mental disorders, and how they change during the process of maturing from childhood to adulthood.

It is easy to describe the difference between the two psychiatric settings. CAP works with psychopathological states of the growing and maturing individual or personality where the psychopathological symptoms change in pace with maturity. GenP, on the other hand, works with adult patients where the process of maturing has, if not ended, at least slowed down.

This means that psychiatrists working with adult patients can work with a system of classification of symptoms over time and states that are not as dependent on age and maturation.

In CAP, great individual differences and gender differences appear which is why symptoms and behavioral disturbances can actually have varying meaning even in children of the same age. A certain symptom can also form an adequate way of expression for children of a certain age, but be considered pathological in other ages.

## BACKGROUND

For more than three decades, Michel Rutter and co-workers [20-22] have periodically reviewed the literature concerning relationships between childhood and adult psychopathology, with particular focus on possible mechanisms involved in the continuities and discontinuities observed between early and late psychopathology, as well as the need for systematic, prospective and long-term longitudinal investigations in this area.

On the whole, the findings on the long-term course of schizophrenia beginning in childhood are broadly similar to that of schizophrenia beginning in adult life. In both cases, the disorder is usually fluctuating with each episode often marked by prodromal, active and recuperative phases, followed by quiescent or residual deficit periods. Like the earlier studies of special groups, the general population prospective studies have confirmed that overt schizophrenia in adulthood is frequently preceded by socio-emotional behavioral disturbances [22]. The long-term course of childhood and adolescent onset schizophrenia is worse than in adulthood schizophrenia, and the patients with manifestation of the disorder below the age of 14 have a very poor prognosis [23].

Nevertheless, early case-control and follow-back studies [24] showed that children who later developed overt schizophrenia were more likely than controls to show social, emotional and behavioral problems in childhood [22]. Various behaviors, in particular, withdrawn and delinquent-aggressive behavior in adolescents at risk of schizophrenia may predict a later onset of the illness. These behaviors, however, are far less predictive of isolated psychotic symptoms prior to a psychosis onset [25]. Schizophrenia-related psychoses can be followed back to early behavioral disturbances [26]. Conduct Disorder is a distinct comorbid disorder that runs parallel to the course of schizophrenia [27]. Early neuroticism may be a precursor to the onset of psychotic symptoms. The mechanisms underlying this association are unclear, but may relate to overlapping features between prodromal phases of psychosis and items that measure neuroticism [28]. Total population epidemiological and longitudinal studies provided a stronger test of the suggestion that abnormalities in childhood constituted precursors of schizophrenia that did not become manifested until early adult life. The precursors include delays in early motor development and impairments in receptive language and cognitive functioning [22]. Findings on CAP clinic attendees who go on to develop either schizophrenia or bipolar disorder, nevertheless, suggests that there may be a degree of diagnostic specificity, with abnormal suspiciousness / sensitivity and relationship difficulties with peers being particularly associated with later schizophrenia [29). Three main queries have yet to be resolved concerning the meaning of the findings on the features in childhood and adolescence that predict the later development of a schizophrenic psychosis. Accordingly, this necessarily raises queries about what is meant by a prodromal phase. Second, all of the findings raise the question of what it is that leads to the translation of precursors or prodromata into overt schizophrenia. The final query concerns the possibility that, despite the early neurodevelopmental abnormalities, there are further changes in both cognitive function and brain structure and function that take place during the course of the schizophrenia spectrum disorder in adult life either as a result of the disease process or of the drugs used in its treatment [22].

## Swedish Child and Adolescent Psychiatry Patients

The population of Swedish CAP patients is heterogeneous, including children who demonstrate problems at school, adjustment/behavioral symptoms and/or psychiatric problems, as well as children with psychosocial, family-related difficulties [30-32]. Those treated prior to 13 years of age often exhibit behavioral symptoms and difficulties with adjustment to peer groups and to school and other members of their families frequently experience psychosocial problems as well. In contrast, adolescents receiving such care appear to develop their "own" more often than do infants and school children, with less common occurrences of parallel psychosocial problems among the rest of the family. The typical CAP patient is either "a troublesome 10-year-old boy" or "a depressed 14-year-old girl" [30-33].

At least a third of all CAP patients, and more often girls than boys, are later seen again as psychiatric patients after reaching adulthood [32, 34-35]. However, the correlation between the nature of the psychopathology requiring CAP care and later diagnosis as an adult is weak. Only a small group of patients require continuous care from childhood to adulthood. Furthermore, the major reasons for which former CAP patients are admitted to GenP care are drug and/or alcohol addiction and/or criminality, rather than symptoms of a psychiatric disorder [31-32, 35-36].

## Previous Longitudinal Studies

In Sweden, we can proudly note that there are prospective and longitudinal studies describing CAP patient materials in different time periods, from 1928 until present, and this may be considered to be unique in the research field. Researchers in the Nordic countries, especially in Finland, also have the opportunity to use registers that allow longitudinal studies of this kind. In the following sections, different longitudinal studies from Sweden and some Nordic studies are reviewed.

## Descriptions of CAP Patients

CAP patients have been described from as early as 1928 when Alice Hellström started her description of psychopathic boys treated at the Mellansjö treatment home. Alice Hellström described all of the children who came to Mellansjö treatment home 1928-1940 under a special research protocol, which she established with the help of Bror Gadelius and Isak Jundell. She then followed her patients for a long time after her retirement and until 1968. However, because of her age, she was not capable of completing her report. The complete research material was bequeathed to the CAP clinic at the St Görans children's hospital in Stockholm, where Ingegärd Fried completed the work in her licentiate's dissertation [37]. Alice Hellström's own words when she was about sixty years, grappling with its materials and the long observation period, are worth considering: ”It is about a child material which, although very different from today's, but to their essential constitutional reactions, is the same human beings as today” [37].

The next study of children treated by CAP was the longitudinal prospective follow up of 2,164 child and adolescent guidance clinic patients (cared for 1953-1955) followed up to 1975. This group was originally studied by Curman and the study was later completed by Nylander [30, 36]. The Stockholm population has been used as a comparison group.

## Different Swedish Risk Groups

Various risk and control groups and children from the general population have been described with prospective longitudinal research from the perspective of several scientific disciplines (see Table 1). This provides a number of opportunities to discuss similarities and differences between patient groups, other groups at risk and children in general.

In addition to the studies named above, there are also descriptions of CAP patients conducted with so called cross-section methods. In 1950, Chief Physician, Svante Nycander at the Erica Foundation presented his thesis ”Personlighetsutveckling på avvägar” (Personality Astray), where 308 boys and girls that were examined and treated at the Erica Foundation Curative Pedagogy Institute in Stockholm were described [33].

**Table 1. Different risk groups as described with longitudinal / prospective methodology**

| Sample | Discipline | Criminality | Alcoholism | Follow-up period |
|---|---|---|---|---|
| Psychopathic boys treated at the Mellansjö-treatment home | CAP | 41% | 28% | 1928-1968 [1] |
| Delinquent boys treated at the Children's Village SKÅ | CAP | 67% | 58% | 1954-1973 [2] |
| Young law-breakers from the general population | CAP, Sociology, Psychology, Criminology | 39% | 46% | 1960-1972 [3] |
| Teenage alcoholics | CAP | 42% | 58% | 1964-1985 1964-1977 [4] |
| Adopted children with heredity for social problems /alcoholism | CAP | 14% | 21% | 1930-1972 [5] |
| Children of alcoholic fathers | CAP | 42% | 35% | 1958-1978 [6] |

Ulf Otto, at the University of Lund, used retrospective longitudinal methods in his thesis from 1972 "Barns och ungdomars självmordshandlingar" (Suicidal acts by children and adolescents) [43] to describe during a period of fifteen years the outcome for 1,727 boys and girls that at the end of the 1950s were treated for attempted suicide. The results have been recovered also in later Swedish studies that indicates that children and youth's suicide acts are a "call for help" that needs treatment, support and help [43]. However, attempted suicide in itself may be a "poor" predictor for later executed suicide. The high risk group that commits suicide before the age of 25 seems to be found among those who develop psychiatric illness or anti-sociality and addiction [32, 34].

During pre-puberty and puberty, behavior problems and mental symptoms are common among children in general. When 222 common Stockholm boys were described during the 1950s, it appeared that every tenth boy in the age of 8-16 years had phobias and compulsive acts. The result of the description of symptoms showed that every fourth schoolboy suffered from some kind of difficulty, nervous symptom or difficulty in adapting to the extent that specialist help or special treatment was needed. However, their prognosis was not decided by the load of symptoms or the behavioral disturbances. The 18-year follow-up assessment showed that the prognosis for most of them was much better than was expected and it was not the load of symptoms but learning ability and home environment that was of importance for the future outcome [38].

## Studies on the Swedish General Population

In addition, different risk and control groups and the general population have been studied with prospective longitudinal research methods from various disciplines during the second half of the 20th century as shown in Table 2.

**Table 2. Different control groups and children from the general population as described with longitudinal / prospective methodology**

| Sample | Discipline | Criminality | Alcoholism | Follow-up period |
|---|---|---|---|---|
| The Lundby-study | Psychiatry | 8% | <br>10% | 1947-1987<br>1947-1972<br>[1, 7] |
| 222 Stockholm boys | CAP | 15% | 19% | 1954-1973<br>[2] |
| Controls/"social twins" to children of alcoholic fathers | CAP | 25% | 20% | 1958-1978<br>[6] |
| The Metropolitan project | Sociology, Criminology | 31% | | 1963-1979<br>[8-9] |
| The Solna Study | Paediatrics, CAP | 35% | | 1955-1988<br>[10-11] |
| The IDA-project | Psychology | 38% | <br>17% | 1965-1985<br>1965-1980<br>[12-13] |

The Lundby Study is a project exceptional and world leading by its prospective design [1]. International reviewers [51] have stated that "the Lundby Study has produced prevalence, incidence and outcome data on depression and anxiety over many years, and is one of the few studies capable of producing reliable data on changes in incidence" [52]. It is a well-known longitudinal survey of the mental health in a total Swedish population during the time period from July 1, 1947, to July 1, 1997. The Lundby population consisting of 3,563 probands was investigated in 1947, 1957, and 1972. Sufficient information was available for 98–99% of the subjects. In 1997–2000, Per Nettelbladt and his research team carried through a fourth field investigation.

In a longitudinal research project, Nylander and Rydelius [42] followed up with the children of male alcoholics from the lowest social class. The results of these studies have shown that when they are still small, the children exhibit signs of mental disturbances and that when they become adults; the boys develop social maladjustment problems and addictions, and have a high rate of both somatic and psychiatric diseases. In comparison to their controls (matched for socio-economic class), the values found for these variables are consistently higher for the probands.

The Stockholm Metropolitan study is a follow-up of 15,000 individuals born in 1953 who were still living in the Stockholm Metropolitan area in 1963. The project was initiated by late professor Carl-Gunnar Jansson and is now conducted by Sten-Åke Stenberg and Denny Vågerö [53]. The study was primarily concerned with sociological issues of social mobility and organization, conformity and deviance, and marital patterns. This study has resulted in over 100 publications [54].

The IDA project is a prospective, longitudinal research program led by Professor David Magnusson from the outset in 1965, investigating three cohorts of subjects: all boys and girls who attended school in a municipality in mid-Sweden, and attended the third, sixth or eighth grade at the time of the first data collection. The main group, encompassing in excess of 1,400 individuals, are the participants in most of the research conducted in the program [55].

The Solna study is a birth-to-maturity study of 212 children born in Stockholm in the mid 1950s. The goal was to acquire a comprehensive picture of individual growth and development by charting the course of physical and psychological development and obtaining reasonably comprehensive life histories that would be useful in many areas of research. The information covers many issues from birth to mid-life. The database is large [56].

## Studies in the Nordic Countries

Thomsen followed up a total of 546 children and adolescents in Denmark, aged 5 to 15 years. They were inpatients in psychiatric hospitals throughout Denmark between 1970 and 1973, and followed up regarding later readmissions and mortality. Approximately one-third of the sample had at least one readmission after the age of 18 years. In total, 24 probands died during the study period. Eight individuals had committed suicide. The SMR was significantly increased [57].

Thomsen also performed a register-based study of 485 children (0-15 years of age) admitted to a child psychiatric hospital from January 1, 1970, to December 31, 1972, who were followed up on December 31, 1986. They showed higher rates of admission to psychiatric hospitals in late adolescence or young adulthood than found in an age-standardized general population [58].

Psychiatric morbidity, expressed as hospital admissions during a 30-year follow-up period, among 322 former child psychiatric patients in a register investigation was studied by Larsen. They were admitted from 1949-1951, and were followed up as of December 31, 1980. By the variables employed, 37% of the sample was judged to have had a good overall outcome, with diagnosis being an inconsistent predictor of outcome [59-60].

An epidemiological study of psychopathology in the first years of life and of the association between mental health problems in infancy and psychiatric disturbances later in life is investigated in a project studying mental health problems and possibilities of intervention from infancy and onward. This Danish study of a general population consists of a birth cohort of 6,090 children born in the year 2000 in the County of Copenhagen, the Copenhagen County Child Cohort (CCCC 2000). Results from this study will add to the knowledge of risk factors and course of mental health problems in childhood and contribute to the validation of the mental health screening made by public health nurses [61].

A Norwegian population of 1,276 former adolescent psychiatric inpatients was followed up on 15 to 33 years after hospitalization by Kjelsberg by record linkage to the national registers of criminality (n=932), disability benefits (n=1,095) and causes of death (n=1,095).

In total, 1,095 patients (53.7% males), representing 85.8% of the original sample could be traced. At follow-up, 52.0% of those investigated had engaged in criminal activity. It was shown that male sex, psychoactive substance use disorder, short hospital stay and poor impulse control remained strong and independent predictors of death [62-66].

The Finnish "From a Boy to a Man study" has an objective to study associations between comorbid psychopathology and long-term outcomes in a large birth cohort sample from age 8 to early adulthood. The sample included long-term outcome data on 2,556 Finnish boys born in 1981 and the aim was to study the impact of early childhood psychopathology types and informant sources on young adult outcomes, based on data from a military registry of psychiatric diagnosis, a police registry on criminal and drug offenses, and self-reported problems in late adolescence and early adulthood. The conclusions in this study were that the subjective suffering and long-term burden to society are especially high among children with comorbid conduct and internalizing problems in childhood. A major challenge for CAP, education, and social services is to develop effective intervention strategies focusing on these children [67].

In a population-based birth cohort in Finland, with the aim of studying the continuity of psychopathology from the age of 3-12 years, children's emotional and behavioral problems were assessed at age 3 using the Child Behavior Checklist 2-3, and at age 12 by parents using the Child Behavior Checklist 11-18, and the Youth Self Report completed by the children. Behavioral ratings were obtained from 800 subjects at both time points and the results showed the complexity of pathways in psychopathology from early childhood to pre-adolescence. In particular, aggressive and destructive behavior in very early childhood predicted later problems and require early recognition and possible intervention at an early age [68].

A Northern Finland 1966 birth cohort has been followed-up on in different studies for 34 and 35 years regarding childhood precursors and risk factors of schizophrenia. The findings supported the longitudinal dimension and life span models of schizophrenia. No powerful risk factor, pre-morbid sign or risk indicator was identified that was useful for the prediction of schizophrenia in the general population [69-72].

## AIM AND QUESTIONS

The aim was to obtain answers to a number of questions concerning a group of former CAP patients diagnosed during child- or adulthood as suffering from schizophrenia, schizotypal disorder, delusional disorders and/or psychotic mood disorders: At what age was the diagnosis made? Was this diagnosis later changed and, if so, in what manner? Were early signs of the disorder detectable prior to or at the time of admission to CAP care? Which CAP patients were later diagnosed as psychotic in GenP? And how did this latter group differ from those who had already received a diagnosis before the age of 18 years?

## MATERIAL AND METHODS
## JÄMTLAND COUNTY COUNCIL

Jämtland County is one of Sweden's 21 counties. It consists of the two provinces Härjedalen and Jämtland and minor parts of Ångermanland and Hälsingland. Jämtland is located in the western part of middle Sweden at the border to Norway. It represents 12% of Sweden's total land mass but only 1.5% of the population. From 1975 – 2003, the total population varied from 133,433 to 127,645 with a peak of 136,301 inhabitants in 1994. Östersund is the only city in the county and the city is a major trade center for the entire county.

The county and the regional hospital in Östersund were well suited for this type of description. In Jämtland County there was one CAP clinic and one GenP clinic under the same health organization giving service to the whole population. Both clinics were located in the same hospital organization at Östersund Hospital.

## THE CHILD AND ADOLESCENT PSYCHIATRY PATIENT GROUP

All 1,420 patients born between 1957 and 1976 and admitted to in- or outpatient CAP care in Jämtland County, Sweden, during the period of 1975-1990 were initially considered for inclusion. Eight individuals not covered by the national registries and twelve who subsequently emigrated during the follows-up period were excluded, leaving a total of 1,400 former CAP patients, including 285 in- and 1,115 outpatient, or 98.6% of the original population. These children and adolescents were referred to CAP by pediatricians or general practitioners (35%), by school or childcare personnel (22%), by social services (12%) or other authorities (2%) or else they themselves and/or their parents sought help (29%). They were all evaluated, in general, treated and terminated their contact with CAP between 1975 and 1990, although some of the youngest patients were readmitted to such care subsequent to 1990.

**Table 3. Index groups for the Stockholm and Jämtland populations**

| Primary Material | Stockholm | | Jämtland | |
|---|---|---|---|---|
| | Number | Percent | Number | Percent |
| | 2364 | | 1420 | |
| Excluded: | | | | |
| Emigrated | 100 | 4,2 | 12 | 0,8 |
| Deceased during follow up | 50 | 2,1 | 38 | 2,7 |
| Unusable data | 50 | 2,1 | 8 | 0,6 |
| Inpatient care | 0 | 0 | 270 | 19 |
| Less than 20 year follow up | 0 | 0 | 484 | 34,1 |
| Index group: | 2164 | 91,5 | 608 | 42,8 |
| Males | 1417 | 65,5 | 325 | 53,5 |
| Females | 747 | 34,5 | 283 | 46,5 |

## A PATIENT GROUP USED FOR COMPARISON

In Table 3, the number of patients not included in the final samples from the comparison group (the Stockholm study) [36] and the corresponding group from Jämtland, and the reasons for the exclusion of these patients are listed as well as the distribution of those assessed in a 20-year follow-up after their CAP care and the distribution of gender.

## EXPERIMENTAL DESIGN AND PROCEDURES

In 1995, a protocol for describing the patients and their histories was established. After identification of patients previously receiving CAP and/or GenP care, both within and outside Jämtland County on the basis of hospital records and linkage to the nationwide Swedish Hospital Discharge Registry (HDR), their gender, present age, reason for initial contact with CAP and/or GenP, and diagnoses, as well as any necessity for inpatient care were noted. During the periods of 1968-1996 and 1987-1996, the ICD-8 and ICD-9 systems, respectively, were employed in Sweden, prior to the introduction of ICD-10 in 1997. To allow comparisons, all diagnoses based on the ICD-8 and ICD-9 categories were converted to ICD-10 [73-74] utilizing the official conversion tables published by the Swedish National Board of Health and Welfare [75-76]. Although the Swedish Association for Child and Adolescent Psychiatry has decided to also apply the DSM system in parallel for clinical practice, obligatory ICD classification is utilized for official registration of diagnoses.

All of the 285 CAP patients admitted to the inpatient care received a diagnosis in connection with their treatment, whereas outpatients were not usually given a diagnosis in cases where their symptoms and problems were developmental in origin or a reaction to their living circumstances. Nonetheless, for 616 of these 1,115 outpatients (55 %), a CAP diagnosis was recorded. In the case of GenP, both in- and outpatients received a diagnosis, so that 524 of the 531 patients (99 %) later admitted to GenP had diagnoses noted in their hospital records and/or in the HDR registry. Specific evaluation of hospital records indicating a diagnosis of psychosis was performed.

Until 1995, combinations of retrospective and prospective approaches were employed, whereas thereafter only prospective methods were used until 2003. The mean observation time was 16.1 (SD 8.5) years, with a range of 12-28 years. A 20-year follow-up was available for 608 of the 1115 outpatients in the study group. Utilizing the t-test for a difference between two proportions the outcomes of these long-term follow-ups have been compared, to published data concerning the occurrence and frequencies of psychotic disorders observed in connection with the 20-year prospective follow-up of 2,164 outpatients treated at the Child Guidance Clinics in Stockholm during the period of 1953-1955 [30, 36].

## Collection of Data

After eliciting the required permission and ethical approval, collection of the data was initiated by examining the CAP hospital records, followed by a prospective survey of a number of these patients later referred to GenP care prior to 2003. Information concerning out- and inpatient GenP care in Jämtland County was obtained by examining local registries, hospital records and the nationwide Swedish Hospital Discharge Registry (HDR) correspondence. Information regarding inpatient care outside of this county was provided by the HDR (which only covers inpatient care). The protocol entailed recording the following information from the CAP hospital records:

- Age at first admission to CAP and age at finishing the care and gender.
- Who referred the patient to the CAP clinic?
- Where or with whom they lived with during period of CAP care (family, foster family, institution, etc.).
- Problems with learning and/or behavior problems at school.
- Information about inpatient or outpatient care at the CAP clinic.
- At the time of admission to the CAP clinic, family circumstances. If the patient's biological parents were living together, this would be described as a complete family and if not, as a split family.
- Any information about adoption.
- Reason for admission to the CAP clinic according to standards established by the Swedish Association for Child and Adolescent Psychiatry.
- Diagnosis.

One-third of the outpatients were not given a formal diagnosis. Outpatients in the CAP clinic did not receive diagnoses when their problems were considered temporary due to growing and maturation.

The retrospective data from CAP hospital records were used as independent variables to the dependent variables mood disorder or not, deceased or alive, suicide or not suicide, convicted of offenses or not and GenP care or not.

The CAP hospital records of those patients who received a diagnosis of schizophrenia and/or psychotic mood disorders at any time during the follow-up were evaluated in greater detail for any early signs of possible psychosis utilizing the Comprehensive Assessment of at-Risk Mental States (CAARMS) developed by Yung and colleagues [77].

The goals of this instrument are two-fold, i.e., to assess psychopathology thought to indicate imminent development of a first-episode psychotic disorder and to determine whether an individual is at ultra-high-risk (UHR) for onset of an initial psychotic disorder.

The diagnostic criteria for UHR have been refined for improved precision by researchers at the University of Melbourne [78-79] and Yale University [80], who have developed sets of criteria based on the presence or onset of one or more of the following: attenuated psychotic symptoms (ideas of reference, magical thinking, perceptual disturbance, paranoid ideation, and odd thinking and/or speech); intermittent psychotic symptoms of too short duration to meet the criteria of the Diagnostic and Statistical Manual of Mental Disorder for psychosis i.e., (symptoms which spontaneously disappear within 1 week); a first-degree family history of a psychotic or bipolar disorder; or a personal history of schizotypal personality disorder, with significant recent functional decline [81].

## Swedish Registers

Sweden and the Nordic countries, especially Finland, are unique concerning official registers. In this chapter, several Swedish national registers were used. The parish registration required by the 1686 Church Ordinance laid the groundwork for future population statistics. Sweden began to keep population statistics in 1749, quite a unique phenomenon.

National registration is the fundamental registration of the Swedish population. In the national registration, it is continuously registered who is living in the country and where they live. The register is based on personal identification numbers.

For a long time it was conducted by the church through parish registration, but since July 1, 1991, the Swedish Tax Authority is responsible for the national registration [82]. Information from the National registration; i.e. personal identification was used as a base for gathering information from all other official registers, which are described below.

From 1987, the National Patient Register covers all public inpatient care in Sweden. Statistics of diseases and surgical treatments of patients have a long history in Sweden.

Data of this kind has been published for more than 100 years and was available during the entire 20th century. In the 1960s, the National Board of Health and Welfare started to collect data on individual patients who had been treated as inpatients at public hospitals. The register built up at that time initially covered all patients treated in psychiatric care and around 16% of patients in somatic care, involving six of the 26 county councils in Sweden [83]. This register has been used to collect data pertaining to inpatient psychiatric care and diagnoses.

The National Causes of Death Register has been used to establish time for death and causes of death. Along with the register, death certificates have been examined. The National Causes of Death Register goes back to 1749 when a nation-wide report system first was introduced.

The National Causes of Death Register is annually updated and based on personal identification numbers and includes all death certificates for the Swedish population. The

National Swedish Board of Health and Welfare has been responsible for publication since 1994 [84].

Statistics of persons convicted of offenses has continuously been recorded since 1972 by SCB. The Swedish NCCP (BRÅ) is, since July 1, 1994, responsible for Sweden's official crime statistics. The Register of Persons Convicted of Offenses has been used to obtain information regarding criminality.

## Analysis of the Data

The findings based on prospective data are descriptive in nature. All data analysis was performed using the SPSS for Windows, release 12.0 (SPSS Inc) software. The chi-square and t-tests were employed to analyze differences between categorical and continuous variables, respectively, with a P-value of <0.05 being considered statistically significant in both cases. Differences between proportions were analyzed utilizing a two-by-two cross table and Students t-test.

Although this t-test is essentially not valid for making such comparisons, extensive studies have shown it to be applicable also in these respects, and, consequently, the student's t-test has been widely and successfully used for analysis of proportional data [85]. There are a number of proposals concerning how to present double-sided probabilities used to compare proportional data [86]. When employing the sum of small (or significant) p-values, all possible tables are generated within given margins, all p-values of the same size or smaller than the point probability are added together to obtain the cumulative p-value, and the resulting value is presented utilizing the notation p (O>=E |O<=E).

In the case of the method of small p-values, the exact point probability for the nil hypothesis that produces the table observed is calculated first. Thereafter, all possible alternative outcomes given the set conditions are generated with a computer program [85].

Since the number of calculations required with exact approaches can easily become excessive (particularly in the case of larger tables), computer programs that provide exact probabilities using the method of small p-values (such as the SPSS) sometimes extract a single sample from all of the possible alternatives and use this to calculate an exact probability value within confidence limits.

## Ethical Considerations

Personal registers are an inalienable part of the research design for longitudinal studies as carried out in this chapter. A comprehensive regulation of research on humans is of national and international nature.

To the extent that personal data is processed in the framework of a research project the Personal Data Act (The Swedish Data Inspection Board 2008) that replaced the out-dated Swedish Data Act from 1973 is applicable. Some personal information is particularly sensitive. These are referred to in the Act as sensitive personal data.

All health information is considered sensitive in the law, regardless of disease. Sensitive personal data may be processed for research purposes under the conditions set out in the Personal Data Act.

The data collection started long before the Act concerning the Ethical Review of Research Involving Humans came into force and, in some cases, before the Personal Data Act. The Ethical Review of Research Involving Humans includes, for example, research on living persons, research on the deceased, research on biological material from humans and research that involves the handling of sensitive personal data.

Accompanying the new law, an authority "Centrala etikprövningsnämnden" (the Central Ethical Review Board) and six regional councils was established. The register study would be implemented within the general register license for health and medical service and the research ethical principles in force at each data collection were carefully followed. An initial application for ethical permission was sent in 1995 and was approved by the ethical review committee of the Medical Faculty of Umeå University: Um document no. 95-051.

The research plan was later amended to include issues of crime and drug abuse. Following a request of the ethics committee, I received notice that the original license (Um document no. 95-051) could continue to apply to the register study on the CAP-patients and future psychiatric morbidity and mortality but that new ethical applications must be submitted for the parts of the project on crime and abuse. Additional applications were therefore sent in for ethical review. In 1999, ethical review committees of the Medical Faculty of Umeå University and the Regional Research Committee at Karolinska Institutet approved the expanded study on crime (Um document no. 99-023 and KI document no. 99-209). Every register search has also been approved by the authority responsible for the register. The chief physician of the CAP clinic and the GenP clinic both respectively approved the reading of medical records within the general register license for health and medical service regularized in the Official Secrets Act.

# RESULTS

## The Child and Adolescent Psychiatry Patient Group at Baseline

- The gender distribution was 733 female (52.4%) and 667 male (47.6%).
- Mean age at admission was 12.1 years of age (S.D. 4.0).
- The patients were referred to CAP by pediatricians or general practitioners (35%), by school or childcare personnel (22%), by social services (12%) or other authorities (2%) or else they by themselves and/or their parents sought help (29%).
- Inpatient care was given to 285 patients (20.4%).
- Over half of the study group (52.5%) lived in a split family.
- Nearly half of the patients (46.5%) had school problems noted in their records.

The most frequently occurring reasons for admission to CAP are shown in Table 4 and diagnoses made at CAP are shown in Table 5.

**Table 4. The ten most frequent occurring reasons for admission to CAP, n = 1389**

| Reason for admission to CAP | Frequency | Percentage |
|---|---|---|
| Behavioral disorder | 292 | 21.0 |
| Relationship problems | 258 | 18.6 |
| Anxiety | 181 | 13.0 |
| Somatic problems and eating disorders | 138 | 9.9 |
| Mental retardation and developmental problems | 80 | 5.8 |
| Suicide attempt, suicide thoughts | 71 | 5.1 |
| Depression | 60 | 4.3 |
| Reaction to stress | 52 | 3.7 |
| Enuresis or encopresis | 47 | 3.4 |
| Abused and/or neglected | 38 | 2.7 |

**Table 5. Diagnoses (blocks) made at CAP according to ICD-10, n = 901**

| Diagnoses (block) | Frequency | Percentage |
|---|---|---|
| Z00-Z99 Factors influencing health status and contact with health services | 321 | 35.6 |
| F90-F98 Behavioral and emotional disorders with onset usually occurring in childhood and adolescence | 196 | 21.8 |
| F40-F48 Neurotic, stress-related and somatoform disorders | 140 | 15.5 |
| X60-X84 Intentional self-harm | 48 | 5.3 |
| F50-F59 Behavioral syndromes associated with physiological disturbances and physical factors | 46 | 5.1 |
| F80-F89 Disorders of psychological development | 39 | 4.3 |
| F30-F39 Mood [affective] disorders | 31 | 3.4 |
| F70-F79 Mental retardation | 27 | 3.0 |
| F10-F19 Mental and behavioural disorders due to psychoactive substance use | 24 | 2.7 |
| F20-F29 Schizophrenia, schizotypal and delusional disorders | 20 | 2.2 |
| F60-F69 Disorders of adult personality and behavior | 4 | 0.4 |
| Other diagnoses | 4 | 0.4 |
| F99 Unspecified mental disorder | 1 | 0.1 |

## The Incidences of Schizophrenia and Psychotic Mood Disorders

By the end of the follow-up period, 62 former CAP patients (36 women and 26 men), which is 4.4% of the entire study population of 1,400, had received an ICD-10 diagnosis of "F20-29: Schizophrenia, schizotypal and delusional disorders" (48 patients) and/or "F30-39: Psychotic mood disorders" (14 patients). The gender distribution among these patients was similar to that among the remainder, who had not been diagnosed as experiencing a psychosis. The various diagnostic groups are presented in Table 6.

Of the one-third [21] of these individuals who received their initial diagnosis of psychosis in connection with CAP care, only two were not considered to have such a condition during later GenP care. The remaining 41 patients were initially diagnosed as psychotic after becoming adults, in connection with GenP care. The overall estimated incidence of first-episode psychosis per 10,000 person-years in the study group was 15.4 (17.1 for females and 13.7 for males).

**Table 6. Diagnoses of psychosis recorded in connection with CAP and GenP care**

| Diagnosis | Number diagnosed in connection with CAP Boys Girls | Number diagnosed in connection with GenP Men Women | | |
|---|---|---|---|---|
| All | 8 | 13 | 23 | 32 |
| *Schizophrenia, schizotypal and delusional disorders* | *7* | *9* | *17* | *26* |
| F20.0 Paranoid schizophrenia | 0 | 0 | 1 | 0 |
| F20.1 Hebephrenic schizophrenia | 0 | 0 | 0 | 1 |
| F20.2 Catatonic schizophrenia | 0 | 0 | 0 | 1 |
| F20.3 Undifferentiated schizophrenia | 1 | 0 | 1 | 8 |
| F20.5 Residual schizophrenia | 0 | 0 | 1 | 0 |
| F20.8 Other schizophrenia | 0 | 0 | 0 | 1 |
| F20.9 Schizophrenia, unspecified | 0 | 0 | 5 | 5 |
| F21 Schizotypal disorder | 1 | 2 | 1 | 0 |
| F22.0 Delusional disorder | 0 | 0 | 1 | 0 |
| F23.0 Acute polymorphic psychotic disorder without symptoms of schizophrenia | 0 | 0 | 0 | 1 |
| F23.9 Acute and transient psychotic disorder, unspecified | 5 | 7 | 2 | 2 |
| F25.0 Schizoaffective disorder, manic type | 0 | 0 | 0 | 2 |
| F25.1 Schizoaffective disorder, depressive type | 0 | 0 | 2 | 1 |
| F25.2 Schizoaffective disorder, mixed type | 0 | 0 | 2 | 1 |
| F25.9 Schizoaffective disorder, unspecified | 0 | 0 | 0 | 1 |
| F29 Unspecified non-organic psychosis | 0 | 0 | 1 | 2 |
| *Psychotic mood disorders* | *1* | *4* | *6* | *6* |
| F30.8 Other manic episodes | 0 | 4 | 0 | 1 |
| F31.0 Bipolar affective disorder, current episode hypomanic | 0 | 0 | 0 | 1 |
| F31.2 Bipolar affective disorder, current episode manic with psychotic symptoms | 0 | 0 | 1 | 1 |
| F31.3 Bipolar affective disorder, current episode mild or moderate depression | 0 | 0 | 0 | 1 |
| F31.5 Bipolar affective disorder, current episode severe depression with psychotic symptoms | 1 | 0 | 0 | 0 |
| F31.6 Bipolar affective disorder, current episode mixed | 0 | 0 | 1 | 0 |
| F31.7 Bipolar affective disorder, currently in remission | 0 | 0 | 1 | 2 |
| F39 Unspecified mood [affective] disorder | 0 | 0 | 3 | 0 |

Notes: No one received a diagnosis of either "F32.3 Severe depressive episode with psychotic symptoms" or "F33.3 Recurrent depressive disorder, current episode severe with psychotic symptoms".

Fourteen patients were diagnosed as psychotic by both CAP and GenP units, providing a total of 76 diagnoses for 62 patients.

## Incidence and Causes of Death by the End of the Follow-Up Period

Three of the 48 patients (6.3 %) who were diagnosed with schizophrenia (one with "F21: Schizotypal disorder" and two with "F23: Acute and transient psychotic disorders") had died by the end of the follow-up period, two by suicide and one from a ruptured cerebral aneurysm. This incidence was similar to that among the patients without a diagnosis of schizophrenia.

## Comparison of the Patients Who Were and Were Not Given an ICD-10 Diagnosis of Schizophrenia and/or Psychotic Mood [Affective] Disorder in Connection with CAP Care

Individuals diagnosed as psychotic in connection with CAP care were older upon initial admission to this care than those without such a diagnosis ($p<0.001$ according to the Pearson Chi-Square two-sided test). Furthermore, those with such a diagnosis were more often in need of inpatient CAP care (46.8% versus 19.2%; $p<0.001$, Pearson Chi-Square two-sided test); were more often admitted to CAP care primarily for symptoms of anxiety (23.0% versus 12.6%; $p = 0.019$, Pearson Chi-Square two-sided test); and more often exhibited confusion/disorientation in connection with their initial examination (21.6% versus 0.7%; $p<0.001$, Pearson Chi-Square two-sided test). Moreover, all of the patients with a CAP diagnosis of psychosis required continued care in GenP, compared to one-third of those without such a diagnosis.

## Age Upon Initial Diagnosis of Psychosis, Including a Comparison between Patients with Schizophrenia and Psychotic Mood Disorder

The mean age at the time of initial diagnosis of psychosis in the patient group was 21.4 years (range 13–41, SD 6.4) and the corresponding median value was 18.0 years. A majority of these (27 = 44%) were diagnosed between the age of 13 and 17, 17 (27%) between 18 and 25 years of age, 10 (16%) between the ages of 26 and 30 and the remaining 8 (13%) were older at this point in time.

A third of those diagnosed as psychotic (21 patients) received this diagnosis in connection with CAP (Table 7) and these patients usually demonstrated more pronounced symptoms. More girls (69.7%) than boys (44.8%) exhibited early onset but this difference was barely statistically significant ($p=0.048$, Pearson Chi-Square two-sided).

Finally, the 48 individuals diagnosed with schizophrenia were significantly younger (mean age 20.3 years; SD 5.2) at the time of the initial diagnosis of psychosis than were the 12 patients with psychotic mood disorders (mean age 26.8 years; SD 8.3) (p-value: 0.0183, Pearson Chi-Square two-sided test).

**Table 7. ICD-10 classification of patients in connection with the initial definitive diagnosis of psychosis**

| Diagnosis according to ICD-10, Chapter V<br><br>Sub-category | Group I<br>CAP diagnosis of psychosis<br><br>total (n = 21) | | Group II<br>GenP diagnosis of psychosis, with certain signs of this condition noted in the CAP record<br>total (n = 15) | | Group III<br>GenP diagnosis of psychosis with no signs of this condition at all noted in the CAP record<br>total (n = 26) | |
|---|---|---|---|---|---|---|
| | n | Percentage of total | n | Percentage of total | n | Percentage of total |
| Schizophrenia, schizotypal and delusional disorders | 16 | 76.2 | 13 | 86.7 | 19 | 73.1 |
| F20 Schizophrenia | 1 | 4.8 | 7 | 46.7 | 5 | 19.2 |
| F21 Schizotypal disorder | 3 | 14.3 | 2 | 13.3 | 1 | 3.8 |
| F23 Acute and transient psychotic disorders | 12 | 57.1 | 2 | 13.3 | 7 | 26.9 |
| F25 Schizoaffective disorders | 0 | - | 2 | 13.3 | 4 | 15.4 |
| F29 Unspecified non-organic psychosis | 0 | - | - | | 2 | 7.7 |
| Mood [affective] disorders | 5 | 23.8 | 2 | 13.3 | 7 | 26.9 |
| F30 Manic episode | 4 | 19.0 | 0 | - | 0 | |
| F31 Bipolar affective disorder | 1 | 4.8 | 0 | - | 6 | 23.1 |
| F 39 Unspecified mood [affective] disorder | 0 | - | 2 | 13.3 | 1 | 3.8 |

## THE CONTINUITY IN DIAGNOSES BETWEEN CAP AND GENP CARE

Of the 531 former CAP patients later admitted to GenP care in adulthood, (38% of the total study population), 20% received a diagnosis within the same ICD-10 category in connection with both types of care, with diagnosis of psychosis at a younger age exhibiting the largest degree of continuity. Thus, of the 27 individuals given such a diagnosis prior to the age of 18, only two were diagnosed differently as adults.

One of these received an unspecified diagnosis of anxiety disorder as an adult; while the other, who had been treated for an acute episodic psychosis as an adolescent, was later diagnosed as experiencing some variety of autism. Of the 21 patients given a diagnosis of psychosis in connection with CAP care, 19 had a psychosis diagnosis in both settings. 12 were placed in the same sub-category of “F20-29: Schizophrenia, schizotypal and delusional disorders” and one in the same sub-category of “F30-39: Psychotic mood disorders” at both time-points.

Three patients with a CAP diagnosis in the sub-category of “F20-29: Schizophrenia, schizotypal and delusional disorders” were later categorized as “F30-39: Psychotic mood disorders” in adulthood. In contrast, three individuals treated during adolescence for “F30-39: Psychotic mood disorders” were later categorized in the sub-category of “F20-29: Schizophrenia, schizotypal and delusional disorders”.

**Table 8. CAP diagnoses for patients who received a diagnosis of psychosis in connection with GenP care, n = 41**

| Diagnosis according to ICD 10<br>All | Number | Percentage |
|---|---|---|
| F90-F98 Behavioral and emotional disorders with onset usually occurring in childhood and adolescence | 15 | 36.6 |
| F40-F48 Neurotic, stress-related and somatoform disorders | 8 | 19.5 |
| Z00-Z99 Factors influencing health status and contact with health services | 6 | 14.6 |
| F30-39 Mood [affective] disorders (non-psychotic) | 3 | 7.3 |
| F70-F79 Mental retardation | 3 | 7.3 |
| X60-X84 Intentional self-harm | 3 | 7.3 |
| F10-F19 Mental and behavioral disorders due to psychoactive substance use | 1 | 2.4 |
| F50-F59 Behavioral syndromes associated with physiological disturbances and physical factors | 1 | 2.4 |
| F80-F89 Disorders of psychological development | 1 | 2.4 |

## Differences in Diagnoses of Psychosis between CAP and GenP Care

The CAP diagnoses for those 41 patients who were later placed in the categories "F20-29: Schizophrenia, schizotypal and delusional disorders" and/or "F30-39: Psychotic mood disorders" in connection with GenP care are documented in Table 8. Most of these individuals (71%) were treated for problems related to the categories "F90-F98: Behavioral and emotional disorders with onset usually occurring in childhood and adolescence", "F40-F48: Neurotic, stress-related and somatoform disorders" or "Z00-Z99: Factors influencing health status and contact with health services". In addition, three were treated for mental retardation and another three for self-harming behavior. These patients received their GenP diagnoses at a mean age of 24.0 years (SD 6.35), 19 within 5 years of completion of CAP care, 6 within 6-10 years, 9 within 11-15 years and 7 patients longer than 15 years following discharge from CAP care.

## Information on Early Signs of Psychosis

Of the three different groups of patients that could be discerned, the first and most distinct (Group I) included the 21 (34%) who exhibited signs and symptoms of psychosis in connection with CAP care and, consequently, received their first definitive diagnosis of psychosis as children. Among this group, 14 demonstrated obvious symptoms of a disorder at their initial contact with CAP care-givers, whereas the diagnosis for the 7 others was established only after an observation period of 1-4 years. Accordingly, the mean period of time that elapsed from first admission to CAP care until definitive diagnosis of a psychosis was 2.0 years, (SD 3.6).

**Table 9. Time period elapsed between completion of CAP care and the first definitive diagnosis of psychosis for patients who received such a diagnosis only in connection with GenP care**

| Signs, symptoms, problems, illness | Time elapsed between completion of CAP care and the initial diagnosis of psychosis | | | | | | |
|---|---|---|---|---|---|---|---|
| | 2 years or less (n= 13) | 3-4 years (n= 6) | 5-6 years (n= 1) | 7-10 years (n= 5) | 11-15 years (n= 9) | 16-23 years (n=7) | Total n= 41 |
| *Signs of psychosis noted, all* | *8* | *2* | *0* | *4* | *1* | *0* | *15* |
| Positive symptoms | 7 | 1 | 0 | 3 | 1 | 0 | 12 |
| Cognitive change in attention/concentration | 4 | 0 | 0 | 2 | 0 | 0 | 6 |
| Emotional disturbance | 2 | 0 | 0 | 0 | 0 | 0 | 2 |
| Negative symptoms | 2 | 0 | 0 | 0 | 0 | 0 | 2 |
| Behavioral change | 5 | 2 | 0 | 4 | 1 | 0 | 12 |
| Motor/psychical changes | 5 | 0 | 0 | 1 | 0 | 0 | 6 |
| *General psychopathology* | *10* | *3* | *0* | *2* | *6* | *5* | *26* |

A second group (Group II) of 15 patients (24%) also showed possible signs of psychosis during their CAP care, but were first diagnosed with such a disorder in connection with GenP care, mostly at a relatively young age.

Their diagnoses were established at a mean of 6.0 years, (SD 5.8) following first admission to CAP care (Table 9, p= 0.0254 compared to Group I; Pearson Chi-Square two-sided test). The CAP records for the third group (Group. III) of 26 patients (42%) contained no notation of signs of psychosis and their definitive diagnosis of this disorder was made following completion of the CAP care.

For these patients, the period from first admission to CAP to first diagnosed onset of psychosis was even longer, mean 12.4 years, SD 7.9 (Table 4; p<0.001 compared to Group I and p=0.0055 compared to Group II, Pearson Chi-square two-sided test). During CAP care, most of this group exhibited unspecific psychopathology, such as behavioral and emotional problems or problems with relationships. Patients placed in the ICD-10 category "F20-29: Schizophrenia, schizotypal and delusional disorders" demonstrated more symptoms of psychosis at an earlier age than did those classified as "F30-39: Psychotic mood disorders" (p-value: 0.0187 Pearson Chi-square two-sided test).

## Causes for Admission of the Patients in Groups I and II to CAP Care

The causes for admission of the 36 patients in Groups I and II, who showed signs of psychosis during their CAP care were as follows: confusion or changes in personality [12]; free-floating anxiety [7]; problems with relationships [4]; behavioral disorder [3]; somatic problems and eating disorders [3]; depression [3]; suicidal [1]; mental retardation and developmental problems [1]; pathological reaction to stress [1]; and request from a physician for an assessment [1]. The symptoms most obviously related to a diagnosis of schizophrenia of some form were confusion or changes in personality ($p<0.001$) and free-floating anxiety ($p=0.020$).

## Changes in Behavior

Changes in behavior e.g., (social isolation, refusal to go to school, loneliness and/or general odd behavior) were the most frequent first signs/symptoms described in the CAP records of the individuals in Groups I and II who eventually received a F20-29 diagnosis, in connection either with CAP (Group I) or GenP care (Group II). Thirty of these 36 patients (83%) showed such behavioral changes and there was no statistically significant difference between the two groups.

## Positive Symptoms

Signs and symptoms related to schizophrenia were present in 75% of these patients and consisted of: unusual thoughts; bizarre ideas, perceptual abnormalities (such as fear of being poisoned, confusion and suspiciousness) and disorganized speech. Again, there was no significant difference in this respect between Groups I and II.

## Motor/Psychical Changes

Both groups contained individuals diagnosed as "F20-29: Schizophrenia, schizotypal and delusional disorders" and "F30-39: Psychotic mood disorders, motor/psychical changes".

Signs and symptoms such as motor restlessness, rituals and poor sleep were present in 44% of these patients and equally common among both groups.

### Cognitive Change in Attention/Concentration

Concentration difficulties and attention deficits, problems with selective attention and forming thoughts, difficulties in comprehension and memory problems were observed in 25% of these cases, somewhat (although not significantly) more often among those classified as schizophrenic. Once again, no difference was found between the groups.

### Emotional Disturbance

31% of the patients in groups I and G II demonstrated impaired emotional functioning or alterations in affect. These features were more frequent among those with psychotic mood disorder and/or belonging to group I, but in neither case were these differences statistically significant.

## Negative Symptoms

Tiredness, listlessness and other negative symptoms were present in 19% of the cases in both Groups I and II, only among those classified as schizophrenic.

## General Psychopathology

The CAP hospital records 67% of those diagnosed with psychotic mood disorders and 60% of those with schizophrenia noted general psychopathology. In 19 of the 36 CAP files for the two groups with early signs (I and II), the symptoms most frequently noted were depression (11 cases), anxiety [8], suicidal intent and self-harm [6] and mania (5). One individual exhibited symptoms of obsessive compulsive disorder and another, mood swings.

## Additional Information, Signs, Symptoms and Problems

A variety of additional information concerning the patients in Groups I and II was present in their records, e.g., descriptions of interpersonal difficulties (14 cases), difficulties in relationships with peers [9], stressful life events [12], physical illness [12], a family history of psychosis [7] or of other psychiatric disorder or alcohol abuse in a close relative [9]; impaired intelligence [4], low socioeconomic status [3], parents who emigrated to Sweden from another country [3], birth following a complicated pregnancy and/or delivery [3] and a history of neglect/child abuse [2].

**Table 10. Comparison of a subgroup of outpatients who were followed-up for a full 20-year period with an earlier longitudinal study in Stockholm [14]**

| | The earlier Stockholm study (n=2.164) | | The subgroup of the present patients (n=608) | | |
|---|---|---|---|---|---|
| | Number | Percentage | Number | Percentage | p-value* |
| Males | 1,417 | 65.5 | 325 | 53.5 | $p < 0.001$ |
| Females | 747 | 34.5 | 283 | 46.5 | $p < 0.001$ |
| Age at the end of the follow up period | | | | | |
| 20-31.5 years | 1415 | 65.4 | 236 | 38.8 | $p < 0.001$ |
| Older than 31.5 years | 749 | 34.6 | 372 | 61.2 | $p < 0.001$ |
| Schizophrenia and or bipolar disorder | 30 | 1.39 | 17 | 2.80 | n.s. |
| Schizophrenia | 21 | 0.97 | 11 | 1.81 | n.s. |
| Bipolar disorder | 9 | 0.42 | 6 | 0.99 | n.s. |

Note: * Fisher Exact Analysis: Two-sided p-values for p(O>=E|O<=E) (the sum of small p's), n.s. = not significant

## Comparison to an Earlier Longitudinal Study in Sweden

An earlier 20-year prospective follow-up study of 2,164 outpatients (1,417 males and 747 females) discharged from the Stockholm Municipal Child Guidance Clinics in 1953, 1954, and 1955 [36] was compared to a sub-group of the study group who had been followed-up for a full 20-year period (325 males and 283 females) with respect to the variables described in Table 10.

The two groups differed with respect to gender and age distribution, since a larger proportion of pre-school and school boys were included in the Stockholm study.

Although the present Jämtland group was older on the averages, there were no differences in the frequency of diagnoses in the categories of schizophrenia and psychotic mood disorders. In both groups, the number of patients receiving a diagnosis of psychosis was small. Only 9 individuals in the Stockholm and 6 individuals in the Jämtland groups, respectively, were recognized as suffering from a bipolar disorder during a 20-year period of CAP and/or GenP care. Most of the subjects with a diagnosis of psychosis were inpatients.

## Reflections on the Findings

As described in the Introduction, the present longitudinal prospective study of CAP patients given a diagnosis of schizophrenia and/or of psychotic mood (affective) disorder either in connection with CAP or later GenP care and followed-up for 12 -28 years after completion of CAP care, was designed to answer a number of specific questions.

The findings can be summarized as follows: 62 of the 1,400 CAP patients (36 females and 26 males) had received an ICD-10 diagnosis of schizophrenia (48 patients = 3.4% of the total population) and/or psychotic mood disorders (14=1%) by the end of the follow-up period. The overall estimated incidence of first-episode psychosis per 10,000 person-years was 17.1. For patients 15-29 years of age, this incidence was lower for males (11.6 versus 16.7) but higher for females (14.2 versus 8.1) than in a study conducted in Australia by Amminger and colleagues [87].

No such gender difference was observed among the 1,338 patients who had not received a diagnosis of psychosis. Three of the 62 patients (4.8%) diagnosed with schizophrenia or mood disorders had died by the end of the follow-up period, two by suicide and one from somatic illness. The corresponding death rate among those without such a diagnosis was similar (2.6%).

The answers to the questions we posed were as follows:

*At what age was the diagnosis of psychosis made?*

The mean age of these patients was 21.4 years (range 13–41 years), with 27 (44%) between 13 and 17, 17 (27%) 18-25 and 18 (29%) older than 25 years of age. No other clinical services for psychotic patients in this age range are provided in the geographical area. Females demonstrated an early onset more often than the males. It is known that a different approach may be required for the early detection and treatment of patients with early-onset psychosis who are more likely to present clinical characteristics associated with a poorer outcome [88-89].

*Was this diagnosis later changed and, if so, in what manner*

Only two of the individuals diagnosed as psychotic before the age of 18 years in connection with CAP care did not receive a diagnosis in the category of schizophrenia or psychotic mood disorders as adults. One of them was later diagnosed with an unspecified of anxiety disorder and the other, who was treated for an acute episodic psychosis during adolescence, received a diagnosis in the area of autism. In 13 cases of the CAP, diagnoses were later altered in connection with GenP to other diagnoses within the same categories: 12 were placed in the same sub-category of "F20-29: Schizophrenia, schizotypal and delusional disorders" and one in the same sub-category of "F30-39: Psychotic mood disorders" at both time-points. Three patients with a CAP diagnosis in the sub-category of "F20-29: Schizophrenia, schizotypal and delusional disorders" were later categorized as "F30-39: Psychotic mood disorders" in adulthood. In contrast, three individuals treated during adolescence for "F30-39: Psychotic mood disorders" were later categorized in the sub-category of "F20-29: Schizophrenia, schizotypal and delusional disorders".

In their 42-year follow-up of 38 patients with childhood-onset schizophrenia and 38 patients with other diagnoses, Remschmidt and co/workers (90) also describe re-diagnosing former CAP patients as adults. Although their findings do indicate diagnostic stability over time in the case of 91% of their patients, 4 of the individuals (11%) with CAP diagnosis of childhood-onset schizophrenia were given another diagnosis as adults.

Schwartz and colleagues (91) propose that such changes in diagnosis, particularly to schizophrenia, rested primarily on the evolution of the illness [91]. Both of these investigators and Schimmelmann and co/workers [92] have established the need for a longitudinally-based diagnostic process for determining incidences, especially with respect to schizophreniform and bipolar disorders.

*Which early signs of disorder were noted prior or upon admission to CAP care?*

Changes in behavior, including social isolation, refusal to go to school, loneliness and odd behavior in general were the initial signs/symptoms most frequently observed prior or upon admission to CAP-care. However, this was only the case with regards to the category of schizophrenia. Among the individuals diagnosed with schizophrenia or psychotic mood disorders, symptoms such as motor restlessness, obsessive rituals and poor sleep were equally common, being observed in 44% of the cases. Patients in both of these groups frequently demonstrated anxiety and depression at the time of admission.

*Which patients received their diagnosis later in connection with GenP care and how did this group differ from those diagnosed earlier during CAP care?*

The patients given diagnoses of psychoses at an age of 25 years or older exhibited unspecific psychopathological symptoms, but no signs of a possible psychotic disorder during their CAP care. However, the shorter the period that elapsed from the completion of CAP care until admission to GenP care, the more frequently symptoms of a possible psychotic disorder were observed at the CAP unit, although these were not specific enough for a diagnosis to be established.

None of these patients were diagnosed with childhood-onset schizophrenia , which by definition, debuts before the age 13 [93]. As described by Rapoport and Remschmidt and their colleagues [23, 94-97], this rare disorder is most probably due to progressive brain degeneration and, it therefore is not surprising that none of the 1,400 CAP patients were afflicted. The scientific literature contains few reports of investigations outside of Scandinavia similar to the present one. In the Nordic countries, findings similar to my own have been reported by Dahl [98] who conducted a 20-year follow-up study of "a child psychiatric clientele with special regard to the diagnosis of psychosis"; by Pedersen and Aarkrog [99-100] who performed a 10- and 20-year follow-up study of child psychiatric patients, and by Strömgren [101] in 1940, when he discussed "Episodic Psychosis in Adolescence". Furthermore, Tyano and co-workers [102] made similar observations concerning "Transient adolescent psychosis" upon monitoring the stability of diagnosis in a cohort of Israeli CAP patients. As discussed above, the current results can be compared to those from a similar 20-year follow-up of CAP patients from the 1950's to the 1970's.

## Methodological Considerations

One disadvantage is that the population of Jämtland County cannot be considered to be representative of the entire Swedish population in all respects. Although comparison with an earlier longitudinal study of outpatients in Stockholm (see above) as well as an unpublished comparison with CAP inpatients in the Stockholm metropolitan area reveals few significant differences, it should be kept in mind that the study group here came from a sparsely populated region. Furthermore, my primary information was obtained from psychiatric hospital records, which are, in many respects, not scientifically rigorous instruments of examination. Although the quality of these records was considered to be satisfactory, they were assessed employing a protocol chosen for the present study and, moreover, also contain information provided by parents, school personnel and other authorities. No concurrent validation of the CAARMS extracted from these files employing personal interviews was carried out. The CAARMS instrument, which is basically a manual for personal interview is not intended for interpretation of hospital records. This lack of validation limits the ability to draw conclusions from the signs noted. In addition, the patients studied here are still relatively young. At the end of the follow-up period, the youngest was 27 years old and had been observed for 12 years, while the oldest was 45 and had been under observation for 28 years. It thus appears likely that additional information of value will emerge from future GenP care concerning the categories "F20-29: Schizophrenia, schizotypal and delusional disorders" and/or "F30-39: Psychotic mood disorders".

## Conclusion

*In summary*, it appears that based on empirical findings during the past 70 years, psychotic disorders have been and continue to be relatively uncommon among patients admitted to CAP care in Sweden. The typical male Swedish CAP patient is "a 10-year-old troublesome boy", while the typical female patient is "a 14-year-old depressed girl".

Both come from families with psychosocial difficulties; have problems at school and risk later delinquency and/or alcohol and/or drug abuse. However, the rate of schizophrenia observed in the group of CAP patients (3,4%) is threefold higher than in the general population, indicating that these individuals run an increased risk for developing severe chronic psychosis and that use of a specific treatment model for early psychosis among children and adolescents might be valuable [87].

The present empirical findings indicate that psychotic disorders debut during the teenage years and, moreover, that disorders in the ICD category "F20-F29: Schizophrenia, schizotypal and delusional disorders" are more common than those classified as "F30-39: Psychotic mood disorders". Clearly, psychotic mood disorders are rare among children and adolescents.

Individuals experiencing early onset of disorders categorized as "F20-F29: Schizophrenia, schizotypal and delusional disorders" may already show typical symptoms upon admission to CAP care at an age of 13-17. In contrast, late-onset disorders appear to be very difficult to anticipate on the basis of information gathered in connection with CAP care. In certain latter cases, the circumstances necessitating CAP care differed from those leading to later admission to GenP care, when symptoms of a psychotic disorder were apparent.

Finally, a handful of the cases appear to have experienced an episodic psychotic disorder during adolescence, as also described previously by Strömgren [101] and more recently by Tyano [102]. For certain subjects, in these other two studies, the symptoms described may reflect the first episode of a psychiatric disorder, usually in the category of F20-29, which returns with full force later in life, whereas in other cases, the psychosis appears to be episodic.

## ACKNOWLEDGMENTS

Professor Per-Anders Rydelius at Karolinska Institutet in his role as supervisor has been very helpful in shaping the design, data collection and compilation of data.

The CAP and GenP units at Östersund Hospital and the Centre for Epidemiology at the National Board of Health and Welfare were all very helpful in supplying me with data. I also want to thank Professor Joseph W DePierre at Stockholm University and Laurie Horowitz at Karolinska Institutet for their skilled help editing the language of the manuscript.

## REFERENCES

[1] Ottosson, J.O.: *Psykiatrin i Sverige*. Stockholm: Natur och Kultur; 2003.

[2] Levander, S., Adler, H., Gefvert, O., Tuninger, E.: *Psykiatri. En orienterande översikt*. Lund: Studentlitteratur; 2006.

[3] Psykiatri [http://www.ne.se/artikel/288196].

[4] Gunnarsson, T.: Psykiatrisk tvångsvård i Sverige–Från medeltida helgeandshus till LPT. *Tidskriften för Svensk Psykiatri Tidskrift för Svenska Psykiatriska Föreningen och Svenska Barn- och Ungdomspsykiatriska Föreningen* 2006 maj 2006.

[5] Qvarsell, R.: *Ordning och behandling: psykiatri och sinnessjukvård i Sverige under 1800-talets första hälft*, Umeå: Umeå University; 1982.

[6] Sjöström, B.: *Kliniken tar över dårskapen: om den moderna svenska psykiatrins framväxt*. Lund: Lund; 1992.

[7] Beckman, V.: *Sinnessjukhuset: bilder ur psykiatrins historia*. Stockholm: Norstedt; 1984.

[8] SOU 1992:73: *Psykiatriutredningen. Välfärd och valfrihet - service, stöd och vård för psykiskt störda*. In: Statens offentliga utredningar; 1992.

[9] SOU 2006:100: *Ambition och ansvar. Nationell strategi för utveckling av samhällets insatser till personer med psykiska sjukdomar och funktionshinder*. In: Statens offentliga utredningar. Stockholm; 2006.

[10] Socialstyrelsen: *Utredning av händelserna i Åkeshov och Gamla stan och dess möjliga samband med brister i bemötande och behandling inom den psykiatriska vården och socialtjänstens verksamhet* (S2003/5291/HS). In. Socialstyrelsen. Stockholm; 2003.

[11] Harding, G.: *Tidig svensk psykiatri*. Lund: Berlingska Boktryckcriet; 1975.

[12] Karlén, K.H.: *Barn- och ungdomspsykiatrin i Sverige: dess historia, problem och patienter*. Uppsala: Uppsala University; 1985.

[13] Schleimer, K.: *Child and adoelscent psychiatry in Sweden*. In: Child and Adolescent Psychiatry in Europe, Historical Development, Current Situation and Future Perspectives. edn. Edited by H R, van Engeland H. Darmstadt/New York: Steinkopff/Springer; 1999: 351-361.

[14] Schubert, J.: Chockökning av sökande till psykvård. In: *Dagens Nyheter*. Stockholm; 1999: A4-5.

[15] SOU 1998:31: *Det gäller livet. Stöd och vård till barn och ungdomar med psykiska problem*. Slutbetänkande av Barnpsykiatrikommittén. Statens offentliga utredningar; 1998.

[16] Wieselgren, I.M.: *Tillgänglighet till insatser för att möta psykisk ohälsa hos barn och ungdomar*. In. Edited by Sveriges kommuner och landsting. Stockholm: Avdelningen för vård och omsorg. Sektionen för vård och socialtjänst; 2007.

[17] Nyberg, L.: Lång väntan för unga i kris. In: *Göteborgsposten*. Göteborg; 2001.

[18] Arbetsgruppen kring översyn av den barn- och ungdomspsykiatriska verksamheten i Jämtlands län: *Översyn av den barn- och ungdomspsykiatriska verksamheten i Jämtlands län*, In. Östersund: Jämtlands läns landsting; 1984.

[19] Engqvist, U.: *Så tänkte man - hur blev det? Beskrivning av barn- och ungdomspsykiatrin i Jämtlands län 1992, åtta år efter översyn av verksamheten*. In. Östersund: Barn och ungdomspsykiatriska verksamheten i Jämtlands län; 1993.

[20] Rutter, M.: Relationships between child and adult psychiatric disorders. Some research considerations. *Acta Psychiatr. Scand.* 1972, 48(1):3-21.

[21] Rutter, M.: Relationships between mental disorders in childhood and adulthood. *Acta Psychiatr. Scand.* 1995, 91:73-85.

[22] Rutter, M., Kim-Cohen, J., Maughan, B.: Continuities and discontinuities in psychopathology between childhood and adult life. *J. Child Psychol. Psychiatry.* 2006, 47(3-4):276-295.

[23] Remschmidt, H., Theisen, F.M.: Schizophrenia and related disorders in children and adolescents. *J. Neural. Transm.* 2005, Suppl.(69):121-141.

[24] Rutter, M., Garmezy, N.: *Developmenatl psychopatology*. In: Handbook of child psychology: Socialization, personality and social development. Volume 4, edn. Edited by Hetherington EM. New York: Wiley; 1983: 775-911.

[25] Miller, P.M., Byrne, M., Hodges, A., Lawrie, S.M., Johnstone, E.C.: Childhood behaviour, psychotic symptoms and psychosis onset in young people at high risk of schizophrenia: early findings from the Edinburgh High Risk Study. *Psychol. Med.* 2002, 32:173-179.

[26] Amminger, G., Pape, S., Rock, D., Roberts, S., Ott, S., Squires-Wheeler, E., Kestenbaum, C., Erlenmeyer-Kimling, L.: Relationship between childhood behavioral disturbance and later schizophrenia in the New York High-Risk Project. *Am. J. Psychiatry* 1999, Apr;156(4):525-530.

[27] Hodgins, S., Tiihonen, J.R.D.: The consequences of Conduct Disorder for males who develop schizophrenia: associations with criminality, aggressive behavior, substance use, and psychiatric services. *Schizophr. Res.* 2005, Oct 15;78(2-3):323-335.

[28] Goodwin, R., Fergusson, D., Horwood, L.: Neuroticism in adolescence and psychotic symptoms in adulthood. *Psychol. Med.* 2003, Aug;33(6):1089-1097.

[29] Cannon, M., Walsh, E., Hollis, C., Kargin, M., Taylor, E., Murray, R.M., Jones, P.B.: Predictors of later schizophrenia and affective psychosis among attendees at a child psychiatry department. *Br. J. Psychiatry Suppl.* 2001, May; 178:420-426.

[30] Curman, H., Nylander, I.: A 10-year prospective follow-up study of 2268 cases at the child guidance clinics in Stockholm. *Acta Paediatr. Scand. Suppl.* 1976, Suppl 260:1-71.

[31] Engqvist, U.: *Om samarbetet mellan barn- och ungdomspsykiatri och vuxenpsykiatri - Personalens kompetens och patienternas behov.* Stockholm: Karolinska Institutet; 2002.

[32] Engqvist, U., Rydelius, P.A.: Barn och ungdomar inom BUP - hur går det för dem? . *Psykisk Hälsa* 2005, 4:39-44.

[33] Nycander, G.: *Personlighetsutveckling på avvägar. Barnpsykiatriska studier.* Stockholm: Tidens Förlag; 1950.

[34] Engqvist, U., Rydelius, P.A.: Death and suicide among former child and adolescent psychiatric patients. *BMC Psychiatry* 2006, 6:51.

[35] Engqvist, U., Rydelius, P.A.: Child and adolescent psychiatric patients and later criminality. *BMC Public Health* 2007, 7:221.

[36] Nylander, I.: A 20-year prospective follow-up study of 2 164 cases at the child guidance clinics in Stockholm. *Acta Paediatr. Scand. Suppl.* 1979, 276:1-45.

[37] Fried, I.: Mellansjo school-home. Psychopathic children admitted 1928-1940, their social adaptation over 30 years: a longitudinal prospective follow-up. *Acta Pediatr. Suppl.*1995, 408:1-42.

[38] Andersson, M., Jonsson, G., Kälvesten, A.L.: *Hur går det för 50-talets Stockholmspojkar? En uppföljning av 222 vanliga skolpojkar och 100 Skåpojkar.* In. Stockholm: Monografier utgivna av Stockholms Kommunförvaltning, no 38 (summary in English); 1976.

[39] SOU 1973:25: *Unga lagöverträdare. 3, Hem, uppfostran, skola och kamratmiljö i belysning av intervju- och uppföljningsdata* : rapport / av Birgitta Olofsson. In: Statens offentliga utredningar. Stockholm: 1956 års klientelundersökning rörande ungdomsbrottslingar; 1973.

[40] Rydelius, P.A.: *Long-term prognosis for the young alcohol abuser.* In: Alcohol and the Developing Brain. edn. Edited by Rydberg U, Alling C, *Engel. J. New York Raven Press Books cop.*; 1985: 187-191.

[41] Bohman, M.: Some genetic aspects of alcoholism and criminality. A population of adoptees. *Arch. Gen. Psychiatry.* 1978, 35(3):269-276.
[42] Rydelius, P.A.: Children of alcoholic fathers. Their social adjustment and their health status over 20 years. *Acta Paediatr. Scand.* 1981, 286(Suppl):1-89.
[43] Otto, U.: Suicidal acts by children and adolescents: A follow up study. *Acta Psychiatr. Scand.* 1972, Suppl 233:1-123.
[44] Öjesjö, L.: *An epidemiological investigation of alcoholism in a total population.* In: The Lundby Study. Lund: University of Lund; 1983.
[45] Jansson, C.G.: *Project Metropolitan, a presentation.* Research report No 1. In: Project Metropolitan. Stockholm: Department of Sociology, University of Stockholm; 1975.
[46] Wikström, P.O.H.: *Patterns of crime in a birth-cohort. Age, sex and class differences.* In: Project Metropolitan Research report No 24. Stockholm: Department of Sociology, University of Stockholm; 1987.
[47] Bohman, M., Wennberg, P., Andersson, T.: Alcohol habits in a suburban male cohort. *Scand. J. Public Health* 2000, 28(4):275-282.
[48] Stattin, H., Klackenberg-Larsson, I.: *Delinquency as related to parents' preferences for their child´s gender.* Reports from the Department of Psychology, University of Stockholm No 686. In: Reports from the Department of Psychology. Stockholm; 1989.
[49] Magnusson, D., Dunér, A., Zetterblom, G.: *Adjustment : a longitudinal study* New York Wiley; 1975.
[50] Stattin, H., Magnusson, D., Reichel, H.: Criminal activity of different ages. A study based on a Swedish longitudinal research population. *British Journal of Criminology* 1989, 29(4):368-385.
[51] MFR (Swedish medical research council*): Swedish psychiatric research 2000.* vol. 7. Stockholm Medicinska forskningsrådet; 2000.
[52] The Lundby Study – 50 years of psychiatric epidemiology [http://www.research.med.lu.se/en_projektdetaljer.php?Proj=398].
[53] Stenberg, S.A., Vagero, D.: Cohort profile: the Stockholm birth cohort of 1953. *International journal of epidemiology* 2006, 35(3):546-548.
[54] Jansson, C.G.: Commentary: The revitalization of the Stockholm Metropolitan Study *International journal of epidemiology* 2006, 35(3):553.
[55] IDA: Individual Development and Adaptation [http://www.oru.se/ templates/oruExtNormal____30650.aspx].
[56] The Solna study [http://www.oru.se/templates/oruExtNormal____30643. aspx].
[57] Thomsen, P.H.: A 22- to 25-year follow-up study of former child psychiatric patients: a register-based investigation of the course of psychiatric disorder and mortality in 546 Danish child psychiatric patients. *Acta Psychiatr. Scand.* 1996, 1996: 94:397-403.
[58] Thomsen, P.H.: The prognosis in early adulthood of child psychiatric patients: a case register study in Denmark. *Acta Psychiatr. Scand.* 1990, 81(1):89-93.
[59] Larsen, F.W.: A 30-year follow-up study of a child psychiatric clientele. II. Psychiatric morbidity. *Acta Psychiatr. Scand.* 1991, 84(1):65-71.
[60] Larsen, F.W., Dahl, V., Hallum, E.: A 30-year follow-up study of a child psychiatric clientele. I. Demographic description. *Acta Psychiatr. Scand.* 1990, 81(1):39-45.
[61] Skovgaard, A., Olsen, E., Houmann, T., Christiansen, E., Samberg, V.; Lichtenberg, A., Jørgensen, T.: The Copenhagen County child cohort: design of a longitudinal study of child mental health. *Scand. J. Public Health* 2005, 33(3):197-202.

[62] Kjelsberg, E.: A long-term follow-up study of adolescent psychiatric in-patients. Part IV. Predictors of a non-negative outcome. *Acta Psychiatr. Scand.* 1999, 99(4):247-251.

[63] Kjelsberg, E.: A long-term follow-up study of adolescent psychiatric in-patients. Part III. Predictors of disability. *Acta Psychiatr. Scand.* 1999, 99(4):243-246.

[64] Kjelsberg, E., Dahl, A.A.: High delinquency, disability and mortality--a register study of former adolescent psychiatric in-patients. *Acta Psychiatr. Scand.* 1998, 98(1):34-40.

[65] Kjelsberg, E., Dahl, A.A.: A long-term follow-up study of adolescent psychiatric in-patients. Part II. Predictors of delinquency. *Acta Psychiatr. Scand.* 1999, 99(4):237-242.

[66] Kjelsberg, E., Sandvik, L., Dahl, A.A.: A long-term follow-up study of adolescent psychiatric in-patients. Part I. Predictors of early death. *Acta Psychiatr.* Scand. 1999, 99(4):231-236.

[67] Sourander, A., Jensen, P., Davies, M., Niemelä, S., Elonheimo, H., Ristkari, T., Helenius, H., Sillanmäki, L., Piha, J., Kumpulainen, K. et al: Who is at greatest risk of adverse long-term outcomes? The Finnish From a Boy to a Man study. *J. Am. Acad. Child Adolesc. Psychiatry* 2007, Sep; 46(9):1148-1161.

[68] Pihlakoski L., Sourander A., Aromaa M., Rautava P., Helenius H., Sillanpaa M.: The continuity of psychopathology from early childhood to preadolescence: a prospective cohort study of 3-12-year-old children. *Eur. Child Adolesc. Psychiatry* 2006, 15(7):409-417.

[69] Isohanni M., Lauronen E., Moilanen K., Isohanni I., Kemppainen L., Koponen H., Miettunen J., Mäki P., Räsänen S., Veijola J., et al: Predictors of schizophrenia: evidence from the Northern Finland 1966 Birth Cohort and other sources. *Br. J. Psychiatry Suppl.* 2005, Aug; 48:4-7.

[70] Isohanni M., Miettunen J., Mäki P., Murray G.K., Ridler K., Lauronen E., Moilanen K., Alaräisänen A., Haapea M., Isohanni I., et al: Risk factors for schizophrenia. Follow-up data from the Northern Finland 1966 Birth Cohort Study. *World Psychiatry* 2006, Oct; 5(3):168-171.

[71] Isohanni M., Murray G.K., Jokelainen J., Croudace T., Jones P.B.: The persistence of developmental markers in childhood and adolescence and risk for schizophrenic psychoses in adult life. A 34-year follow-up of the Northern Finland 1966 birth cohort. *Schizophr. Res.* 2004, Dec 1; 71(2-3):213-225.

[72] Jääskeläinen E., Miettunen J., Veijola J., McGrath J., Murray G., Jones P., Isohanni M.: Associations between early development and outcome in schizophrenia--A 35-year follow-up of the Northern Finland 1966 Birth Cohort. *Schizophr Res.* 2008, Feb;99((1-3)):29-37. .

[73] World Health Organization (WHO): *The ICD-10 Classification of Mental and Behavioural disorders - Clinical descriptions and diagnostic guidelines*; 1992.

[74] World Health Organization (WHO): *The ICD-10 Classification of Mental and Behavioural disorders - Diagnostic criteria for research.*; 1993.

[75] Translator ICD-8 to ICD-9 [http://www.socialstyrelsen.se/NR/rdonlyres/ 35188CBA-9FF9-4F76-A321-BA2675BE3A4C/0/8TO9.pdf].

[76] Translator ICD-9 to ICD 10 [http://www.socialstyrelsen.se/NR/ rdonlyres/0FC3412B-6D56-4B66-9A06-F5D52DF8808F/0/ 9TO10.PDF].

[77] Yung A.R., Yuen H.P., McGorry P.D., Phillips L.J., Kelly D., Dell'Olio M., Francey S.M., Cosgrave E.M., Killackey E., Stanford C., et al: Mapping the onset of psychosis: the Comprehensive Assessment of At-Risk Mental States. *Aust. N. Z. J. Psychiatry* 2005, 39(11-12):964-971.
[78] Yung A.R., McGorry P.D.: The prodromal phase of first-episode psychosis: past and current conceptualizations. *Schizophr. Bull.* 1996, 22(2):353-370.
[79] Yung A.R., Phillips L.J., Yuen H.P., McGorry P.D.: Risk factors for psychosis in an ultra high-risk group: psychopathology and clinical features. *Schizophr. Res.* 2004, 67(2-3):131-142.
[80] Miller T.J., McGlashan T.H., Rosen J.L., Cadenhead K., Cannon T., Ventura J., McFarlane W., Perkins D.O., Pearlson G.D., Woods S.W.: Prodromal assessment with the structured interview for prodromal syndromes and the scale of prodromal symptoms: predictive validity, interrater reliability, and training to reliability. *Schizophr. Bull.* 2003, 29(4):703-715.
[81] Wood S.J., Pantelis C., Velakoulis D., Yucel M., Fornito A., McGorry P.D.: Progressive changes in the development toward schizophrenia: studies in subjects at increased symptomatic risk. *Schizophr. Bull.* 2008, 34(2):322-329.
[82] Statistiska Centralbyrån (SCB): *A brief history of Statistics Sweden.* 2006.
[83] The National Patient Register [http://www.socialstyrelsen.se/en/ Statistics/statsbysubject/The+Swedish+Hospital+Discharge+Register.htm].
[84] Dödsorsaksregistret [http://www.socialstyrelsen.se/Statistik/statistik_ amne/dodsorsaker/Dodsorsaksregistret.htm].
[85] SISA Binomial [http://www.quantitativeskills.com/sisa/distributions/ binomial.htm].
[86] Agresti A.: A survey of exact inference for contingency tables. *Statistical Science* 1992, 7(1):131-177.
[87] Amminger G.P., Harris M.G., Conus P., Lambert M., Elkins K.S., Yuen H.P., McGorry P.D.: Treated incidence of first-episode psychosis in the catchment area of EPPIC between 1997 and 2000. *Acta Psychiatr. Scand.* 2006, 114(5):337-345.
[88] Ballageer T., Malla A., Manchanda R., Takhar J., Haricharan R.: Is adolescent-onset first-episode psychosis different from adult onset? *J. Am. Acad. Child Adolesc. Psychiatry* 2005, 44(8):782-789.
[89] Schimmelmann B.G., Conus P., Cotton S., McGorry P.D., Lambert M.: Pre-treatment, baseline, and outcome differences between early-onset and adult-onset psychosis in an epidemiological cohort of 636 first-episode patients. *Schizophr. Res.* 2007, 95(1-3):1-8.
[90] Remschmidt H., Martin M., Fleischhaker C., Theisen F.M., Hennighausen K., Gutenbrunner C., Schulz E.: Forty-two-years later: the outcome of childhood-onset schizophrenia. *J. Neural. Transm.* 2007, 114(4):505-512.
[91] Schwartz J.E., Fennig S., Tanenberg-Karant M., Carlson G., Craig T., Galambos N., Lavelle J., Bromet E.J.: Congruence of diagnoses 2 years after a first-admission diagnosis of psychosis. *Arch. Gen. Psychiatry* 2000, 57(6):593-600.
[92] Schimmelmann B.G., Conus P., Edwards J., McGorry P.D., Lambert M.: Diagnostic stability 18 months after treatment initiation for first-episode psychosis. *J. Clin. Psychiatry* 2005, 66(10):1239-1246.
[93] Nicolson R., Rapoport J.L.: Childhood-onset schizophrenia: Rare but worth studying. *Biological Psychiatry* 1999, 46:, 1418-1428.

[94] Arango C., Moreno C., Martínez S., Parellada M., Desco M., Moreno D., Fraguas D., Gogtay N., James A., Rapoport J.: Longitudinal brain changes in early-onset psychosis. *Schizophr. Bull.* 2008, Mar;34(2):341-353.

[95] McKenna K., Gordon C.T., Lenane M., Kaysen D., Fahey K., Rapoport J.L.: Looking for childhood-onset schizophrenia: the first 71 cases screened. *J. Am. Acad. Child Adolesc. Psychiatry* 1994, Jun. 33(5):636-644.

[96] Remschmidt H.: Early-onset schizophrenia as a progressive-deteriorating developmental disorder: evidence from child psychiatry. *J. Neural. Transm.* 2002, 109(1):101-117.

[97] Sporn A.L., Greenstein D.K., Gogtay N.J.N., Lenane M., Gochman P., Clasen L.S., Blumenthal J., Giedd J.N., Rapoport J.L.: Progressive brain volume loss during adolescence in childhood-onset schizophrenia. *Am. J. Psychiatry* 2003, Dec;160 (12):2181-2189.

[98] Dahl V.: A follow-up study of a child psychiatric clientele with special regard to the diagnosis of psychosis. *Acta Psychiatr. Scand.* 1976, Aug;54(2):106-112.

[99] Pedersen, J., Aarkrog, T.: A 10-year follow-up study of an adolescent psychiatric clientele and early predictors of readmission. *Nord J. Psychiatry* 2001, 55(1):11-16.

[100] Pedersen, J., Aarkrog, T.: A 20-year study of an adolescent psychiatric clientele, with special reference to the age of onset. *Nord J. Psychiatry* 2001, 55(1):5-10.

[101] Strömgren, E.: *Episodiske Psykoser* (Monograph in Danish). Köbehavn: Ejnar Munksgarard; 1940.

[102] Valevski, A., Ratzoni, G., Sever, J., Apter, A., Zalsman, G., Shiloh, R., Weizman, A., Tyano, S.: Stability of diagnosis: a 20-year retrospective cohort study of Israeli psychiatric adolescent inpatients. *J. Adolesc.* 2001, Oct;24(5):625-633.

In: Psychosis: Causes, Diagnosis and Treatment
Editor: Xenia Anastassiou-Hadjicharalambous
ISBN: 978-1-62081-516-8


*Chapter 5*

# CHILDHOOD TRAUMA AND PSYCHOSIS

***Theodora Koulenti***
***and Xenia Anastassiou-Hadjicharalambous****
Psychology Program, University of Nicosia, Nicosia, Cyprus

## ABSTRACT

During the last decade there has been an increase of interest in the study of the plausible link between childhood trauma and psychotic symptomatology.

A considerable body of empirical evidence revealed that many patients with psychotic symptoms have indeed experienced childhood traumas but because of methodological weaknesses no causal relationship was managed to be established. These studies however despite their methodological weaknesses gave rise to the argument that psychotic symptomatology cannot solitarily be viewed as purely in the terms of genetic and biological aetiologies.

Over the last decades a series of systematic reviews of previous studies, gave rise to new, large-scale studies that aim to clarify previous evidence, in a more accurate and methodology-consistent manner. Even though the new attempts brought to the light new empirical evidence and a stronger relationship between childhood trauma and psychosis has been established, we still need a much more detailed understanding of the underlying mechanisms which connect the two.

## INTRODUCTION

Psychotic symptoms have been considered to emerge as a result of trauma or negative impact of negative life events and aversive environmental conditions. This suggestion was initiated from the high rates of childhood sexual abuse and other traumas among patients with psychotic symptoms [1]. Investigating whether childhood trauma is related to mental health problems in adulthood has crucial clinical implications in terms of the accuracy of formulations and the comprehensiveness of treatment planning [2].

* E-mail: hadjicharalambous.x@unic.ac.cy

The term 'childhood trauma' refers to a range of negative life experiences, such as sexual, physical and emotional abuse, as well as physical and emotional neglect [3]. Childhood abuse has been linked, over the years to various adult psychiatric disorders, including depression, anxiety disorders, substance abuse, eating disorders, post-traumatic stress disorder (PTSD), personality disorders, sexual dysfunction, dissociation and suicidality [3].

However, the link between childhood trauma and psychotic disorders was, until recently, overlooked in favour of the dominant biogenetic factor [3]. Potential social causes of psychosis, have been neglected in favour of the advancement of genetic and biological etiologies [3]. The possible reasons for this selective attention and the denial of possible social and environmental factors involve a firm devotion to a rather simplistic biological paradigm, inappropriate fear of being accused of 'family blaming', avoidance of explicit traumatisation on the part of the clinicians and the researchers and issues of re-diagnosing from psychosis to PTSD once abuse is discovered [4].

Nevertheless recent empirical evidence asserts that psychotic experiences in disorders, such as schizophrenia, cannot be seen detached from the normal functioning of the individual, therefore the role of adverse environmental and social factors need be taken into account [5]. A number of case studies of psychiatric inpatients and outpatients, who were diagnosed with a psychotic condition, suggest that the majority of them reported that they had experienced childhood traumas, such as sexual or physical abuse. This finding abetted researchers to search deeper whether this relationship is causal [4].

Furthermore, empirical evidence suggests that lifetime prevalence of PTSD is significantly higher in patients with severe mental illnesses than in the general population, allowing the assertion that a causal relationship could exist [1]. Child abuse and child sexual abuse seem to be consistently related to scales indicative of psychosis, and particularly schizophrenia. Studies, in clinical settings, have revealed that among child psychiatric patients, 77 % of those who experience child sexual abuse were diagnosed with psychotic symptoms. Women inpatients, diagnosed as schizophrenic, 60% had suffered child sexual abuse or incest [2].

It wasn't until recently that the crucial relationship between childhood trauma and psychosis started being recognized in the circles of scientific literature. During the last few years there have been a number of debates among clinicians and researchers suggesting that child abuse can be a cause for psychotic disorders, such as schizophrenia [6]. Research interest has started to be directed on the possible relationship between childhood trauma and the risk of developing psychotic experiences later in life [7]. Researchers raised the question whether there can be a causal relationship between the two, something which could create considerable implications for the professional practice of psychologists and treatment procedures [3].

A recent debate at the Maudsley Institute of Psychiatry in London proposed the motion that child abuse could be a cause for schizophrenia [8]. Later on, the British Medical Journal published the work of David Kingdon, underlining the failure of antipsychotic medication to hit the problem of psychosis to its root and suggesting the revolving to psychological factors in interventions, such as childhood physical and mental trauma [8]. Moreover, Acta Psychiatrica Scandinavica, published in 2005 the first full literature review of a big number of studies, suggesting a significant causal relationship between childhood trauma and psychosis [4].

## INITIAL RESEARCH AND SOCIAL VIEWS OF TRAUMA AND PSYCHOSIS

In the last few years there is an increased concern about the issue of over-medicalization for treatment of mental disorders, perhaps because of financial incentives, and the devaluation of psychotherapy and psychosocial treatments [6]. This concern gave the motive to researchers to examine whether childhood trauma can be a causal factor to the onset of psychotic disorders, by reviewing the historical context in which the problem was developed and, later on, by seeking new empirical evidence examining a potential relationship between the two [6].

During the decade of 1970, long before being able to investigate the relationship between childhood trauma and psychosis, there was a need, in the social context, to provide evidence that child abuse was existent, common and had devastating consequences for the victims [6]. This point of view that seemed to be denied by society at the time and any attempts for relevant publications were contradicted, by the excuse that this scenario was incredibly rare. However, in the passing of time, the responses started changing, by admitting that abuse did exist but its consequences were minimal [6].

After that the view that long term physical and psychological problems were associated with childhood trauma started being more widespread. At the same time though, there was a tendency of blaming the victims for what they had experienced by being provocative, prematurely sexual and partly guilty for their abuse [9]. Blame kept shifting from the victims to the mothers and from there to the therapists who were accused for planting false memories to the patients' minds. After this long process of changing views and debates, a few years ago, a general consensus was established, suggesting that child abuse is clearly related to psychiatric illness and specifically depression, anxiety, substance misuse, eating disorders, sexual dysfunction, personality disorders and PTSD [10]. However, there was still no acceptance of the relationship between childhood trauma and psychosis, since psychiatry insisted in the underlying role of genetic and biological vulnerability [11].

There were a few studies at the time which attempted to provide empirical evidence about the plausible link between childhood trauma and psychosis [1]. In 1984, an in-depth study of 188 individuals in a psychiatric hospital has revealed that more than 50% of the women residents were physically or sexually abused in previous years [12]. Three years later, in a study of 66 women inpatients, there was an attempt to correlate childhood abuse experiences with severity of adult psychiatric symptoms. It was found that 72% had histories of sexual or physical abuse and 59% had histories of sexual or physical abuse in childhood [13]. In 1989, an influential study conducted by Romme and Escher, found that 70% of voice hearers developed their hallucinations after experiencing a traumatic event [14]. It was speculated that hallucinations could be a coping process for dealing with traumas of the past [14]. Another study, revealed interesting findings concerning patients with borderline disorder, after being in depth interviewed: 81% of patients gave histories of major childhood trauma experiences, 68% had been sexually abused, 71% physically abused and 62% witnessed serious domestic violence. These results demonstrated a strong association between a diagnosis of borderline personality disorder and a history of abuse in childhood [15].

## Development in Trauma Theory and Current Research Focus on the Relationship between Childhood Trauma and Psychosis

During the decade of 1990's, even though there were many attempts to establish, scientifically, a relationship between childhood trauma and psychosis, they suffered from methodological inconsistencies and lack or resources [16]. For example, Honig et al (1998), compared, in their study, the form and content of chronic auditory hallucinations in patients with schizophrenia, patients with dissociative disorder and non-patient voice hearers. The study revealed that, in most patients, the onset of auditory hallucinations preceded a traumatic event or an event which triggered the memory of an earlier trauma [16]. However, in this study, the sample was not random and issues of lack of generalization were raised [1]. Moreover, in the study of the first 89 indivuiduals referred to an intensive case management psychiatric program, revealed substantial previously undetected physical and sexual abuse. However, none of those patients had even been asked about their abuse histories [17]. The same study reveals that, at the time, childhood trauma was a factor which seemed to be invisible within adult mental health services. Most of the times there was absence of routine inquiry about abuse history, abused histories were often ignored, often leading to misdiagnosis or mistreatment [17].

More recently, Read et al (2003) reviewed 200 case notes of community patients. It was found that those who had experienced sexual abuse, either as children or adults, were more likely to experience two, or more, characteristic symptoms of schizophrenia [2]. This finding suggests that many individuals with psychotic symptoms may have endured trauma experiences prior to the onset of psychosis, even though the measurement of sexual abuse rely on self-reports and case notes [1]. Moreover, this study also revealed that childhood abuse predicted hallucinations in adult life. More specifically, patients who were physically abused as children were twice as likely to experience hallucinations. Those who were sexually abused were three times as likely to experience hallucinations. Moreover, auditory hallucinations, in patients, were more strongly associated with child abuse [2]. Consequently, even though there are methodological inconsistencies characterizing research attempts, in this period, they formed the beginning for a new perspective and gave the rise to more consistent and recent major studies on the subject [6]. Particularly, there was a focus on the functions of psychotic symptoms: it was found that there was a complex relationship between dissociation and psychotic symptoms, delusions often formed patients' attempts to make sense of severe trauma symptoms, through flashbacks, and there was often dissociation of regulating negative affect of abuse memories [2].

Furthermore, research evidence of the last decade, has shown that more than 2/3 of patients initially hospitalized for psychosis, experienced at least one traumatic event in their lifetime, almost ½ were exposed to life-threatening trauma and 1/3 has been victimized in childhood [18]. The same study suggests that the magnitude of the trauma history in childhood, such as rape, sexual molestation, sexual and physical abuse, also increases the vulnerability to patients with psychosis, placing them in high risk for PTSD [18].

A number of significant reviews of the literature, examining the possible causal relationship between childhood trauma and psychosis, have been published in the last few years. A review by Read et al (2005) summarized research studies and examined review papers on psychiatric inpatients and outpatients who were diagnosed with a psychotic condition [4]. Even though it is generally believed that the rates in this review are generally underestimated because child abuse is generally underreported, still the majority of the sample reported experiencing either physical or sexual abuse [4]. Even though this review paper suggested a relationship between childhood trauma and abuse, methodological issues did not allow deciding whether this relationship is causal or not [3]. The mass of the evidence studied in this review was from studies using cross-sectional designs or uncontrolled group comparisons. This allows the authors to provide useful estimates of the prevalence of childhood trauma in clinical populations but not adequate to determine whether the relationship between childhood trauma and psychosis is causal [18].

A big general population study, conducted by Bebbington and colleagues (2004), gave rise to new empirical evidence. The sample was assessed for psychiatric disorders and then asked whether they had experienced any kind of 'victimization experiences', as defined by the researchers: sexual abuse, bullying, running away from home, time in local authority care, time in childhood institution, expulsion from school, homelessness, violence at work, serious injury or assault [19]. The study suggested that there was a significant relationship between the trauma and psychosis, with the strongest association being sexual abuse [19]. However, a limitation of this study was the fact that the participants were not required to provide information about the timing or the severity of their adverse life events, living the possibility that some of those abusive experiences may have occurred in adult life [3].

Another big sample study in Holland, gave a new perspective concerning the methods used. The sample was interviewed about their childhood experiences, while being 'psychosis free' and after three years they were reassessed [20]. Results revealed that people who had been abused were much more likely to develop psychosis, than those who were not, during the study period, even after controlling the genetic predisposition factor [20].

However, another research study conducted at about the same time, gave a different perspective than the previous ones. The sample involved individuals who experienced severe abuse and they were followed up as adults [21]. They were then compared with a general population group. The results did not show a significant relationship between childhood trauma and schizophrenia, contradicting previous empirical evidence. However, concerns of accuracy of the sample's self-reports, the methodology and the sample were raised [21].

Finally, another research study, conducted by Hammersley et al (2007), tested the risk of experiencing adult hallucinations, a common psychotic symptom, if experiencing a childhood trauma [6]. Childhood traumas, in this case, involved physical, sexual and emotional abuse, neglect, and certain adverse childhood events, such as witnessing the mother's abuse. The results suggested that those who had experienced the greatest number of types of childhood trauma were 4.7 times likely to have experienced hallucinations [6].

## The Balance of Evidence

In the years following the review of Read et al (2005), there was an attempt to balance and clarify the evidence, related to childhood trauma and psychosis, through new, large-scale research studies [3].

One study conducted by Spauwen et al (2006), aimed in examining associations between self-reported psychological trauma and psychotic symptoms as a function of psychosis proneness [22]. The sample involved 2524 adolescents and young adults who provided self reports on psychological trauma and were interviewed to assess any potential presence of psychotic symptoms. Those who reported psychotic trauma were 2.6 times more likely to experience psychotic symptoms at follow up, with the higher risk being those who had experienced sexual abuse [22].

Even when possible interfering factors such as gender, socioeconomic status, cannabis use, mental disorders and urbanicity were controlled, still the association between trauma and psychotic symptoms was obvious. The connection between the two increased in a positively graded fashion with the number of traumatic events [22]. Even though this paper establishes a close link between trauma and psychotic symptoms, one limitation was the fact that the measure of the trauma utilized in this study, was basic and the participants were not asked to provide detailed information concerning the timing, severity or duration of the trauma [3]. There is a possibility that traumatized participants could be included in the non-traumatized group, reducing, in this way, the prospective of the study to assess the strength of the association between trauma and psychotic symptoms [3].

The results of the study of Spauwen et al (2006) were also sustained by another general population study conducted at about the same time. The sample involved 1290 adolescents [23]. After controlling factors, such as age, gender and socioeconomic status, results showed that sexual trauma and bullying were associated with non-clinical psychotic experiences. The frequency of the trauma was positively related to psychotic experiences, suggesting causality between bullying and sexual trauma and psychotic symptoms [23]. The results of this study reveal similarity with the results of Spauwen et al (2006), with the authors suggesting that the association between victimization in childhood and non-clinical psychotic experiences in adolescence may imply risk for psychotic disorders later in life [3].

Furthermore, another research study which used data from the National Comorbidity Survey and the British Psychiatric Morbidity Survey, also attempted to study the effect of cumulative traumatic experiences on psychosis [24]. The results of this study indicated that experiences, of two or more types of trauma, significantly predicted psychosis and a causal relationship between the two was evident [24].

As with previous studies, this research study suggested that multiple trauma exposure increases the risk for developing psychosis. For the National Comorbidity Survey sample the results showed that sexual molestation and physical abuse were stronger predictors of psychosis, while the sample results from the British Psychiatric Morbidity Survey, sexual abuse was more predictive of psychosis [24]. Moreover, in another research paper of the same group, using again data from the National Comorbidity Survey, also demonstrated that childhood molestation and rape, before the age of 16, were predictive of visual, auditory and tactile hallucinations [24].

Recently, research evidence of a large scale study, 10641 adult respondents from the Australian National Survey of Mental Health and Wellbeing, added to previous research projects that endorsement of any delusional experience was significantly more likely in those who experienced traumatic events during their lifespan [25].

Research evidence was consistent with previous studies, revealing that there was a strong link between traumatic experiences associated with childhood, such as sexual molestation and rape, and delusional experiences [25].

However, one limitation of the specific study was the fact that there were not any time details concerning the trauma, making it impossible to identify whether the trauma preceded the delusional experiences or not [3].

## CONCLUSION

Since the major review of 2005 and the large-scale studies followed in the next years, scientific evidence accumulated that established a systematic link between numbers of traumas experienced and being at risk for psychotic symptoms [3]. There is also evidence for predictiveness of child abuse on hallucinations specifically. Most evidence suggests that childhood trauma, and more strongly sexual abuse is a strong predictor of psychosis, [3].

Despite significant advancements in the field there are still only a small number of well-designed studies, controlling for possible confounding variables, with large samples [4]. Moreover, another important issue in the studies reviewed, is the reliability of self-report of abuse, raising concerns about the accuracy of child abuse disclosures by psychiatric patients. Furthermore, many of the studies conducted so far are either correlational or uncontrolled group comparisons, telling us little about whether the relationship child abuse and psychosis is a causal one. Other factors may account for the relationship, such as other adverse events or circumstances in childhood.

Additionally, another issue is the categorization of symptoms. Certain symptoms which may be categorized as psychotic by clinicians, before the identification of the trauma, may be re-categorized as non-psychotic when the trauma has been identified (e.g. symptoms of PTSD) [4]. In this case, the symptom has not changed but the observer's perception has changed, illustrating problems of diagnosis to patients. All these raise the need for future designs to overcome the limitations [4].

The investigation of the relationship between childhood trauma and psychosis raises a huge responsibility towards the people who experience psychosis. If scientific literature aims in contributing to the improvement of therapy and intervention methods, researchers need to incorporate individuals' life experiences to their attempts for investigation [6]. Unless we start searching for people's distressing life experiences and make sense of them, instead of simply trying to suppress the psychotic symptoms with pills, patients will be condemned to live their lives controlled by medication [6]. By not considering the causal role that childhood experiences might have on psychosis, it means that professional practice will keep exposing patients to the unnecessary side effects of neuroleptic medication and denying them the chance to receive appropriate psychological treatment [7].

The research studies described above, mainly involve schizophrenia spectrum disorders with common symptoms hallucinations and delusions. However, certain mood disorders, such as bipolar disorder and unipolar psychotic depression may also have psychotic features. Nevertheless, there are no systematic investigations of the life experiences of people who suffer from psychotic mood disorders, something which raises the need for further research studies in the future [6].

To conclude even though there is a huge progress concerning the studying of the association between childhood trauma and psychosis, there is still need for methodologically rigorous investigations that will attempt a more detailed understanding of the underlying mechanisms linking trauma and psychosis.

## REFERENCES


[1] Morrison, A.P., Frame, L. and Larkin, W. 2003, Relationships between trauma and Psychosis: A review and integration, *British Journal of Clinical Psychology,* vol. 42, pp. 331–353.

[2] Read. J., Agar, K., Argyle, N. and Aderhold, V. 2003, Sexual and Physical Abuse during childhood as predictors of hallucinations, delusions and thought disorder, *Psychology and Psychotherapy: Theory, Research and Practice*, vol. 76, pp. 1-22.

[3] Larkin, W. and Read, J. 2008, Childhood Trauma and psychosis: Evidence, pathways, and implications, *Journal of Postgraduate Medicine*, vol. 54, pp. 287-293.

[4] Read, J., Van Os, J., Morrison, P. A. and Ross, C.A. 2005, Childhood Trauma, Psychosis and Schizophrenia: A literature review with theoretical and clinical implications, *Acta Psychiatrica Scandinavica*, vol.112, pp. 330-350.

[5] Bentall, R. P. 2006, *The Environment and Psychosis, Rethinking the Evidence*. In: Larkin W., Morrison, A.P., editors, Trauma and Psychosis: New Directions for theory and therapy, London: Routledge, 2006.

[6] Hammersley, P., Read, P., Woodall, S. and Dillon, J. 2008, Childhood Trauma and Psychosis: The genie is out of the bottle, *Journal of Psychological Trauma*, vol. 6, no. 2-3.

[7] Read, J. 1997, Child Abuse and Psychosis: A Literature Review and Implications for Professional Practice, *Research and Practice*, vol. 28, no. 5, pp. 448-456.

[8] Kingdon, D. 2006, Psychological and Social Interventions for Schizophrenia, *British Medical Journal*, vol. 333, pp. 212-213.

[9] Armstrong, L. 1996, *Rocking the cradle of sexual politics: What happened when women said incest*, Reading, MA: Addison-Wesley Publishing Company.

[10] Read, J., Goodman, L., Morrison, A., Ross, C., and Aderhold, V. (2004). *Childhood trauma, loss and stress*. In J. Read, L. Mosher, and R. Bentall (Eds.), Models of madness: Psychological, social and biological approaches to schizophrenia. London: Routledge.

[11] Read, J., Mosher, L., and Bentall, R. (2004). *Models of madness: Psychological, social and biological Approaches to schizophrenia*. London: Routledge.

[12] Carmen, E.H., Rieker, P.P.and Mills, T. 1984, Victims of Violence and Psychiatric illness, *American Journal of Psychiatry*, vol. 141, pp. 378-383.

[13] Bryer, J.B., Nelson, B., Miller, J. B. and Krol, P. 1987, Childhood Sexual and Physical Abuse as Factors in Adult Psychiatric Illness, *American Journal of Psychiatry*, vol. 144, pp. 1426-1430.

[14] Romme, M. and Escher, A., 1989, Hearing Voices, *Schizophrenia Bullettin*, no. 15, pp. 209-216.

[15] Herman, J.L., Perry, J.C. and van der Kolk, B.A. 1989, Childhood Trauma in borderline personality disorder, *American Journal of Psychiatry*, vol. 146, pp. 490-495.

[16] Honig, A., Romme, M. A., Ensink, B. J., Escher, S. D., Pennings, M. H. and deVries., M. W. 1998, Auditory Hallucinations: A Comparison between patients, *Journal of Nervous and Mental Disease*, no. 186, pp. 646-651.

[17] Rose, M. S., Peabody, G. C. and Stratigeas, B. 1991, Undetected Abuse Among Intensive Case Management Clients, *Hospital Community Psychiatry*, vol. 42, pp. 499-503.

[18] Neria, Y., Bromet, E. and Sievers, S. 2002, Trauma Exposure and Posttraumatic Stress Disorder in Psychosis: Findings from a first – admission cohort, *Journal of Consulting and Clinical Psychology*, vol. 70, no. 1, pp.246-251.

[19] Bebbington, P., Bhugra, D., Brugha, T., Singleton, N., Farrell, M., Jenkins, R., et al., 2004, Psychosis, victimization and childhood disadvantage: Evidence from the second British national survey on psychiatric morbidity, *British Journal of Psychiatry*, 185, 220-226.

[20] Janssen, I., Krabbendam, L., Bak, M., Hanssen, M., Vollebergh, W., de Graaf, R., et al, 2003, Childhood abuse as a risk factor for psychotic experiences, *Acta Psychiatrica Scandinavica*, vol. 109, pp. 38-45.

[21] Spataro, J., Mullen, P. E., Burgess, P. M., et al, 2004, Impact of child sexual abuse on mental health: prospective study in males and females, *British Journal of Psychiatry*, vol. 184, pp. 416 -421.

[22] Spauwen, J., Krabbendam, L., Lieb, R., Wittchen, H.U. and Van Os, J., 2006, Impact of psychological trauma on the development of psychotic symptoms: Relationship with psychotic proneness, *The British Journal of Psychiatry*, vol. 188, pp. 527-533.

[23] Lataster, T., Van Os, J., Drukker, M., Henquet, C., Feron, F., and Gunther, N. 2006, Childhood victimization and developmental expression of non-clinical delusional ideation and hallucinatory experiences, *Social Psychiatry and Psychiatric Epidemiology*, vol. 41, no. 6, pp. 423-428.

[24] Shevlin, M., Dorahy, M. and Adamson. G. 2007, Childhood Traumas and hallucinations: An analysis of the National Comorbidity Survey, *Journal of Psychiatric Research*, vol. 41, pp. 222-228.

[25] Scott, J., Chant, D., Andrews, G., Martin, G. and McGrath, J. 2007, Association between trauma exposure and delusional experiences in a large community-based sample, *The British Journal of Psychiatry*, vol. 190, pp. 339-343.

In: Psychosis: Causes, Diagnosis and Treatment
Editor: Xenia Anastassiou-Hadjicharalambous
ISBN: 978-1-62081-516-8


*Chapter 6*

# STAGES, COURSE AND PROGNOSIS OF PSYCHOSIS

***Theodora Koulenti and Xenia Anastassiou-Hadjicharalambous****
Psychology Program, University of Nicosia, Nicosia, Cyprus

## ABSTRACT

Psychosis usually erupts early during development and can be disabling for life. Symptoms are more common in young people and the majority of patients remain symptomatic for their whole lifespan. Identifying psychosis in early stages is of major importance in terms of treatment.

Recent developments on medication have had positive results on problematic symptoms; however, unwanted side effects and non-compliance of patients' to their doctors' descriptions often contribute to the decrease of recovery odds.

Early stages of psychosis can be very distressing for both the patient and the closed environment. There is often a delay of time for treatment, after experiencing the first symptoms of psychosis. The longer this delay is, the poorer the treatment outcomes are, in terms of symptoms. During the early stages of psychosis, the symptoms are not always obvious from the beginning.

However, they can begin to develop and increase in number, severity and rate of recurrence during the $2^{nd}$ and $3^{rd}$ phase. Patients may lose touch with reality or their capacity to function in an organized integrated manner. The continuity among the stages makes it more difficult to define when a person has slipped to psychosis, however, early identification and treatment is more likely to reduce the burden of the disease. Relapses are also common and unfortunately, treatment of subsequent episodes of psychosis is less pleasing than the first.

Consequently, since the developmental progression is partly based on early identification and intervention , on timely therapy is therefore essential so that the patient develops techniques to identify, monitor and reduce possible relapses.

* E-mail: hadjicharalambous.x@unic.ac.cy

## Introduction

Psychosis is characterized by delusions and hallucinations and is a common symptom in people with schizophrenia spectrum disorders, mood disorders and dementia [1]. The narrowest definition of psychotic is constrained to delusions or outstanding hallucinations, with the hallucinations occurring in the absence of insight into their pathological nature (DSM Manual). A broader definition also includes positive symptoms of schizophrenia (i.e. disorganized speech, grossly disorganized or catatonic behavior [2]. Scientists use, in the psychiatric literature, the term 'Psychosis – Risk Syndrome' to describe early signs, symptoms and disabilities preceding the full onset of the illness. The term is also used to describe early signs of reversion to people who already have psychosis and are in a remitted phase [3]. Empirical evidence suggests that psychotic disorders often emerge gradually in a prodromal period, ranging from several weeks to several years or more [1]. Recent research studies reveal that, in psychosis, both gene-environment interactions are likely to play a role [4] and a long duration of untreated psychosis may result in a worse recovery prognosis [1]. Patients suffering from psychotic disorders are often characterized by pronounced deficits on their functioning, such as cognitive processes, working memory and response inhibition, at all stages of their illness and therefore treatment procedures must be applied from early signs, where possible [4].

## Course and Development of Psychosis

Psychotic Disorders, such as schizophrenia, have been observed worldwide. Prevalence of schizophrenia among adults is often reported to be in the range of 0.5% to 1.5%. Annual incidences are most often in the range of 0.5 to 5.0 per 10,000, even though birth group studies suggest some geographic and historical variations in prevalence [2]. Schizophrenia and psychotic disorder usually erupt early during development and can be disabling for life. The expression of psychosis is much more common in young people and usually declines with age [4]. According to the *Diagnostic and Statistical Manual of Mental Disorders*, the median age at onset for the first psychotic episode of schizophrenia is in the early to mid-20s for men and in the late 20s for women [2]. Empirical evidence asserts that schizophrenia affects, average, 1% of any population worldwide and the risk is higher for men. The peak period for onset in men is 15-25 years of age and 25-35 for women. Onset in the teenage years is also common [3].

The onset may be unexpected or insidious, but the majority of individuals exhibit some type of prodromal phase marked by the slow and gradual development of a variety of signs and symptoms, such as social withdrawal, loss of interest in school or work, deterioration in hygiene and grooming, unusual behavior and sudden occurrences of anger. Family members may find this behavior difficult to understand, however, the manifestation of some active-phase symptom marks the disturbance as schizophrenia [2]. The age of onset may have both pathophysiological and predictive implication. Individuals with an early age at onset are more often male and have a poorer premorbid adjustment, lower educational achievement, more evidence of brain abnormalities, more prominent negative signs and symptoms, more evidence of cognitive impairment and a worse outcome. On the contrary, individuals with a later onset are more often female, have less evidence of brain abnormalities or cognitive impairment and present a better outcome [2].

Schizophrenia is considered to be a serious psychiatric disorder because it disables early in life and its attendant deficits can last to old age, often for a lifetime [3]. Many studies on course and outcome of schizophrenia propose that the path to the disorder may be variable, with some individuals displaying exacerbations and remissions, while others remain chronically ill. Full remission to complete premorbid functioning is not frequent in this disorder. Of those who remain ill, some appear to have a comparatively steady course, while others demonstrate a progressive deterioration associated with severe disability [2].

Even though treatments for schizophrenia have improved to the point that patients have the ability to live in the community, still, the majority of patients remains symptomatic and struggle with deficits in self-care, work capacity and interpersonal relationships [3]. Latest treatment procedures control the positive symptoms of the disorder, such as hallucinations, delusions, and disorganized thought, speech and behavior but their disruptive capacity is always a danger. Moreover, experts assert that central nervous system neurobiological processes, which are responsible for generating psychosis, precede its onset by months or years and are irreversible by the time of onset. For this reason, identifying psychosis in early phases is of major importance [3]. In the early stages of the, negative symptoms may be obvious, appearing primarily as prodromal features, therefore, positive symptoms appear as well. However, because positive symptoms are particularly responsive to treatment, they usually diminish, but in many individuals negative symptoms persevere [2].

Even though in the previous decades serious mental health problems seemed to be untreatable, in the last few years this picture started changing. Researchers started investing in a more humanitarian and anti-institutionalization way of thinking [3]. They suggested that there was noteworthy evidence that disorders, such as psychosis, were not necessarily lifelong and incurable [3]. Numerous studies have indicated a group of factors that are associated with a better prognosis. These include, 'good premorbid adjustment, acute onset, later age at onset, absence of anosognosia (poor insight), being female, precipitating events, associated mood disturbance, treatment with antipsychotic medication soon after the onset of illness, consistent medication compliance, brief duration of active-phase symptoms, good interepisode functioning, minimal residual symptoms, absence of structural brain abnormalities, normal neurological functioning and no family history of schizophrenia'[2].

Even though with new medication problematic symptoms seemed to be partly controlled, helping in this way patients to function in the broader society, nobody could dispute the power of unwanted side effects, leading patients to non-compliance with their doctor's prescriptions [3]. Specifically, concerning psychosis, statistics show that 90% who suffer psychotic first episode will be in remission, at the end of one year of treatment only 1/3 seems to have a good functional outcome. This happens partly because the recent psychotropic medication reduce significantly the positive symptoms of the disorder, such as delusions and hallucinations, but have not helped significantly in controlling the rest sets of symptoms, such as negative and mood symptoms and cognitive deficits. These unwanted side effects make for patients medication compliance very difficult, therefore the chances for recovery decrease [3].

Furthermore, along the passing of time, there were several debates concerning issues of reliability and validity of diagnoses or issues of stigmatization of patients and its harm on their mental health, bringing confusion on whether or not diagnosis of schizophrenia could be seen as useful if led to accurate predictions of patients' positive respond to neuroleptic medication [4].

## THE EARLY STAGES OF SCHIZOPHRENIA AND PSYCHOSIS

The early stage of psychosis is highly distressing for both the individual and family and friends. It may take a considerable length of time to reach treatment after experiencing the first symptoms of psychosis. Empirical evidence reveals that treatment fluctuates from 6 months – 2 years, while others may experience delays of several years [5]. This delay is known as DUP (duration of untreated psychosis) and is often during this stage that patients may experience paranoia, voices, hallucinations or unusual ideas which disrupt their lives. During this period the risk of self-harm is high and specialist help is needed without further delays. Research studies concerning the prognosis of patients who experience a longer DUP has shown that these patients also experience poorer outcomes in terms of symptoms, quality of life, and social functioning, even 6-12 months after receiving treatment. It is therefore vital to seek professional help timely [5]. Moreover, DUP has been found to be associated with longer time until remission, less remission and more psychotic relapse [6]. On the other hand, early implementation of intensive psychosocial intervention, along with medication, has been reported to improve the patients' social functioning and self-esteem, and therefore have a better prospect for long-term prognosis [6].

The early stages of schizophrenia or first – episode psychosis include a premorbid, a prodromal phase and a first psychosis stage. The premorbid phase is a period of normality for people who eventually develop the disorder. Even though deficits exist they are not obvious or seriously disabling for the individual. However, during the 2$^{nd}$ phase, usually around pruberty, the psychosis-risk symptoms begin and develop with increasing number, severity and rate of recurrence [3]. During this phase, a prolonged period of symptoms and increasing disability occurs before the onset of severe and continual positive psychotic symptoms become adequate to allow the diagnosis of schizophrenia or first – psychosis episode. The psychosocial harm that is often caused, at that time, is often difficult to reverse [7]. Moreover, during the prodromal phase, the mental stage of the patient is changed, compared to the person's pre-morbid functioning, up until the onset of frank psychotic symptoms [8]. This phase has been reported to last around 2-5 years average [7]. Finally, during the 3$^{rd}$ phase, symptoms are reported to be more obvious. People feel that their hallucinations and delusions are real and they behave accordingly. The patient loses its insight and perspective, as well as the capacity to function in an organized integrated manner [7]. There are often prolonged delays in initiating effective treatment for first-episode psychosis, even though any sufficient delay is associated with poorer response and outcome because early identification and treatment during the first stages of psychosis is more likely to reduce the burden of disease while it is active [7].

Even though empirical evidence asserts 3 main phases of schizophrenia or first-episode psychosis that patients go through, it is not always easy to define or say precisely when a person has slipped into psychosis [8]. The pre-morbid phase often blends with the first non specific psychiatric symptoms and the prodromal phase often mingled with the onset of first-episode psychosis. There is continuity among the 3 stages and because many issues are interrelated, factors, such as the degree of deviation from normality, the frequency of the experience and the length of time in which symptoms are present, should be taken into consideration [8].

According to the model of McGlashan and Hoffman (2000) for the development of psychosis, in normal human development, synaptic connectivity expands and wanes according to the stages of human development [9]. Specifically, synaptic connections flourish and grow from birth to age five, and then they continue to expand until adolescence and finally start reducing during adult cognitive development. However, in some cases, synaptic connectivity is less than normal because of genetics, pregnancy and birth complications, etc. In these cases, children may develop deficits in social, academic and cognitive functioning and during adolescence synaptic connectivity may be reduced [9]. This model suggests that, in other cases with a pathway to psychosis, the childhood dissemination of synaptic connectivity is normally vigorous, but the pathogenic prospective for psychosis lies in an abnormally intensified rate of synaptic pruning during adolescence and young adulthood. These cases may also lead to the onset of psychosis as previous hypothesized pathways; however timing to psychosis may differ [9]. In other words, there are cases that disabilities are already present and precede adolescent changes, providing premonitory signals of upcoming problems. There are also cases of no warning signals because of a normal adolescence, and when symptoms arrive, with no obvious warning, there are often ignored and denied until the psychosis becomes a fact. In these cases the advantages of early detection and treatment are lost [9].

During the first signs of the disorder, the patients are usually functional and do not demonstrate any obvious symptoms. However, they start developing new accelerating deficits in their social and intellectual functioning as well as on their organizational abilities [1]. Psychosis 'risk-symptoms' usually appear, in most of the cases, six months to three years before the onset of psychosis. Aberrant salience, meaning the unusual or incorrect assignment of salience to unimportant stimuli has been considered to be a central mechanism in the development of psychosis [1]. During the onset of the symptoms, innocuous stimuli become more significant and capture the attention of the patient. Sharpened senses, feelings of being at the verge of some important breakthrough, high sense of emotionality and anxiety of uncontrolled changes are often reported at the beginning of the process [1]. Negative symptoms have been reported to develop first and positive symptoms follow [3]. During the last few months, before the onset of psychosis symptoms increase in number and intensity. Symptoms of schizophrenic behavior, such as ideas of reference, paranoid ideation, unexplained sights and sounds, become more apparent, even though elements of reality exist in the forms of doubt. When these characteristics become adequately attenuated, psychosis arises [3].

Emotional recovery and relapse are interlinked. Empirical evidence asserts that the 2 years period after the first episode appears to be a critical period in determining possible long-term outcomes. Relapse occurs in 20-35% at 1 year, 50-65% at 2 years and 80% at 5 years [10]. Consequently, relapses are common during the first 5 years after the first episode. For this reason, this phase is known as 'critical period'. Young people often find it difficult to adjust and accept so many life changes, such as taking daily medication, especially if they have substantially recovered. Poor obedience often results to one or more relapses which are risky, disruptive and may consequence in an increased chance of treatment resistance [10]. Moreover, results of various research studies reveal that, 5 years after onset, 70% of the group has experienced a psychotic relapse and by 9 years the rate was 85%, with no relapsing patients after this, suggesting that a safety point has been reached. Other studies found similar relapse rates (70-80%), even though different criteria were adopted [7].Treatment of subsequent episodes of psychosis is less pleasing than the first with patients less likely to recover from psychosis. Inability to prevent relapse often forms the basis for developing depression and anxiety. These negative feelings work as a chain to cause further psychotic experiences, more involuntary admissions, stigmatization and loss of social status and friendships [10]. However, relapse rates may also be influenced by critical and hostile home environments, particularly in the absence of antipsychotic medication. The same applies for negative social attitudes and responses towards patients with psychosis, considering that productive social relationships promote recovery [4]. Moreover, as Morrison et al (2004) assert, when working with patients a big challenge is to help them develop strategies to identify and therefore minimize and resolve relapse. Self-monitoring and establishing a normalizing rationale for why relapse may occur, as well as awareness of the stages that are part of the relapse process, are major steps for relapse prevention [11]. For start, patients should be able to identify possible stressors and triggers that could be strong enough to cause a possible relapse. In this way, patient and therapist are able to explore the relation between events and consequences and establish the development of first symptoms. Afterwards, the patient is in the position of identifying how his/hers psychotic symptoms were developed and what can trigger this process [11]. Therefore, the patient is now capable to monitor the events that could activate his/hers core beliefs, which are responsible for psychotic symptoms. After this stage, the therapist may teach the patient alternative strategies of dealing successfully with these stressors or problems, providing the patient with a feeling of positivism about the future [11]. In cases in which patients do not manage to spot indicators responsible for their relapse, individuals of the patients' close environment, such as family and friends, can play a vital role. In many cases, families are able to identify psychotic symptoms which indicate the onset of relapse, making it possible for the application of early interventions [11]. In cases which early warning signs are observed self-monitoring is appropriate, while others monitor observable behaviors that the patient may not be aware of. The importance of monitoring signs of relapse is the employment of strategies to prevent the effects of relapse to patients, since the earlier the application of interventions, the greater the chances of positive results [11]. The future of patients with psychosis is of major interest. Psychological interventions are more successful for patients with early psychosis. These treatments are more possible to play an important role in the optimal recovery of patients if offered during the early stages. Optimal recovery is less possible to be achieved in the absence of psychological interventions, along with proper medication [7].

## DEVELOPMENT OF PSYCHOSIS AND ASSOCIATED FEATURES ON EVERYDAY FUNCTIONING

One of the main issues with patients suffering from psychotic disorders and schizophrenia in particular, is the lack of insight of their illness and their need for treatment, probably because of neuropsychological deficits [12]. Scientific evidence suggests that psychotic symptoms are clearly related with worse daily functioning, even among those who do not meet the diagnostic criteria for a disorder or when the symptoms do not reach the clinical threshold for a psychotic disorder (Nuevo et al, 2010). Patients are frustrated with the people around them and their doctors who insist that they have a serious mental illness exactly because they are certain that they do not. For this reason, they often refuse any possible help or treatment, except in cases that it's their only option to gain their freedom from hospitals. This severe unawareness of illness is damaging to the patients' relationships but also to their chances of recovery because of their incompliance with possible treatments [12]. Personal confessions of patients with psychotic illnesses reveal that when symptoms start appearing, often during days or weeks, stress is becoming really intense. If neither the patient nor the individuals surrounding the patient notice on time, it gets more difficult to ease the symptoms [14]. However, if it is noticed early enough, it is easier for the patient to implement a number of techniques to alleviate the problems. Diary planning, prioritizing events and time management are techniques often used by patients to ease the problems, and therefore stress and symptoms, along with sharing of findings with health professionals and medication, until the patient manages to make sense of things again [14].

Patients with psychotic illnesses often demonstrate symptoms of paranoia as well. Even though suspiciousness is a common feeling, up to a certain range, to many people, paranoia, in the sense of mistrust and suspiciousness, in the case of psychotic illnesses, can reach the level of unrealistic and exaggerated distrust of others [14]. Patients may 'lose touch' with reality, they can be over-suspicious of other peoples' motives and they often fear that other people may want to harm them. When people develop these ideas it is often extremely difficult to realize that their fears are not reasonable or realistic and cognitive behavioral therapy is essential in order to help them to step back and think their possibilities [14].

Delusions are also considered to be a common feature of psychosis. Delusions are conceptualized as rationalization of experiences, particularly atypical or anomalous perceptions of events, for which an explanation is not evident [15]. A better understanding of the cognitive processes and the deficits on reasoning processes, which underlie symptoms of delusions, can lead to improvements in cognitive behavioral therapy for psychosis [15].

Moreover, patients with psychotic illnesses often admit that they often experience hallucinations, such as hearing voices, clearly and realistically [14]. Hallucinations are described as the experience of a sensory perception in the absence of a corresponding external stimulus [15]. For many patients auditory hallucinations are a common feature of psychosis and are highly distressing for the individual. Often this symptom persists, despite the efficacy of medication [16]. Health professionals suggest to the patients to keep a diary recording these experiences, and afterwards try to reduce the activities associated with the periods hearing the voices, as a measure of control [16]. Cognitive behavioral therapy is useful in this case as well. Along with the positive symptoms (e.g. paranoia and hallucinations) people with psychotic illnesses also experience a series of negative symptoms which have a number of effects on their personal and social life. Alogia, anhedonia, emotional blunting, attention and concentration deficits are only a few of the examples that patients may experience [14].

Considering all the above, for some psychotic individuals medication is an important part of managing psychosis since symptoms of psychosis are caused by a chemical imbalance in the brain and specifically in the limbic region. Antipsychotic medications vary and some of them are more effective than others, while some of them may have intense side effects. Different people may need different doses of medication because everyone's body reacts differently with medication [17].

## Conclusion

Even though there is an expanding interest in the study of psychosis, there is still a growing need in research to study patients' experiences in the context in which they are occurring. Considering that psychotic experiences and symptoms, such as delusions, hallucinations, flat affect, anhedonia and asociality can be found in the interaction between the person and its environment, a future direction of research could involve validation of experimental and questionnaire findings in the realm of daily life, relating laboratory findings to real life functioning [18]. Furthermore, future research could further validate score interpretations in measuring in measuring psychosis proneness, with longitudinal studies, in order to see if scores can predict conversion to psychosis [1].

The importance of timely treatment is an unquestionable fact on the developmental progression of psychosis [6]. However, since psychotic disorders, such as schizophrenia, are considered to be the most expensive psychiatric disorders, there is a constant need for intervention research and improvement of treatments. From a public health perspective a focus on better pharmacological and more specific psychotherapeutic, cognitive, behavioral, psychososial and rehabilitative interventions is necessitated [19]. A multipronged effort focusing on better pharmacological treatments along with more specific psychotherapeutic, cognitive, behavioral, psychosocial and rehabilitative interventions is warranted [19].

Finally, there is a need for future research direction concerning preventive interventions of psychosis, in the context of treatment. Since the developmental progression of psychosis is often based on fast and efficient treatment procedures, preventive interventions can be directed towards reducing the risk of relapse or recurrence and toward minimizing excessive or inappropriate levels of disability [20]. Preventive studies can also be directed towards eliminating the development of the illness in those at risk, and especially youth, by designing prevention models which will engage a wide spectrum of fields, such as treatment research, service systems and services research, and be based upon models of etiology, patho-physiology and risk [20].

## References

[1] Cicero, C. D., Kerns, G. J. and McCarthy, M. D. 2010, The Aberrant Salience Inventory: A New Measure of Psychosis Proneness, *Psychological Assessment*, vol. 22, no. 3, pp. 688-701.

[2] American Psychiatric Association: Diagnostic and Statistical Manual of Mental Disorders, Fourth Edition, Text Revision. Washington, DC, American Psychiatric Association, 2000.

[3] McGlashan, H. Th., Walsh, C. Barbara and Woods, W. Scott. 2010, *The Psychosis Risk Syndrome – Handbook for Diagnosis and Follow-Up*, Oxford University Press, New York.

[4] Horgan, C., McKenzie. K. and Fearon, P. (eds) 2008, *Society and Psychosis*, Cambridge University Press, New York.

[5] French, P., Smith, J., Shiers, D., Reed, M. and Rayne, M. (eds) 2010, *Promoting Recovery in Early Psychosis – A practice manual*, Wiley – Blackwell, Oxford.

[6] Haan, L., Linszen, H. D., Lenior, E. M., Doderlein, de Win, E. and Gorsira, R. 2003, Duration of Untreated Psychosis and Outcome of Schizophrenia: Delay in Intensive Psychosocial Treatment Versus Delay in Treatment With Antipsychotic Medication, *Schizophrenia Bulletin*, vol. 29, no.2.

[7] Gleeson, F.m. J. and McGorry D. P. (eds) 2004, *Psychological Interventions in Early Psychosis – A Treatment Handbook*, John Wiley and Sons Ltd, England.

[8] Yung, R. A., McGorry, D. P., McFarlane, A. C., Jackson, J. H., Patton, C. G. and Rakkar, A. 2004, Monitoring and Care of Young People at Incipient Risk of Psychosis, *FOCUS*, vol. 2, no. 1.

[9] McGlashan, H. T. and Hoffman, E. R. 2000, Schizophrenia as a Disorder of Developmentally Reduced Synaptic Connectivity, *Arc. Gen. Psychiatry*, vol. 57, pp. 637-648.

[10] Gumley, A., Braehler, C., Laithwaite, H., McBeth, A. and Gilbert, P., 2010, A Compassion Focused Model of Recovery after Psychosis, *International Journal of Cognitive Therapy*, vol. 3, no. 2, pp. 186-201.

[11] Morrison, P. A., Renton, C. J., Dunn, H., Williams, S. and Bentall, P. R. 2004, *Cognitive Therapy for Psychosis – A Formulation Based Approach*, Brunner – Routledge, New York.

[12] Amador, D. and David, A. (2004), *Insight and Psychosis – Awareness of Illness in Schizophrenia and Related Disorders*, Oxford University Press, New York.

[13] Nuevo, R., Chatterji, S.,Verdes, E., Naidoo, N., Arango, A. and Ayuso-Mateos, J.L. 2010, The Continuum of Psychotic Symptoms in the General Population: A Cross-national Study, Schizophrenia Bulletin, Available Online at: http://schizophreniabulletin.oxfordjournals.org/ content/early/2010/09/13/schbul.sbq099.full

[14] Turkington, D., Kingdon, D., Rathod, S., Wilcock, S., Brabban, A., Cromarty, P., Dudley, R., Gray, R., Pelton, J., Siddle, R. and Weiden, P. (eds) 2009, *Back to Life, Back to Normality*, Cambridge University Press, New York.

[15] Garety, A. P., Freeman, D., Jolley, S., Dunn, G., Beddington, E. P., Fowler, G. D., Kuipers, E. and Dudley, R. 2005, Reasoning, Emotions, and Delusional Conviction in Psychosis, *Journal of Abnormal Psychology*, vol. 114, no. 3, pp. 373-384.

[16] Van Lieshout, R. and Goldberg, O. J. (2007), Quantifying Self-Reports of Auditory Verbal Hallucinations in Persons with Psychosis, *Canadian Journal of Behavioural Science*, vol. 39, no. 1, pp. 73-77.

[17] McGorry, D. P. and Jackson, J. H. (eds) 2004, *The Recognition and Management of Early Psychosis - A Preventive Approach*, Cambridge University Press, Cambridge.

[18] Oorschot, M., Kwapil, T., Delespaul, P. and Myin-Germeys, I. 2009, Momentary Assessment Research in Psychosis, *Psychological Assessment*, vol. 21, no. 4, pp. 498-505.

[19] Jeste, V. D. and Glick, D. I. 2000, Editor's Introduction: Intervention Research in Psychosis: Past, Present and Future, *Schizophrenia Bullentin*, vol. 26, no. 3.

[20] Lebowitz, D. B. and Pearson, L. J. 2000, Intervention Research in Psychosis: Prevention Trials, *Schizophrenia Bulletin*, vol.26, no.3.

In: Psychosis: Causes, Diagnosis and Treatment
Editor: Xenia Anastassiou-Hadjicharalambous
ISBN: 978-1-62081-516-8


*Chapter 7*

# SEMANTIC MEMORY AND SYMPTOMATOLOGY IN SCHIZOPHRENIA: A REVIEW

***Keith R. Laws,*** [1,*] ***Verity C. Leeson,*** [2]
***Mohammed M. Al-Uzri*** [3,4] ***and Tejinder K. Kondel*** [1,5]
[1]School of Psychology, University of Hertfordshire, UK
[2]Centre for Mental Health, Imperial College London, UK
[3]Division of Psychiatry, University of Leicester, UK
[4]Leicestershire Partnership NHS Trust, Leicester, UK
[5]Parent-Infant Psychology Service, Whittington, UK

## ABSTRACT

This chapter reviews the past twenty years of research on semantic memory function in schizophrenia. This now substantial body of work has consistently documented abnormal semantic memory in most schizophrenia patients across a range of tasks (including priming, semantic fluency, picture naming) and which, varies from being quite mild through to some cases being indistinguishable from the impairment seen in Alzheimer's disease. Furthermore, although some patients have problems accessing intact semantics, others – possibly with longer illness duration - show an apparent loss of knowledge from the semantic store itself. While the abnormalities of semantic memory i.e. knowledge, offer a potential candidate of explanation for some symptoms, little work has examined the relationship between semantic memory and symptomatology.

In a manner of speaking
Semantics won't do…
I just want to say
That just like you I should find a way
To tell you everything
By saying nothing
(*In a Manner of Speaking,* Tuxedo Moon, 1985)

* E-mail: k.laws@herts.ac.uk

## INTRODUCTION

What is the meaning of the word 'love'? What is the capital of Peru? If we know the answers to these questions (or believe we know the answers), then that information resides within our semantic memory. Since the seminal work of [1], one of the most important distinctions in human memory is arguably that between episodic and semantic memory (see Table 1).

Episodic memory is autobiographical and assumed therefore, to vary between individuals, reflecting their differing personal experience e.g., I recall that I had scrambled eggs for breakfast.

By contrast, semantic memory is more invariant, shared across individuals and incorporates '...an organized body of knowledge involving words, concepts, their meanings, their associations, and the rules for manipulating these symbols and concepts' [2, p.377].

For example, that paella consists of rice, prawns, calamari, and mussels and so on, it is served in a large bowl and a staple food of many Spaniards, the word *Paella* derives from the Latin word *Patella* meaning 'pan' and so on. The basic units of semantic information are concepts referring to things such as animals or furniture, or ideas or facts (which are generated in the course of exposure to the environment).

These units comprise a series of exemplars grouped together into categories according to salient shared features: for instance, chair, table and sofa can be categorized as furniture.

**Table 1. Differences between Episodic and Semantic Memory (Modified from [1])**

| Episodic | | Semantic |
|---|---|---|
| Information | | |
| Source | Sensation | Comprehension |
| Units | Events, episodes | Facts, ideas, concepts |
| Organisation | Temporal | Conceptual |
| Reference | Personal | Universe |
| Veridicality | Personal belief | Social agreement |
| Operations | | |
| Retrieval query | Time? Place? | What? |
| Retrieval report | Remember | Know |
| Recollective experience | Remember past | Actualised knowledge |
| Registration | Experimental | Symbolic |
| Inferential capacity | Limited | Rich |
| Context dependency | More pronounced | Less pronounced |
| Affect | More important | Less important |

The organisation of this information is conceptual rather than temporal, so categorisation provides the structure of semantic memory. In a highly complex environment like ours, categorisation helps us to adapt and cope with the complexity of our surrounding [3]. Investigations of semantic memory developed along two main directions. First, experimental cognitive psychology informing us about semantic memory in the healthy individual and second, the neuropsychology of semantic memory, typically outlining what may be inferred from abnormal function in patients with neurological (typically individual case studies) and potentially psychiatric disorders, such as schizophrenia – in the case of the latter, being more recent and more contentious.

## A Case Study of Semantic Memory Impairment in Schizophrenia [4]

Within neuropsychology, semantic memory has traditionally been examined using single case studies, though far less in the study of people with schizophrenia. Nonetheless, a small number of in-depth case studies of semantic memory function in schizophrenia have been published.[4] reported a patient named DH, a 38-year-old single man with a diagnosis of schizophrenia, but who appeared to have a classic visual agnosia affecting his semantic knowledge and particularly for living things – a so-called category-specific deficit [see 5].

Patient DH

DH first presented to psychiatric services at the age of 24, where he was thought to be simply introverted and socially isolated. Twelve years later, however, he presented again with bizarre persecutory and referential delusions, third-person auditory hallucinations and other 'first rank' schizophrenic symptoms (thought broadcasting, thought insertion and thought withdrawal). His positive symptoms responded well to antipsychotic medication, but he remained severely impaired by negative symptoms. After spending time in a rehabilitation service, he eventually moved into hostel accommodation where he has lived ever since.

There was no significant medical history; DH has never had a head injury, and no history of drug or alcohol abuse. A CT scan revealed no gross abnormality, with DH's ventricles and sulci being within normal limits for his age; and a SPECT scan revealed no perfusion abnormality and temporal lobe perfusion that was within normal limits. DH was well-oriented and scored 29/30 on the Mini Mental State Examination [6]. His estimated premorbid NART IQ [7] was 81 and his current full-scale WAIS-R IQ was 69[8].

As assessed by the Visual Object and Spatial Perception Battery [9], DH's apperceptive and spatial perceptual skills were intact. Despite often reporting not knowing what a picture represented, DH copied line drawings with reasonable accuracy, even when the structural characteristics were quite complex (see Figure 1) and again, accords with his having intact apperceptive and spatial-perceptual skills and hence, his ability to form stable percepts.

By contrast, DH was impaired on all tasks requiring item recognition and this extended to his ability to name to verbal descriptions (correctly naming only 6/24 descriptions), indicating that his object identification problem extends beyond the visual modality.

DH was asked to name 260 line drawings and again, was severely impaired, naming less than 50% (119/260); however, it was notable that his naming of living things e.g. animals and fruits and vegetables (21% : 21/98) was much worse than for naming nonliving things (60.5%: 98/162).

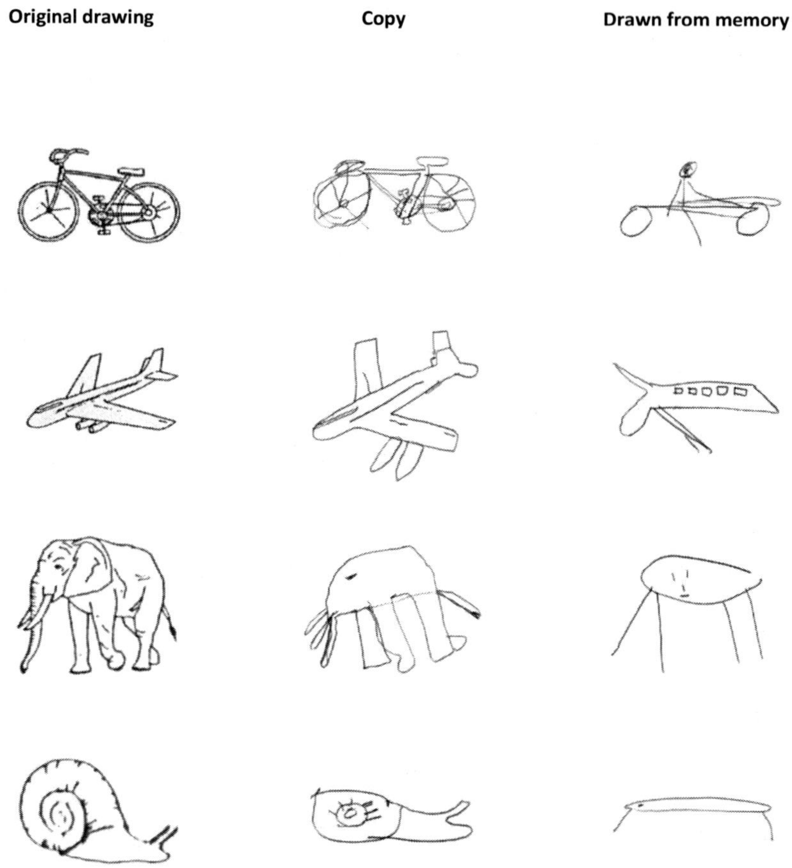


Figure 1. Examples of DH's Copy Drawing and Drawing from Memory.

He was further asked to name 3-dimensional models of animals to see if the additional visual information would aid recognition; however, he named only 2/16 (cow and dog) models; and his errors included: Panda →*dog*; Lion →*dog*; Giraffe →*different sort of horse*; Monkey →*horse*; and responding *don't know* for various animals including Horse, Elephant and Pig. DH also performed poorly on a less cognitively demanding word-picture matching task (i.e. not requiring name retrieval, but simply pointing to a named target amongst 5 pictures from the same category).

Again, DH showed much better performance with nonliving (42/60: 70%) than living (24/60: 40%) things. Hence, DH's problem extends to the simple task of matching a name with a target picture (amongst related distractors). DH was also asked to describe named items. Examples of his descriptions appear in Table 2. Manifestly, DH's definitions of living things were less detailed than for nonliving things and that DH's difficulty was not restricted to visual input.

**Table 2. Examples of DH's Descriptions to the Names of Living and Nonliving things**

| Living | Nonliving |
|---|---|
| Alligator – never heard of it. | Accordion – oh yeah, buttons. Piano. Played in pubs. Music sounds like folk music. (*Can you tell me anything else?*)... You put it over your neck with a strap. |
| Rhino - never heard of it. | Helicopter – flies in the air. |
| Swan – swims in the water (*anything else, what does it look like?*) no (*what colour is it?*) white. | Rolling pin – to do with cookery. For making pastry. |
| Lobster – fish. | French horn – musical instrument. |
| Fox – 4 legs. | Motorcycle – drives and wears a helmet. Makes a noise. Has wheels. |
| Penguin – bird or chocolate (*can you describe the bird called penguin?*)... no, nothing. | Spinning wheel – goes round |

Overall, DH's deficit shows striking similarities with the type of central semantic impairment observed in visual agnosias following neurological damage to the temporal lobes.

Moreover, the deficit has a category-specific profile [see 3] consistently affecting one category (living things) more than another (nonliving things). A recent review of the neuroanatomical loci relating to such category effects, [10] identified bilateral damage to the inferior temporal lobes and medial structures (hippocampus, amygdala, parahippocampal gyri) as common in such disorders.

Indeed, the most consistent findings to emerge from a recent meta-analysis of 15 voxel-based morphometry (VBM) studies in schizophrenia[1] [11] was a relative reduction in the volume of the left superior temporal gyrus and the left medial temporal lobe - largely confined to the left medial temporal lobe (in nine of 13 studies) rather than the right medial temporal lobe (three of 13 studies).

Using a case-study approach, [12] examined the extremely thought disordered patient TC (for examples of speech, see Table 3), who showed a significant semantic memory impairment. Looking at TC's speech, the presence of an abnormality in semantics seems inescapable. On neurocognitive testing, TC's naming ability was inconsistent across both time and modality (i.e. to-picture and to-description).

[1] VBM is a technique for estimating the density or volume of grey matter (or white matter) and typically, involves a voxel–by-voxel comparison of grey matter for two groups of subjects or a correlation between volume and task performance.

## A Case Study of How Semantic Memory Relates to Formal Thought Disorder

> Patient TC
>
> TC is a 38-year-old man who has suffered from schizophrenia from his late teenage years. His birth and early life were normal and he did quite well academically at school (achieving four 'O' levels). Shortly afterwards, however, he began to do poorly and failed his 'A" levels. By the age of 19 he had become withdrawn, was unable to work, and was admitted to hospital, where he showed persecutory and grandiose delusions, delusions of control and third-person auditory hallucinations. He had a number of relapses and remissions, but never recovered fully. Ultimately, he became chronically hospitalised. The patient has been in a stable clinical state for 7-10 years. His presentation is dominated by grossly thought-disordered speech, associated with ill-formed delusional preoccupations revolving around heaven and John Lennon; he also alludes to auditory hallucinations from time to time and these are superimposed on a moderately severe negative symptom "defect state"

He also showed a severe comprehension deficit that was highly variable across time. Further testing revealed that the comprehension deficit did not reflect a disorder of working memory, but stemmed directly from impaired access to word meaning. They concluded that a central semantic memory deficit would most parsimoniously account both for TC's expressive and receptive language problems and that this deficit reflected a disorder of semantic *access* rather than a degradation of the semantic knowledge base itself. Five years later [13], TC showed a remarkable improvement in his thought disorder symptoms. Having previously produced grammatically well-formed, but completely incoherent speech, TC had had begun to speak rationally without immediately drifting off into unrelated topics [13] therefore administered the same battery of tests to TC and his comprehension of language showed a marked and significant improvement with the remitting of his major symptom. Although TC's naming did not improve, it did become more consistent and finally, he showed a residual tendency to accept false information in silly sentences tasks. Crucially then, at least *some* of the semantic problems appear to be causally related to the symptom – possibly affecting comprehension more than any other aspect of semantic processing.

Moreover, these findings indicate that while *some* aspects of the semantic disorder are state related (to the symptoms) others may be traits of schizophrenia *per se*. While case studies of cognitive function are almost the main method for studying cognitive problems in neurological patients, such case studies are infrequent in the study of psychiatric disorders. Nonetheless, these two cases patently document – in the case of DH, a profound and highly specific (category-specific) semantic agnosia; and in the case of TC, a clear link and moreover, the breaking of the link between semantic memory deficits and thought disorder symptoms.

The next section of this chapter surveys the evidence for semantic memory deficits in schizophrenia and the final section outlines a new study examining the relationship between a wide range of semantic memory tests and symptoms in a relatively high functioning group of patients.

**Table 3. Examples of TCs Responses to Silly Sentences**

| | |
|---|---|
| Forks have windows | Yes they do. Augmented pretension. Four plus four equals sixteen. It's a larger element, it's photographic and phototropic, but it's a higher number, higher course-work. It grows through evaporation or nocturnalism, it's sleepy, you rediscover it and I suppose forks could have windows through evaporation. |
| Forks are used for fuel | Yes, they add up and kind of like a solution. It's say, it's an equine or equinox, like fungi. Something in the brain tells you it's a high number. Bacteriology, a numerate number, it's a particle, therefore it contains solution is to answer the right question. A fork is a solution, an aqueous solution. Fork in a kettle, something brittle, do hairs bristle on a comb or fungi? It could be naval or positive solution ratified, like a kettle, if kettle is the right answer. It could be 8th or 7th one right? Brown aqueous solution inside the kettle |
| Cups have a head | Yes, but a faulty one, there's nothing there. It's like latent vaporism, it could be there or not. Like a con-layer, a further learning primate |

## NAMING

Picture naming has been the most common test used to assess the intactness of semantic knowledge in various pathological groups e.g. Alzheimer's disease [14]. In a recent meta-analysis, [15] reported that only 13 of 22 (59%) studies documented naming impairments in schizophrenia patients. Despite apparent inconsistencies, however, the overall effect size across studies was extremely large ($d$ = 1.45) "*...even if performance had been reported to be preserved*" [15]. Translating this effect size into the so-called 'Common Language Effect Size' [16] reveals that 85% of schizophrenia patients name fewer items than controls. The contrast between statistical significance and effect size points to a considerable number of studies with small samples that undoubtedly lack sufficient power to detect real differences. In the two largest studies [4, 17] examining 55 patients and 22 controls in the former and 54 patients and 24 controls in the latter, the effect sizes were large at 1.32 and 1.49 respectively (following Cohen's nomenclature 0.2 = small; 0.5 = medium and 0.8 = large). Examining naming of 120 colour pictures, [4] found as many as three-quarters of the schizophrenic sample showed impaired naming (scoring $<5^{th}$ percentile of healthy controls); and moreover, in 15% of cases, the deficits were category-specific (i.e. significantly greater in one category than another). Indeed, in six patients, the category deficit was highly selective and produced a *classical* dissociation i.e. patients were impaired in one category and within the normal range for the other category [see 18]. Moreover, all of the patients showing category effects continued to show the same effect when re-tested 2-4 months later. This evidence is, if anything, stronger than that often presented in neurological cases with category deficits [19].

**Table 4. Example Responses to the Silly Sentences Test [from 20]**

| Sentences | Explanation |
|---|---|
| Rats have teeth (replied false) | *'Because I don't think they do have teeth'* |
| Owls have blades (replied true) | *'To fly with'* |
| Beefsteaks crawl on their bellies (replied true) | *'A cow is still alive before it's slaughtered, so it could be true, they could crawl on their bellies a bit'* |
| Admirals have fins (replied true) | *'Because they go on the ocean where fish are'* |
| Crows are in charge of ships (replied true) | *'In the crow's nest'* |

Hence, a proportion of schizophrenic patients presenting with such deficits parallel the findings documented in the context of neurological pathology (e.g. herpes simplex encephalitis, dementia of the Alzheimer's type and so on) who present with category deficits. This level of specificity suggests that, in some schizophrenia patients (as many as 15%) lexical-semantics are not compromised in a generalized fashion, but that some semantic categories are affected more than others – a category-based disorder such as this one is difficult to reconcile with anything other than a semantic disorder.

## Silly Sentences

[20] used the "silly sentences" test [after 21] to assess semantic memory in their cohort of schizophrenics. This task involves either accepting or rejecting various statements such as "rats have teeth" and "grapes are people". Not only did the patients prove to be slower than the normal group with over 60% falling outside of the normal range altogether, they also tended to make more errors in their verifications. Nearly one-quarter of the sample made three or more errors and the trend was towards verifying false statements as true rather than rejecting true statements (see Table 4 for example responses). By contrast, using 143 silly sentences, [22] somewhat surprisingly reported no differences in overall accuracy between 63 schizophrenic patients and 66 controls. Why the general null finding contrasts with several previous reports, [20, 23, 24], is unclear, but one possibility relates to the high levels of education (mean 13.9 years) and intelligence (mean 113.9) in their patient group. Indeed, Rossell and colleagues had screened-out patients with lower IQ. Importantly, however, they did find that deluded patients were more likely to accept sentences congruent (and reject sentences incongruent) with the themes of their abnormal beliefs (classified as persecutory, grandiose, political, religious, relationships and somatic).

## Fluency: Problems with Semantic Disorganisation

Models designed to account for the semantic deficit evident in schizophrenia (and in particular, thought disordered speech) rely on long established network theories of semantic memory [25]. Such models assume that semantic knowledge is organised as a network of associated concepts, which represent memory as nodes, and relations as the associative pathways between the nodes. In a similar vein, schizophrenia patients may have semantic networks that are, in some way, different from that seen in healthy individuals. Idiosyncratic organisation within the network or an abnormal pattern of spreading between nodes would also account for the incoherent, tangential speech observed in individuals with FTD. [26] proposed that unfocussed activation and disorganisation distinguish the networks of schizophrenic patients and Goldberg and colleagues have more recently championed this notion as an explanation for FTD [e.g. 27]. One common method to investigate the structure of semantic networks in schizophrenia patients has been through verbal fluency, which appears to be both impaired *and* anomalous for both semantic (category) and phonemic (letter) tasks ([28-34]). Beyond the poverty of output, it is also possible to say something about the organisation of responses in fluency tasks in schizophrenia patients. Patients often produce inappropriate words during semantic fluency [35] e.g. *potato* for the category of fruits, possibly indicating abnormal semantic boundaries in schizophrenia [see also 36].

Further, [35] estimated the size of the lexicon to be intact in schizophrenic patients, suggesting inefficient retrieval and search strategies, rather than a loss of semantic knowledge itself. An attempted replication by [37]; however, produced quite contrary results with patients and controls producing comparable numbers of inappropriate semantic fluency items and moreover, they concluded that the lexicon size was indeed compromised in patients. Fluency in patients with schizophrenia has produced one of the largest effect sizes amongst neurocognitive tests [38]. [39] meta-analysed 30 studies using both phonemic and semantic fluency in a total of 1633 schizophrenics, with large effect sizes emerging for both ($d$=0.95 and $d$=1.12 respectively and semantic fluency being significantly more impaired). Similarly, [40] reported effect sizes of $d$ =0.99 and 1.27 respectively in 13 studies and over 900 schizophrenic patients. [39] also reported that both fluency effect sizes were highly correlated with WAIS IQ. Furthermore, longer illness duration was associated with worse semantic fluency (but not phonemic fluency). Interestingly negative symptoms (Scale for the Assessment of Negative Symptoms [SANS] [41]) and not positive symptoms (Scales for the Assessment of Positive Symptoms [SAPS] [41]) correlated with phonemic, but not semantic fluency - which is consistent with proposed links between negative symptoms and frontal lobe dysfunction [see 42].

Studies have often, although not always, reported significant correlations between negative symptom scores and impairment on a range of executive tests [e.g. 43], and the correlation is substantiated by a meta-analysis of 40 studies of various fluency measures revealing a correlation of -.27 [44]. Finally, a meta analysis of 8 semantic fluency studies comparing relatives of schizophrenics with unrelated controls [45] revealed a large effect size (*Hedges' g* =0.87), thus pointing to semantic fluency being a potential familial trait characteristic [see also 46]. Some evidence also suggests that fluency problems in schizophrenia might act as an endophenotype manifesting itself even in those who are not ill, but who are first-degree relatives of the affected. Various studies have reported impaired semantic fluency in the healthy siblings of people with schizophrenia, suggesting that that poor fluency may be a familial trait characteristic. A meta-analysis of eight semantic fluency studies comparing siblings of schizophrenics with controls [46] reported a large effect size (*hedges g*=.87). While several meta-analyses have documented various cognitive deficits in the first degree relatives of patients [46 and 47], unfortunately no other aspects of semantic memory have been examined. Some have reported that while fluency performance in schizophrenic patients is worse than controls, both groups perform better on the semantic fluency than the phonological fluency [31, 48, 49]. Others, however, have reported that schizophrenics show the reverse pattern whereby phonological fluency performance is superior to semantic fluency performance [30, 31, 50].

In addition, the magnitude of the *difference* between semantic fluency and phonological fluency may significantly correlate with global FTD ratings [51], indicating that greater difficulty searching through semantic memory is associated with increased FTD. [31], however, did not find that semantic fluency was associated with FTD ratings although the authors concede that [51] used a more comprehensive FTD measure. [40] carried out a meta-analysis of studies examining phonological and semantic fluency, of which five studies had examined this phenomenon in relation to FTD. They report that, out of these, three did not support a correlation between disproportionately impaired semantic fluency and FTD. These differing results make it impossible to draw any conclusion from these studies; however, the authors comment that " ...these results must be considered in light of restriction in range of thought disorder, difficulty in its reliability rating, and the rather small cohorts in the studies that assess the relationship" [40,p.76]. While semantic fluency impairments often exceed those for phonemic fluency in schizophrenia and other conditions such as Alzheimer's disease [14], the same pattern emerges in normal healthy ageing [14,52-54]. Therefore, directional differences in semantic and phonemic fluency may be less informative than previously suspected; rather the patients are showing some exaggeration of the normal profile rather than a qualitatively different profile.

Another methodological approach to detecting semantic abnormalities has been with multidimensional scaling and clustering techniques, which examine the 'distance' between word pairs in a semantic fluency paradigm. In semantic fluency tasks, individuals typically report exemplars in subgroup clusters e.g. pets, wild animals, exotic animals, birds, insects and so on [55]. The clustering patterns are typically analysed using multi-dimensional scaling (MDS) and consistently reveal less coherent semantic clusters in schizophrenia patients than healthy controls [33,56-60]. For example, [56] found that goodness of fit measures were high for healthy individuals, suggesting category exemplars (animals) were generated in an organised manner along two semantically organised dimensions - domesticity and size. Conversely, schizophrenics had low goodness of fit scores and appeared not to be using semantically organised dimensions for generation in the same way as normal subjects. They concluded, "...patients with schizophrenia...appear to lack organisation and logical associations within their semantic network" (p.271). In an identical paradigm, [33] also reported the same two dimensions of domesticity and size in healthy individuals, while for schizophrenics, the dimension of size was not evident in the networks of many of the patients [see also 61]. In a unique attempt to dissociate symptoms and semantic memory deficits, [62] employed a double-blind crossover study. Hence, some patients started medication free and then went onto receive medication, while others received a placebo. No significant changes in performance occurred for the Boston Naming test, word and semantic fluency, the Peabody word-picture matching task and the Token Test of comprehension. Nonetheless, on an intra-categorical priming task, clinically rated FTD symptoms correlated inversely to performance, with the degree of improvement for highly related intra-categorical prime-target pairs correlating with improvement in TD symptoms. Interestingly, symptom improvement was associated only with performance on an automatic, implicit task and not on those requiring conscious, explicit responses. The authors suggest that this reflects the fact that the patients who showed the most reduction in FTD became more able to capitalise on semantic relatedness to improve RT.

## Battery Approaches

One widely held view of semantics proposes that the input from different sense modalities is stored in a unitary system in which all information, regardless of the modality of access or acquisition, is stored together [63]. Although some have argued for separate but interconnected modality-based stores of knowledge [64], the often striking item-to-item correspondence of errors across modalities (e.g. on tests of naming-to-definition versus picture naming), the loss of an item from a single semantic store for all modalities would seem more parsimonious. Hence, studies will inevitably be limited in conclusions when using single rather than multiple tasks. Indeed, we will argue below that converging evidence is required from a variety of tests in order to determine if, for example, patients have difficulty accessing semantics or a disorder of the semantic store itself. Using a comprehensive battery, [65] assessed semantic memory in patients with schizophrenia. The *Cambridge Semantic Memory Test Battery* (CSM) consists of five tests [66 see Table 5]. Three of the tests (picture naming, picture sorting, and word-picture matching tests) employ one consistent set of stimuli, designed to assess input to and output from central representational knowledge about the same group of items through visual and verbal modalities; and the remaining two are naming to definition and category fluency. [65] found that, on many of the semantic tests, a group of elderly schizophrenics performed at a level similar to that of patients with mild to moderate Alzheimer's disease. Two further groups of schizophrenics - a mild group who had relapsing and remitting episodes (but were able to live independently) and a core group who were younger (but had unremitting illness) - also showed semantic memory deficits.

As expected, the deficits were less severe in the mild group, with the core group displaying impairment intermediate between the elderly and mild groups, thus highlighting the potentially crucial role played by severity and chronicity of illness in the level of semantic memory impairment.

Additionally, they showed that the semantic deficits were not a simple facet of intellectual functioning (current or estimated premorbid), stating that "...significant impairment on the semantic memory test battery could be found in patients with *preserved intellectual function, no matter how strictly this was defined*" (our italics).

Employing the CSM battery, [68] reported significantly worse category fluency and naming-to-description in younger schizophrenics (mean age =34.9) patients than controls. The remaining tests (picture naming, word-picture matching and sorting) failed to reveal significant differences; however, at least for picture naming, this may reflect low power as the effect size was 0.73.

Further, no significant correlations emerged between severity of symptoms (using the Brief Psychiatric Rating Scale [69]) and performance on any aspect of the semantic memory battery, though this may well also reflect the small sample size. In a further study using the CSM, [70] compared a group of 20 schizophrenia patients with 22 Alzheimer's Dementia (AD) and 15 elderly healthy controls. The profile of semantic memory performance for the AD group indicated marked impairment on all tests, whereas the profile for chronic schizophrenia was more uneven.

Based on this, the authors argued that, unlike the AD group, the semantic impairment in schizophrenia patients did not result from a degraded store. On subordinate sorting and the Camel and Cactus pictures and words[2], schizophrenic patients produced error rates significantly greater that healthy controls, but did not differ from the AD group.

By contrast, for picture naming, word–picture matching and superordinate category sorting, AD patients made significantly more errors than schizophrenic patients (Cohen's *d* >.8). Indeed, schizophrenics performed at a level similar to that of the healthy controls; however, this finding may reflect the influence of substantial ceiling effects on these tests[3]. Doughty and colleagues propose that such an uneven profile (in the schizophrenia group) does not accord with a degraded semantic store disorder (as per the consistent and widespread impairment in the AD group).

**Table 5. Cambridge Semantic Memory Battery [67] (CSM)**

| | |
|---|---|
| 1. | Category fluency. Subjects generate as many items as they could from the category of animals in one minute. |
| 2. | Picture naming. Subjects asked to name line-drawn items on 48 cards. |
| 3. | Word to picture matching. The subjects point to a named item from an array containing six items from the same category. |
| 4. | Naming to description. Subjects hear descriptions of 24 different living and man made items and are asked to give the name. |
| **5.** | Picture sorting. Subjects asked to sort the same 48 cards (used in the 2nd and 3rd tests) into: (a) Level one (superordinate) - living (24 items) vs. manmade (24 items). (b) Level two (categories) - the living items into land animals, birds, and water creatures, the manmade items into household items, musical instruments and vehicles. (c) Level three (subordinate) - the land animals into native vs. foreign to Britain, and the household items into electrical vs. non-electrical items |

Nevertheless, this seems a somewhat premature conclusion given the ceiling effects on several tests preventing the finding of any impairment on those tests. At a general level, the problem of ceiling effects on such tasks stems inevitably from their being primarily devised

[2] This task is similar to the Pyramids and Palm Trees test – requiring participants to match a target picture or name with one of two distracters e.g. Camel goes with Cactus or Fir Tree.

[3] Indeed, the authors removed control data from their analyses for this reason; and used a log-linear transform of the patient data.

for use with those who have dementia[4]. Nevertheless, when comparisons are required with controls (which is almost always) or with less severely impaired patients, then analyses will be detrimentally affected by the ceiling effect (regardless of transforming the data) and the use of nonparametric statistics generally reduces power and makes the use of covariates complex. One solution, however, is to use boostrapping techniques and we will return to these later.

## Biased or Distorted Semantic Memory Rather than a Loss of Knowledge?

Semantic memory functioning may not simply be impaired, characterised by low scores on relevant tasks, but it may also be anomalous. As indicated in [71], it may be necessary to "take the unprecedented step of beginning to think in terms of a neuropsychological function that is heightened, biased, distorted or otherwise deranged rather than being merely compromised" (p. 170). In the context of anomalous semantics, [72,73] first examined the notion of overinclusiveness in the thinking of people with schizophrenia. Cameron had patients sort objects into groups and noted that they exhibited "*an inability to maintain the boundaries of the problem and to restrict their operation within its limits*". The result was the expression of ideas that appeared vague and could cause the mental set of the speaker to cease to correspond to that of the listener. Payne and co-workers followed up this work with a range of experimental paradigms examining overinclusion [74]. They used tasks such as requiring synonyms for words and sorting pictures into conceptual categories, which revealed that schizophrenics were significantly more overinclusive than healthy controls and non-psychotic psychiatric controls. Of additional interest was the finding that acute schizophrenics were more overinclusive than those with established schizophrenia. This finding stands out against the vast majority of studies proposing that established schizophrenia is associated with more severe deficits. Studies reporting overinclusiveness in schizophrenia patients [76, 75] imply a *qualitative* abnormality in how semantics information is accessed and so, goes beyond any simple *quantitative* changes in semantic activation.

Disorganisation of the semantic system may allow insight into how thought disorder manifests as deviant understanding as well as abnormal speech production since it implies that the associative pathway between semantic nodes are not stable or reliable. [76] examined the time taken by schizophrenics to decide whether an item is a member of a conceptual category (i.e. is a robin a bird?). Not only were the patients slower to make this type of judgement than controls, but they took the longest to process related items that were outside of the category (e.g. aeroplane for the bird category), while controls took the longest over borderline, atypical category members (e.g. penguin for the bird category). Furthermore, the schizophrenic group were more likely to verify non-category members as belonging to that category, indicating an outward shift of the category boundary. An attempted replication and extension of the original study [77], however, failed with schizophrenic patients exhibiting normal representations of category boundaries for words and picture stimuli. Although

[4]Even this assumption is unwarranted given that neuropsychologists are typically looking at a performance profile across a range of tests and so, it is crucial to know if the pattern mirrors or deviates from that expected in healthy normal individuals (see Laws 2005 for striking examples).

Elvevåg and colleagues gave no specific reason for the difference across studies, they proposed that semantics is intact, while ‘movement’ between concepts is impaired. The notion of overinclusion also fails to receive support from [78] in their word search study, where participants searched for a target word or member of a category within lists. Using a search list with words that were either semantically related or unrelated to the target item, Gurd and colleagues found that patients made most errors when the non-target words were semantically unrelated to the target item. By contrast, performance was better when the non-target words were drawn from a related superordinate category (for example, search for *any boat* amongst trailer, tank, helicopter, *canoe*, coach). They propose a selective lexical-semantic parallel processing deficit underpins word-finding aberrations in schizophrenia.

## Semantic Priming

Most semantic memory research paradigms rely upon so-called “off-line” tasks that require conscious, strategic semantic processing (see Figure 3). In other words, individuals need consciously to generate the semantic information on tasks such as naming items, giving descriptions, generating exemplars from a given set, drawing from memory and so on. By contrast, so-called “on-line” tasks assess semantic knowledge in ways that does not require the conscious accessing of that knowledge.

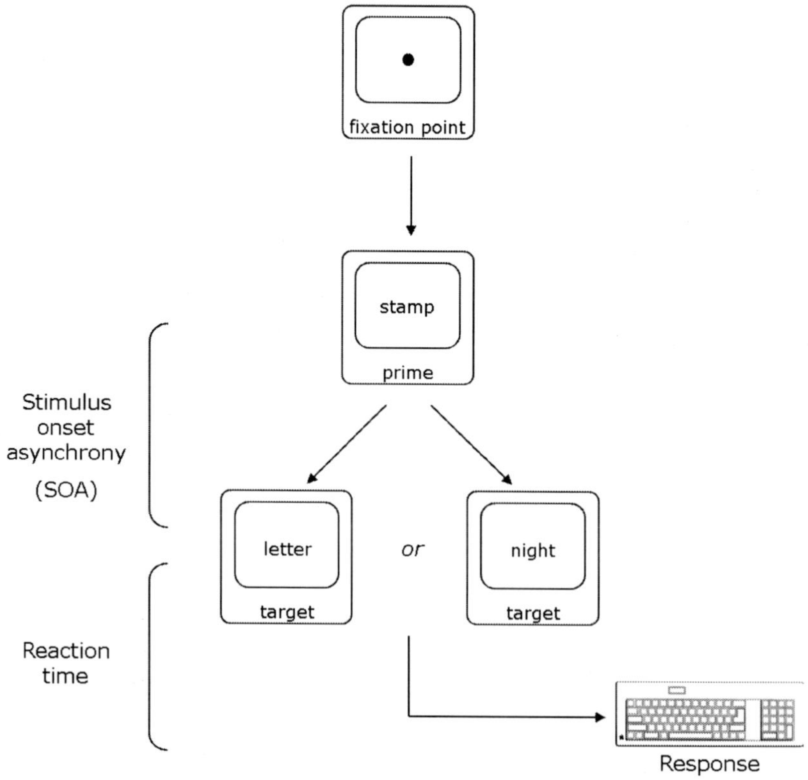


Figure 3. Standard Lexical Decision Task.

To achieve this end studies typically employ priming techniques. Priming involves assessing the level of assistance that one word (the prime) imparts to the processing of another word (the target) - and this *assistance* is viewed as a measurement of their proximity within semantic space.

Typically participants are asked to perform a lexical decision task (is the word real or not?) or simply asked to pronounce sequences of presented words. The facilitation effect is the decrease in reaction time to pronounce a word or recognise a string of letters as a real word, when a semantically related prime is presented compared with an unrelated prime. For example, the prime-target pairing *lemon-sour* would result in faster responding than *lemon-bus*. Additionally, because of the assumed associations of concepts within networks, activation may spread, not only to directly related concepts, but also to concepts that are more distant.

Some studies have utilised this and employed an indirect priming condition whereby, for example, the word *lemon* activates the related concept *sour*, which, in turn activates *sweet* resulting in *lemon* priming *sweet* (see below).

Since the earliest investigation by [79], more than 30 studies of semantic priming in schizophrenia have emerged. These studies have investigated whether semantic priming is altered in schizophrenia per se, as well as focussing specifically on patients with the symptom of thought disorder. Recent meta-analyses have agreed that semantic priming is not significantly impaired in schizophrenia – [80] reported $d$= 0.07 (in 36 studies in direct priming) and [13] reported $d$ = 0.028 (in 81 studies combining direct and indirect priming – see below). Reviewing 23 schizophrenia studies, [81] remarked that studies had described increased, normal *and* reduced semantic priming, and further that '*it is presently unclear how semantic priming disturbances (should they be reliably demonstrated) may be related to thought disorder as manifested clinically*'. They also noted that few studies had corrected for a well-recognised psychometric artefact produced by general slowing of reaction times in schizophrenia – if schizophrenics are simply slower to respond on both the unprimed and primed versions of the task, this will inflate priming - even if the proportional change is the same. To take an example, owing to a simple arithmetical artefact: the difference between a mean reaction time of, say, 900 ms in the unprimed condition and 600 ms in the primed condition is numerically greater than that for the difference between, say, values 600 ms and 400 ms in controls, even though the proportional increase is the same. [80] directly examined the latter point in their meta-analysis of 29 priming studies in schizophrenics, where they reported that general slowing was a significant moderator of effect size ($Z$=2.82, $p$=0.004), with the greater the slowing the greater the amount of priming. This also held true in the comparison between patients with thought disorder and controls (for 16 studies $Z$=3.23, $p$=0.001). In their original study, [79] used a short prime–target interval or stimulus onset asynchrony (SOA) of 250 ms, designed to capture the 'automatic' process of spread of activation in semantic memory. Nonetheless, it is now recognized that slower, so-called 'controlled' processes, also contribute to the phenomenon of semantic priming; and the basic priming design has been subjected to many variations with some studies employing long (>400ms) SOAs (see Table 7). In their meta-analysis, [13] found a significant difference between the studies that used short SOAs ($d$ =0.17, n=34,) and the studies that used long SOAs ($d$=0.06, n=22), although both effect sizes were clearly very small.

## Table 6. Main findings from Semantic Priming Studies

| Study | Task | Prime (ms) | ISI (ms) | Direct priming | Indirect priming | Number of Participants |
|---|---|---|---|---|---|---|
| | | SOA | | | | |
| Aloia et al, 1998 [56] | WP | Terminated by saying | 350 | TD group showed less priming than NTD and NC. | - | 9TD, 11NTD, 21NC |
| Barch et al, 1996 [86] | WP | 100 | 200-950 | All groups showed at short SOA, but only controls showed at long SOA | - | 34TD, 56NTD, 10PC, 28NC |
| Barch et al, 1999 [119] | WP<br>LD | 100 | 200/850 | For WP found in NC, but not sz at short and long SOA For LD found in sz and NC at short SOA but only NC at long SOA. | - | 56sz, 25NC |
| Besche-Richards and Passerieux, 2003 | LD | 250 | 250 | Found in TD and NC when high number of related pairs but only in NC for low number of related pairs | - | 15sz, 15NC |
| Besche et al, 1997 [87] | LD | 250 | 250 | Found in NTD and NC but not in TD. | - | 24TD, 10NTD, 15PC, 40NC |
| Blum and Freides 1995 [88] | LD | 100 | 250 | Found in TD, NTD and NC. | - | 10TD, 10NTD, 11HC |
| Chapin et al, 1989 | LD | 3500 +TARGET | | Found in sz, PC and NC | × | 12sz, 12PC, 12NC |
| Chapin, et al, 1992 [94] | LD | 3500 +TARGET | | Found in NC and sz. | × | 45sz, 15NC |
| Gouzoulis-Mayfrank et al, 2003 | LD | 200 | 500 | Found in NC, TD and NTD but greater in TD | All groups including TD showed no evidence | 60sz, 20NC |
| Henik et al, 1992 [96] | LD | 140 | 100/ 1700 | Found in NC and TD at long SOA. TD showed reduced priming at short SOA. | - | 22sz, 17NC |
| Henik et al, 1995 | LD | 140 | 100/ 1700 | Increased in sz compared to NC | - | 16sz, 16NC |
| Manschreck et al, 1988 | LD | 250 | - | Found in TD, NTD and NC. TD fastest overall | - | 12TD, 6NTD, 9PC, 11NC |
| Moritz et al, 2001a | LD | 200 | 0 | Found in TD, NTD and NC. | TD showed enhanced indirect priming compared to NC and NTD | 16TD, 28NTD, 36PC, 30NC |
| Study | Task | Prime (ms) | ISI (ms) | Direct priming | Indirect priming | Number of Participants |
| | | SOA | | | | |
| Moritz et al, 2001b | WP | 200 | 0 | TD showed greater priming than NC or PC. | - | 15TD, 30NTD, 30NC |

| Study | Task | Prime (ms) | ISI (ms) | Direct priming | Indirect priming | Number of Participants |
|---|---|---|---|---|---|---|
| | | SOA | | | | |
| Moritz et al, 2002 | WP | 200 | 0 | Found in NC, NTD and TD when neutral baseline used. Only in TD and NC when unrelated baseline used | TD showed enhanced indirect priming compared to NC and NTD | 12TD, 20NTD, 65NC |
| Ober et al, 1995 [95] | LD<br>WP | 50 | 200 | Found in sz and NC. | - | 19sz, 22NC |
| Ober et al, 1997 | LD | 60 | 200/ 940 | Found in NC in both conditions. Found in sz when high number related pairs and long SOA only. | - | 31sz, 20NC |
| Passerieux et al, 1995 | LD | 64/240 | - | No sig priming found in any group or condition | - | 17sz, 11NC |
| Passerieux et al, 1997 [89] | LD | 450 | 50 | Found in NTD and NC but not in TD. | - | 11TD, 11NTD, 11HC |
| Spitzer et al, 1993a [90] | LD | 200 | 0/500 | Found in TD, NTD and NC. | Found in all groups at long SOA but only TD at short SOA | 29TD, 21NTD, 32NC |
| Spitzer et al, 1993b [93] | LD | 200 | 0/500 | Found in sz and NC. | Found in sz and NC, but only sz at short SOA | 32sz, 32NC |
| Spitzer et al, 1994 [91] | LD | 200 | 0/200/ 500 | Found in NTD and NC, greater in TD. | - | 36TD, 34NTD, 44NC |
| Vinogradov et al, 1992 | LD<br>WP | 50 | 200 | Found in NC for LD and WP. Only found in sz for WP. | - | 50sz, 50NC |
| Weisbrod et al, 1998 [92] | LD | 250 | 0 | Found in TD, NTD and NC. Greater in TD group. | Found in TD only | 16TD, 24NTD,38NC |

*Note.* LD: lexical decision WP: word pronunciation ISI: inter stimulus interval SOA: stimulus onset asynchrony NC: normal controls PC: psychiatric controls TD: thought disordered NTD: non-thought disordered sz: schizophrenic ×: not examined ✓: examined SOA is time between the presentation of the prime and the presentation of the target (i.e. prime presentation time + inter stimulus interval).

## Indirect Semantic Priming

An alternative to the traditional priming paradigm, widely used in the schizophrenia literature, is indirect priming. In this version of the semantic priming paradigm the target and prime words are only indirectly related, typically via a mediating word; e.g., lemon → sweet (mediating word *sour*), black → chalk (mediating word *white*). This experimental design aims to examine the hypothesis that activation of associations is not just greater than normal in schizophrenia, but that it extends to associations that are far more distant. This paradigm has been used particularly to examine whether the odd speech displayed by thought-disordered patients reflects overactive semantic networks, which would therefore be more sensitive to indirect priming.

Turning to the relationship with symptoms, Spitzer argues that the priming paradigm shows "conclusive evidence that FTD schizophrenic patients suffer from an increased activation and/or decreased inhibition of the semantic network" [82].

Furthermore, when [83] manipulated the stimulus onset asynchrony (SOA: the interval between onsets of prime and target) thought disordered patients showed an advantage at short SOA, whereas controls and non thought-disordered patients showed an effect at the longer SOA. This finding suggests that semantic activation in thought disorder may occur through normal networks, but reaches distant concepts more quickly since non-thought disordered patients and normal controls experienced the same priming effect when more time was allowed for the semantic activation to spread further. In their review of all priming in FTD [84] identified eight studies examining priming in FTD, and reported a small effect that is in the opposite direction to that predicted by the increased spreading activation hypothesis.

Indeed, five studies reported hypopriming (i.e. less facilitation on trials using related pairs than in the comparison group: [85-89] and three reported hyperpriming (i.e. more facilitation on trials using related word pairs than in the comparison group:[90-92]).

A more recent meta-analysis of nine studies, [80] found $d$ =0.19 (95% CI 0.03 to 0.36), which although small does represent a significant increase. Crucially however they further examined six of the nine studies involving comparisons of thought disordered patients and controls, and in these the effect size was much larger ($d$=0.56 [95% CI 0.31 to 0.80]). A fundamental question addressed specifically by the priming literature is whether the semantic abnormality affects automatic, controlled processing or both.

Crucially, of course, priming studies bypass issues relating to effort or motivation, as responses are implicit rather than explicit. A myriad of methodological issues surround this type of task and may influence performance, however.

Therefore, despite the large number of published studies using priming tasks with schizophrenic patients, drawing any unassailable conclusions from the results is a difficult venture given the range of objectives, cohorts and methodologies employed. While some support exists for the notion that automatic, preconscious processing is selectively more affected [89,93] others have failed to find evidence in favour [94,95].

Nonetheless, since spreading semantic activation theories of language production propose that speech relies mostly on unconscious, automatic activation, it follows that a symptom characterised by abnormal speech i.e. FTD, is more likely to be associated with abnormal automatic semantic memory processing.

Indeed, the studies reported above do provide stronger evidence for a selective impairment of automatic processing in FTD patients [96,83] than schizophrenia *per se*.

## Access Versus Storage Disorders

Researchers into the neuropsychology of semantic memory have used a model proposed by [97], which proposes two distinct patterns of semantic memory impairment: firstly, degraded stores type disorder (knowledge is lost), and secondly, impaired accesses type disorder (knowledge exists, but the retrieval process is compromised).

The criteria for both models are summarised in Table 7. The validity of this distinction has been occasionally disputed [98]; however, these two patterns of semantic memory impairment in neurological disorders have achieved wide acceptance in the literature. For instance, in a study of semantic memory deficit in Alzheimer's disease, [67] concluded that Alzheimer's disease is a degraded store type disorder. These conclusions were based on observation of consistency across different tests (modalities) and level of superordinate knowledge affected. The access-storage distinction has both theoretical and clinical implications. A degraded store type disorder will imply loss of the representation, which means that interventions will be, more or less, damage limitation; and the best one can hope for is to prevent further loss of the representation.

**Table 7. Access and Store Disorders Criteria [after 97]**

| Store disorder | Access disorder |
|---|---|
| High consistency with the same items across time and different tests. | Inconsistent pattern of performance across different testing times and task. |
| Ineffectiveness of priming and cueing techniques to aid retrieval'. | Improved performance with cueing and priming |
| Less familiar/frequent items are lost first; more frequent items presumably have a larger representation, which make them last to be affected. | Item familiarity/frequency effects are less apparent; as the representation exists for both familiar and less familiar items, there is less apparent difference between assessing frequent and non-frequent items than in store disorder. |
| Subordinate, or attribute information is especially affected; as it represents the most specific and potentially unique information. By contrast, superordinate information will be the least and last affected, as it represents the most general information processed and the most represented. | Subordinate attribute knowledge is likely to be less affected; after obtaining the superordinate information, obtaining subordinate information should be not as much problem as it is in store disorder, because the representation still intact. |

By contrast, in access type disorder the representation is intact and interventions should target enhancing the access to the representation. Consequently, knowing the type of the disorder would be very useful in planning interventions for those patients to enable them to function at their optimal level.

Several studies have described the type of the deficit seen in schizophrenia as one of accessing semantic information [35,49,90], with patients sometimes being able and at others are unable to access information. By contrast, others report an actual loss of semantic knowledge (also-called store type: [37, 99, 100]). A common denominator that emerges is that studies of relatively young patients point to access type disorder, while studies of older patients with longer illness duration suggest a picture of degraded store disorder (see Table 8). Of particular interest in this regard, [35] examined verbal fluency consistency across five times to determine the numbers of shared and unique words to generate an estimate of lexicon size. Compared to depressed patients and healthy controls, schizophrenics generated fewer clusters of related words and more words outside of the specified category; however, the number of variable words did not differ from controls and [35] concluded that the schizophrenics had impaired access to an *intact* semantic store.

In relation to symptoms, lower levels of fluency were associated with negative features and incoherence was associated with the production of inappropriate words – neither of which is surprising given that the symptoms and measures are, to some extent, synonymous. By contrast, in a replication, [37] reported a reduced size for the lexical-semantic store. Interestingly, the patients examined by [35] were somewhat younger than those examined by [37] (mean age 35 vs. 42) and also had a shorter duration of illness – thus raising the possibility that problems of accessing the lexicon may evolve into problems with store itself as the disorder progresses.

In addition, [101] studied the performance of thirty schizophrenic patients on a lexical decision task in a semantic priming paradigm. They reported that the length of illness was associated with reduced priming effect, which is an access criterion. This important observation raises the possibility that a *process* may occur by which aging and increased chronicity alter the clinical picture from meeting the criteria of an access disorder into one that meets the criteria for a degraded store disorder.

While it remains possible that access and storage disorders exist separately and do not change across time in patients with schizophrenia, reports consistently point to a store disorder in older chronic samples and an access disorder in younger less chronic samples (see Table 8). The possibility that the two types of disorders might represent different stages of the illness, arguably gains some support from a previous report of a mixed picture of access and store – like profiles that related to overall level of cognitive impairment [102]. They suggested that, specifically in schizophrenia, patient performance might vary along a dimension of deficit severity rather than a dichotomous separation of access and store disorders. This picture of variable performance across a continuous dimension accords more with a gradual *process* than a dichotomy model, which indicates two separate categories.

Analysing naming consistency across 2 - 4 months, [17] used a two parameter stochastic Markov chain model [103] to estimate probabilities for an individual having a named stored (s) and then for being able to retrieve (r) the item from store[1]. Interestingly, for the patients,

---

[1] For each subject, two probabilities [r] and [s] were calculated using the stochastic model (Faglioni and Botti, 1993). Probability [r] signifies the likelihood that a stored representation would be accessed and probability [s]

intelligence (IQ) significantly influenced storage but not retrieval. Patient length of illness also significantly influenced both storage and retrieval, indicating a small reduction in the semantic store in patients with longer illness duration (estimated at approximately 1% store loss every three years and an additional 1% retrieval loss every 5 years). These findings indicate that storage and retrieval decline in parallel and in proportion over the course of the illness rather than, for example, supporting a transition from retrieval problems to storage problems.

**Table 8. Studies of Type of Semantic Memory Deficit in Schizophrenia according to Age**

| Study | Test | Type | Mean age (years) |
|---|---|---|---|
| Spitzer et al, 1993 [93] | Priming | Access | 27 |
| Al-Uzri, Laws and Mortimer 2004 [68] | Picture naming | Access | 34.9 |
| Allen, Liddle and Frith, 1993 [35] | Fluency | Access | 35 |
| Joyce, Collinson and Crichton 1996 [49] | Fluency | Access | 36 |
| Rossell and David 2006 | Definitions, categorising, Semantic priming, synonyms and word associations | Store | 36.4 |
| Laws, McKenna and Kondel, 1998 [102] | Picture naming, consistency, cueing, familiarity | Access or storage depends on level of deficit | 41 |
| Chen et al 2000 [37] | Fluency | Store | 42.3 |
| Laws, Leeson and McKenna, 2006 [4] | Picture naming across consistency after 2-4 months | store | 43.1 |
| Laws, Al-Uzri, Mortimer, 2000 [106] | Picture naming, frequency, consistency | Largely store | 46 |
| Doughty et al, 2008 [70] | Picture Naming, Sorting, Word-Picture Matching, Camel and cactus test | Access | 51 |
| McKay et al, 1996 [65] | Fluency, Picture Naming, Sorting, Word-Picture Matching, Definitions | Similar to Alzheimer i.e. Store | 64-72 |
| Kondel et al 2006 [99] | Relearning names with cueing over 2 months | Store | 75 |

reflects the integrity of the semantic store itself. A probability of 1 indicates no impairment. Values for [s] and [r] probabilities were calculated using the following formulae: Retrieval probability [r] = 2S2/S1+2S2; Storage probability [s] = S1+2S2 /2r.

[4] examined the relationship between formal thought disorder (FTD) and picture naming. They tested picture naming in 16 schizophrenic patients with high FTD ratings, 16 schizophrenic patients with low FTD ratings and 16 healthy controls. As expected, the two patient groups had impaired naming, but the impairment was significantly greater in high than low FTD patients. Moreover, the high FTD patients showed a profile that differed from both the low FTD patients and the healthy controls insofar as their naming was inconsistent across time, characteristic of an access disorder. They calculated storage and retrieval probabilities based on the model outlined earlier[103]. Analysis of the relationships between specific FTD symptoms and naming revealed several positive FTD symptoms associated with the probability of name retrieval - including derailment, tangentality and incoherence (with higher symptom ratings predicting greater difficulties accessing the lexical–semantics in each case). Intriguingly, all three symptoms relate to aspects of FTD where words, phrases or ideas occur in an oblique or unrelated manner. The two other symptoms of FTD (illogicality and pressure of speech) that were not associated with retrieval probability - are distinct in that they do not appear to reflect speech that contains words, phrases or ideas that show reduced associations. Pressure of speech was the only variable that significantly predicted the estimated number of names stored - such an association is not readily explained by existing theories of lexical–semantic dysfunction in FTD such as disorganised activation of the semantic memory network [62] or increased activation of this network [104]. The authors speculate that the relationship between pressure of speech and certain lexical–semantic processes may be more relevant to another aspect of psychopathology, for example, elevated mood and it may be that elevated mood is associated with poorer encoding at storage or even a permanent loss of representations from the lexical–semantic store. So, it seems that different aspects of thought disorder symptoms may be underpinned by quite different, albeit related, lexical-semantics deficits.

With this in mind, models of disorganised activation of the semantic network in patients with FTD [26,105] may provide an explanation for the findings. [105] describe the erroneous performance of thought-disordered schizophrenics as "the result of local biases that change on a moment to moment basis." Disorganisation that is not static would probably present as access disorder-like performance and thus, the access disorder characteristics reported in high FTD patients [4] accords with this notion of disorganised semantic activation. Moreover, if one were to attempt to predict the abnormalities in speech that would result from disorganised activation within the semantic memory network, those where words, phrases or ideas occur in an oblique or unrelated manner would be obvious candidates.

Access and storage disorders may also map onto the ability of patients to live and function independently in the community. In the [106] study, which is suggestive of access type disorder, the sample was largely community dwelling and even the inpatients were in community-based rehabilitation units, while in the [100] study, a largely store disorder emerged in the more chronically hospitalised patients. Furthermore, [102] reported that all the chronically hospitalised patients displayed a store-like profile, and the community dwelling-patients showed an access profile or a mixed picture.

The significance of the access-storage dimension may have important implications for tailoring care profiles to different *types* of patients. It also raises a related issue, which is the possibility that appropriate and speedy intervention in community-dwelling and quite well patients may impede or stop any transition from access to store like disorder.

## Executive Function and Inhibition

Several authors have suggested that the boundary knowledge and categorisation anomalies reported in schizophrenia may reflect a dysexecutive problem rather than a semantic disturbance *per se* [51,107]. Executive function is an umbrella term to cover a huge array of cognitive and behavioural factors. Executive function unquestionably plays a significant role in both the searching and retrieval of information from semantics. Nowhere is this clearer than in the studies of fluency (as noted above), where phonemic fluency deficits are associated with unilateral left frontal damage, and semantic fluency is impacted by both temporal and frontal lesions, being somewhat larger in the former than the latter [108]. Two particular aspects of executive functions that may be relevant to semantic functioning here - rather than an impairment of the semantic representations themselves (e.g., [107, 109, 111]) - are both the ability to *shift* between semantic categories and the ability to *inhibit* inappropriate responses. Whilst *inhibition* describes a multitude of processes, cognitive and indeed otherwise (e.g. behavioural), it is pivotal to the control of undesired responses, and this obviously includes verbal responses – as is most apparent on tasks such as the Stroop and the Hayling Sentence Completion task. In a direct examination of the role of executive function on categorisation, [110] found that schizophrenia patients performed worse on a variety of semantic tasks - including sorting - when compared not only to healthy controls, but crucially to individuals with acquired brain injury (ABI) who showed prominent executive dysfunction. The schizophrenia patients were matched to the ABI group for level of executive dysfunction and so, [110] argue that the semantic impairment in schizophrenia does not result from an executive dysfunction. They reported no significant differences between the ABI and control group on semantic measures and concluded "People with acquired brain injury (ABI) and a prominent executive dysfunction …showed intact semantic memory ability" (p.177). Despite this, the brain-injured group was clearly much worse than the control group with large effect sizes[2] and nonsignificant inferential statistics pointing to the study being underpowered to detect semantic problems in the brain-injured group. We cannot therefore (from this study) conclude that executive dysfunction plays little or no role in semantic memory problems.

A large literature, normally viewed as more relevant to executive function than semantic in schizophrenia, is that involving the Stroop task. While the Stroop task is typically viewed as a measure of executive function, it undoubtedly involves the inhibition of heightened automatic lexical-semantic responses; and as such, has relevance to models suggesting that schizophrenia may be associated with overactive semantic networks (e.g [112]). A recent meta-analysis of 36 schizophrenia studies revealed a *Hedges' g* of 0.62 for accuracy and 0.43 for response time [113] indicating moderate interference effects. The inhibition of prepotent or salient lexical-semantic responses are clearly abnormal in schizophrenia and potentially related to symptoms including hallucinations [114] and thought disorder[112]. Using a novel Stroop-like paradigm [111] examined the relatedness of prepotent and required responses in patients with high and low FTD and healthy controls. Participants viewed two visual stimuli and were required to respond to each with a newly learned name (see Figure 2 below). Six conditions were examined, with four necessitating the *inhibition* of a prepotent semantic

[2] Naming 0.9; word-picture matching 0.5; sorting -1.0; semantic associations (pictures) 0.97; and semantic associations (words) 1.0).

response while varying the relatedness of prepotent and required responses i.e., identical, semantically related, or unrelated. Two further conditions examined working memory demands by requiring the naming of 'real' or 'abstract' pictures that do and do not necessitate inhibition, respectively. Both the control and the low-FTD groups were significantly slower when the prepotent response was identical or semantically related to the (incorrect) required response compared to when they were unrelated.

| **Condition** | **Working memory** | **Inhibition** | **Prepotent and incorrect required response** | **Response choice** | **Primes** | **Required response** |
|---|---|---|---|---|---|---|
| INH1 | Yes | Yes | Identical | Semantically related | | *"sun"* *"moon"* |
| INH2 | Yes | Yes | Identical | Unrelated | | *"book"* *"car"* |
| INH3 | Yes | Yes | Semantically related | Unrelated | | *"fork"* *"chair"* |
| INH4 | Yes | Yes | Unrelated | Unrelated | | *"tree"* *"cat"* |
| MEM | Yes | No | - | - | | *"fox"* *"dog"* |
| NAM | No | No | - | - | | *"cup"* *"plate"* |

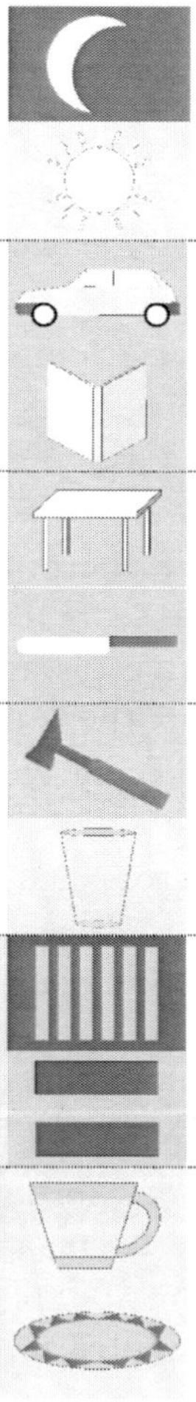

Figure 2. Inhibition conditions developed by [111].

By contrast, high-FTD patients showed no difference in RT between the identical, semantically related, or semantically unrelated conditions but made significantly more errors in the semantically related condition. The pattern of errors shown by high FTD suggested that they experience the automatic activation – or 'pop-up' of semantically related representations [cf. 115] and [111] interpreted their findings as supporting the notion that *increased* inhibition underpins the disorganised access to semantic memory in patients with FTD.

Crucially, the findings of [111] were extended by [116] using the same paradigm in a sample of 41 chronic patients and 25 healthy controls. [116] similarly found that schizophrenia patients were impaired when inhibiting a semantically associated response. Moreover, they reported that semantic memory performance correlated significantly with psychomotor poverty (negative) more than disorganisation or reality distortion symptoms [117]. Indeed, abnormal inhibition underpins models proposing both semantic disorganisation and increased spreading of activation in schizophrenia. These two models, however, occupy opposing perspectives - with disorganisation believed to reflect *increased inhibition* and increased spreading activation putatively reflecting *reduced inhibition*. Neither has a clear outcome, since studies examining inhibition have returned conflicting results with reports of increased inhibition [118], reduced inhibition [119] and indeed, no evidence for impaired inhibition at all [120,121]. Reduced cognitive inhibition has long been thought to contribute to the development of positive symptoms [122] and the *filter deficit* theory of schizophrenia, proposed that the deficiency was with the mechanism that "*controls and limits the contents of consciousness*" (p. 225). Nonetheless, when specific symptoms, such as FTD have been examined, the link to abnormal inhibition has been reported by some [e.g.119] and not others [114]. Similarly, we could view auditory hallucinations as intrusive thoughts that arise because of some difficulty with inhibition; however, the role of inhibitory processes in auditory hallucinations has also failed to receive support from studies using negative priming [123] and interference [124] paradigms. Nonetheless, others have documented a relationship between auditory hallucinations and inhibition. For example, [114] used the Hayling Sentence Completion task, where individuals have to complete the last word of a sentence but using a word that does not make sense e.g. the cat sat on the …[light bulb] – the task requires voluntarily suppressing active mental representations in semantic memory (i.e. mat). In a later study employing directed forgetting and updating working memory paradigms, [125] found a highly specific association between inhibition and hallucinations. They reported no correlations between their indices of intentional inhibition and either negative or positive symptoms per se, but did with hallucinations; and they propose that hallucinations reflect problems in suppressing mnestic representations. The varied findings might relate to the conceptual distinction drawn between automatic and intentional forms of inhibition [126], Therefore, any failure of previous studies to establish a relationship between inhibition and symptoms may be because they have used paradigms assessing automatic inhibition. For example, hallucinations are clearly consciously experienced mental events and as such, may reflect abnormal functioning of intentional inhibition processes. This of course contrasts with priming and the link with symptoms, where automatic effects are seen to link with symptoms– especially FTD. Interestingly [127] had also demonstrated that while FTD was associated with no difference between related and unrelated priming conditions, patients with hallucinations showed normal priming. Hence, different symptoms may correspond with different kinds of inhibition difficulties.

As noted above, a key issue concerns the relationship between semantic memory and the striking symptomatology associated with schizophrenia (including *positive* symptoms such as hallucinations, delusions and thought disorder as well as the *negative* symptoms of withdrawal, lack of volition, lack of speech and so on). For some time it has been argued that individuals with schizophrenia have disturbed knowledge about the world [128] and that some of their symptoms would seem to be prime candidates to be linked to disorders of knowledge i.e. a semantic memory abnormality. As outlined above, support for this link does exist with symptoms such as thought disorder [12, 20, 31,129] and delusions [22, 130]. The number of studies examining the relationship has been surprisingly few and some of the strongest evidence comes from in-depth single case studies examining associations between semantic measures and specific symptom types [12,130].

## REFERENCES


[1] Tulving, E. Episodic and semantic memory. In E. Tulving and W. Donaldson (Eds.), Organization of memory, (pp. 381–403). New York: Academic Press (1972).

[2] Nebes, R.Semantic memory in Alzheimer's disease. *Psychological Bulletin*, 106 (3), 377-394 (1989).

[3] Chen E, McKenna P J, and Wilkins A. Semantic Processing and Categorisation in Schizophrenia In: Sims A. (ed). *Speech and Language Disorders in Psychiatry.* Gaskell, The Royal College of Psychiatrists, 126-137 (1995).

[4] Laws KR, Leeson VC and McKenna PJ. Domain-specific deficits in patients with schizophrenia. *Cognitive Neuropsychiatry,* 11, 537-556 (2006).

[5] *Laws*, KR, Adlington, R.L., *Moreno*-Martínez F.J. and *Gale*, T.M. *Category-Specificity: Evidence for Modularity of Mind.* Nova. (2011).

[6] Folstein, M.F., Folstein, S.E., and McHugh, P.R. "Mini-mental state". A practical method for grading the cognitive state of patients for the clinician. *Journal of Psychiatric Research,* 12(3), 189-198 (1975).

[7] Nelson, H. E. *National Adult Reading Test (NART).* Windsor: NFER Nelson (1982).

[8] Wechsler, D. *Manual for the Wechsler Adult Intelligence Scale—Revised.* Psychological Corporation, New York (1981).

[9] Warrington EK, James M. *The Visual Object and Space Perception Battery.* Thames Valley Test Company. Bury St Edmunds. (1991).

[10] Gainotti, G. What the locus of brain lesion tell us about the nature of the cognitive defect underlying category-specific disorders: a review. *Cortex,* 36, 539-559 (2000).

[11] Honea R, Crow TJ, Passingham D, Mackay CE.. Regional deficits in brain volume in schizophrenia: a meta-analysis of voxel-based morphometry studies. *American Journal of Psychiatry.* 162, 2233–2245 (2005).

[12] Laws, K.R., Kondel, T.K., McKenna, P.J. Receptive and Expressive language Disorders in Schizophrenic Thought Disorder: Impaired Semantic Access and Monitoring. *Cognitive Neuropsychiatry,* 4, 89-106 (1999).

[13] Leeson VC, McKenna PJ, Murray G, Kondel TK, Laws KR "What happens to semantic memory when formal thought disorder remits? Revisiting a case study." *Cognitive Neuropsychiatry* 10(1):57-71 (2005).

[14] Laws, KR, Duncan, A and Gale, T.M 'Normal' semantic-phonemic fluency discrepancy in Alzheimer's disease? A meta-analytic study. *Cortex,* 46, 595-601 (2010).

[15] Doughty OJ, Done DJ. Is semantic memory impaired in schizophrenia? A systematic review and meta-analysis of 91 studies. *Cognitive Neuropsychiatry*;14:473–509 (2009).

[16] McGraw, K. O., and Wong, S. P. A common language effect size. *Psychological Bulletin,* 111, 361-365 (1992).

[17] Leeson, V.C., McKenna, P.J., and Laws, K.R Storage and Access Procedures in Schizophrenia: Evidence for a Two Phase Model of Lexical Impairment. *Journal of Clinical and Experimental Neuropsychology*, 27 (6):700-701 (2005).

[18] Shallice, T. (1998). *From Neuropsychology to Mental Structure*. Cambridge: Cambridge University Press.

[19] Laws, KR. Illusions of Normality: A Methodological Critique of Category-Specific Naming. Cortex, 41, 842-851 *[Lead article with peer commentaries]* (2005).

[20] Tamlyn, D., McKenna, P.J., Mortimer, A. N., Lund, C. E., Hammond, S., and Baddeley, A.D. Memory impairment in schizophrenia: It's extent affiliations and neuropsychological character. *Psychological Medicine*, 22: 101-115. (1992).

[21] Collins, A. M., and Quillian, M. R. Retrieval Time from Semantic Memory. *Journal of Verbal Learning and Verbal Behavior*, 8, 240-247 (1969).

[22] Rossell, S.L., Shapleske, J., and David, A.S. Sentence verification and delusion: a content specific deficit. *Psychological Medicine*, 28, 1189-98 (1998).

[23] Clare L, McKenna P J, Mortimer A M, and Baddeley A D. Memory in Schizophrenia: what is impaired and what is preserved. *Neuropsychologia* 31(11), 1225-1241 (1993).

[24] Duffy L and O'Carroll R. Memory Impairment in Schizophrenia – A Comparison with that observed in the Alcoholic Korsakoff Syndrome. *Psychological Medicine,* 24(1), 155-65 (1994).

[25] Collins, A.M. and Loftus, A.S. A spreading activation theory of semantic processing. *Psychological Review*, 82, 407-428. (1975).

[26] Hoffman, R.E.. Computer simulations of neural information processing and the schizophrenia/mania dichotomy. *Archives of General Psychiatry*, 44, 178-187 (1987)

[27] Goldberg, T.E. and Weinberger, D.R. Thought disorder in schizophrenia: A reappraisal of some older formulations and an overview of some recent studies. *Cognitive Neuropsychiatry*, 5, 1-19. (2000).

[28] Arango, C. Bartko, J.J. Gold J.M. and Buchanan, R Prediction of neuropsychological performance by neurological signs in schizophrenia. *Am. J. Psychiatry*, 156 1349–1357. (1999).

[29] Egan, M.F. Goldberg, T.E. Gscheidle, T. Weirich, M. Rawlings, R. Hyde, T.M. Bigelow L. and Weinberger, D.R. Relative risk for cognitive impairments in siblings of patients with schizophrenia. *Biol. Psychiatry*, **50** 98–107. (2001).

[30] Feinstein, A., Goldberg, T.E., Nowlin, B. and Weinberger, D.R. Types and characteristics of remote memory impairment in schizophrenia. *Schizophrenia Research*, 30, 155-163. (1998).

[31] Kremen, W.S., Seidman, L.J., Faraone, S.V. and Tsuang, M.T. Is there disproportionate impairment in semantic or phonemic fluency in schizophrenia? *Journal of the International Neuropsychological Society*, 9, 79-88. (2003).

[32] Laurent, A Biloa-Tang, M. Bougerol, T. Duly, D. Anchisi, A.-M. Bosson, J.-L. Pellat, J. d'Amato T. and Dalery, J. Executive/attentional performance and measures of schizotypy in patients with schizophrenia and in their nonpsychotic first-degree relatives. *Schizophr. Res.*, 46 269–283(2000).

[33] Paulsen, J.S., Romero, R., Chan, A., Davis, A.V., Heaton, R.K., and Jeste, D.V. Impairment of the semantic network in schizophrenia. Psychiatry Research, 63(2-3), 109-121. (1996).

[34] Zakzanis, K.K. Troyer, A.K. Rich J.B. and Heinrichs W., Component analysis of verbal fluency in patients with schizophrenia. *Neuropsychiatry Neuropsychol. Behav. Neurol.*, **13** 239–245 (2000).

[35] Allen, H. A., Liddle, P.F., and Frith, C.D.. Negative features, retrieval processes and verbal fluency in schizophrenia. *British Journal of Psychiatry,* 163, 769-775 (1993).

[36] Moelter ST, Hill SK, Hughett P, Gur RC, Gur RE, Ragland JD. Organization of Semantic Category Exemplars in Schizophrenia. *Schizophrenia Research* 78: 209–217 (2005).

[37] Chen, R.Y.L., Chen, E.Y.H., Chan, C.K.Y., Lam, L.C., and Lieh-Mak, F.. Verbal fluency in schizophrenia: reduction in semantic store. *Australian and New Zealand Journal of Psychiatry*, 34 (1), 43-48. (2000).

[38] Heinrichs, R.W., Zakzanis, K.K. Neurocognitive deficits in schizophrenia: a quantitative review of the evidence. *Neuropsychology* 12, 426– 445 (1998).

[39] Henry J.D., and Crawford J.R. A meta-analytic review of verbal fluency deficits in schizophrenia relative to ther neurocognitive deficits. *Cognitive Neuropsychiatry* 10, 1-33 (2005).

[40] Bokat C.E., and Goldberg, T.E. Letter and category fluency in schizophrenic patients: a meta-analysis, *Schizophrenia Research* **64** 73-78 (2003).

[41] Andreasen N.C. and Olsen S. Negative vs positive schizophrenia. *Archives of General Psychiatry,* 39, 789-794. (1982).

[42] Ziauddeen H, Dibben C, Kipps C, Hodges JR, and McKenna PJ Negative schizophrenia symptoms and the frontal lobe syndrome: one and the same? *Eur Arch Psychiatry Clin Neuroscience* 26 1:59-67. (2010).

[43] Donohoe G, Robertson IH. Can specific deficits in executive functioning explain the negative symptoms of schizophrenia? A review. *Neurocase* 9:97–108 (2003).

[44] Dibben CR, Rice C, Laws K, McKenna PJ Is executive impairment associated with schizophrenic syndromes? A meta-analysis. *Psychological Medicine*, 39:381–392 (2009).

[45] Szöke A, Schurhoff F, Mathieu F, Meary A, Ionescu S, Leboyer M. Tests of executive functions in first-degree relatives of schizophrenic patients: a meta-analysis. *Psychological Medicine*, 35: 771–82. (2005).

[46] Snitz BE, Macdonald AW III, Carter CS. Cognitive deficits in unaffected first-degree relatives of schizophrenia patients: a meta-analytic review of putative endophenotypes. *Schizophrenia Bulletin* 32:179-194. (2006).

[47] Sitskoorn MM, Aleman A, Ebisch SJ, Appels MC, Kahn RS. Cognitive deficits in relatives of patients with schizophrenia: a meta-analysis. *Schizophrenia Research*, 71(2-3):285-295. (2004).

[48] Elvevåg, B., Weinstock, D.M., Akil, M., Kleinman, J.E. and Goldberg, T.E. (A comparison of verbal fluency tasks in schizophrenic patients and normal controls. *Schizophrenia Research*, 51, 119-126. (2001).

[49] Joyce EM, Collinson S L and Crichton P. Verbal Fluency in Schizophrenia: Relationship with Executive Function, Semantic Memory and Clinical Alogia. *Psychological Medicine,* 26(1), 39-49. (1996).

[50] Gourovitch, M., Goldberg, T.E. and Weinberger, D.R. Verbal fluency deficits in patients with schizophrenia: Semantic fluency is differentially impaired as compared with phonological fluency. *Neuropsychology*, 6, 573-577. (1996).

[51] Goldberg T E, Aloia M S, Qourovitch M L, Missar D, Pichard D, and Weinberger D R.Cognitive Substrates of Thought Disorder, 1: The Semantic System. *American Journal of Psychiatry*, 155(12), 1671-1676. (1998).

[52] Crossley, M., D'arcy, C., and Rawson, N. S. B. Letter and category fluency in community-dwelling Canadian seniors: A comparison of normal participants to those with dementia of the Alzheimer or vascular type. *Journal of Clinical and Experimental Neuropsychology*, 19, 52–62. (1997).

[53] Kozora E and Cullum CM. Generative naming in normal aging: Total output and qualitative changes using phonemic and semantic constraints. *The Clinical Neuropsychologist*, 9: 313–320, (1995).

[54] Tomer R and Levin BE. Differential effects of aging on two verbal fluency tasks. *Perceptual and Motor Skills*, 76: 465–466, 1993.

[55] Troyer, A. K. Normative data for clustering and switching on verbal fluency tasks. *Journal of Clinical and Experimental Neuropsychology*, 22, 370-378. (2000).

[56] Aloia, M.S., Gourovitch, M.L., Weinberger, D.R., and Goldberg, T.E. An investigation of semantic space in patients with schizophrenia. *Journal of the International Neuropsychological Society,* 2(4), 267-273. (1996).

[57] Moelter, S.T., Hill, S.K., Ragland, J.D., Lunardelli, A., Gur, R.C., Gur, R.E., and Moberg, P.J. Controlled and automatic processing during animal word list generation in schizophrenia. *Neuropsychology,* 15(4), 502-509. (2001).

[58] Rossell, S.L., Rabe-Hesketh, S., Shapleske, J., and David, A.S. Is semantic fluency differentially impaired in schizophrenic patients with delusions? *Journal of Clinical and Experimental Neuropsychology,* 21(5), 629-642. (1999).

[59] Sumiyoshi, C., Matsui, M., Sumiyoshi, T., Yamashita, I., Sumiyoshi, S., Kurachi, M.Semantic structure in schizophrenia as assessed by the category fluency test: effect of verbal intelligence and age of onset. *Psychiatry Research*, 105, 187– 199. (2001).

[60] Sumiyoshi C, Sumiyoshi T, Nohara S, Matsui M, Kurachi M, Niwa S. Disorganization of semantic memory underlies alogia in schizophrenia:An analysis of verbal fluency performance in Japanese subjects. *Schizophrenia Research*, 74, 91-100 (2005).

[61] Tallent, K.A., Weinberger, D.R. and Goldberg, T.E. Associating semantic space abnormalities to formal thought disorder in schizophrenia: Use of triadic comparisons. *Journal of Clinical and Experimental Neuropsychology*, 23, 285-296. (2001).

[62] Goldberg, T.E., Dodge, M., Aloia, M., Egan, M.F. and Weinberger, D.R. Effects of neuroleptic medications on speech disorganisation in schizophrenia: biasing associative networks towards meaning. *Psychological Medicine*, 30, 1123-1130. (2000).

[63] Caramazza A., Hillis A E., Rapp B C. and Romani C. The multiple semantic hypotheses: multiple confusion? *Cognitive Neuropsychology*, 7, 161-189. (1990).

[64] McCarthy R A and Warrington E K. Evidence for modality-specific meaning systems in the brain. *Nature*, 334, 428-430. (1988).

[65] McKay, A.P., McKenna, P.J., Pentham, P., Mortimer, A. N., Holbery, A. and Hodges, J.R. Semantic Memory is Impaired in Schizophrenia. *Biological Psychiatry*, 39: 929-37. (1996).

[66] Adlam AL, Patterson K, Bozeat S, and Hodges JR. The Cambridge semantic memory test battery: detection of semantic deficits in semantic dementia and Alzheimer's disease. *Neurocase* 16,193–207. (2010).

[67] Hodges J R, Sellman D P and Butters N. Semantic Memory Impairment in Alzheimer'sDisease: failure of Access or Degraded Knowledge? *Neuropsychologia*, 30 (4), 301-314. (1992).

[68] Al-Uzri MM, Laws KR and Mortimer AM An early marker for semantic memory impairment in patients with schizophrenia. *Cognitive Neuropsychiatry,* 9(4), 267-279. (2004).

[69] Overall J E and Gorham D R The Brief Psychiatric Rating Scale. *Psychological Reports*, 10, 799-812. (1962).

[70] Doughty, O.J., Done, D.J., Lawrence, V.A., Al-Mousawi, A., Ashave, K., Semantic memory impairment in schizophrenia — deficit in storage or access of knowledge? *Schizophrenia Research* 105, 40–48 (2008).

[71] McKenna P J, Mortimer A M and Hodges J R. Semantic Memory and Schizophrenia. In: David A S and Cutting J C (eds), The Neuropsychiatry of Schizophrenia Lawrence Erlbaum Associates Ltd.163-178. (1994).

[72] Cameron, N. Schizophrenic thinking in a problem solving situation. *Journal of Mental Science*, 85, 1012-1035. (1939).

[73] Cameron, N. Language and thought in schizophrenia. In Kasanin, J.S. (Eds.), *Language and thought in schizophrenia* (pp.50-63). Berkeley: University of California Press. (1954).

[74] Payne, R.W. Handbook of abnormal psychology. In Eysenck, H.J. (Eds.), *Handbook of abnormal psychology* (pp.420-483). London: Pitman (1973).

[75] Harrow, M., and Quinlan, D. *Disordered Thinking and Schizophrenic Psychopathology.* New York, NY: Gardner Press (1985).

[76] Chen E, Wilkins A, and McKenna P J. Semantic memory is both impaired and anomalous in Schizophrenia. *Psychological Medicine,* 24(1), 193-202 (1994).

[77] Elvevåg, B., Weickert, T., Wechsler, M., Coppola, R., Weinberger, D.R., Goldberg, T.E. An investigation of the integrity of semantic boundaries in schizophrenia. *Schizophrenia Research*, 53, 187-198 (2002).

[78] Gurd, J.M.M., Elvevåg, B. and Cortina-Borja, M. Semantic category word search impairments in schizophrenia. *Cognitive Neuropsychiatry*, 2, 291-302. (1997).

[79] Manschreck, T.C., Maher, B.A., Milavetz, D.A., Weisstein, C.C. and Schneyer, M.L.Semantic priming in thought disordered schizophrenic patients. *Schizophrenia Research*, 1, 61-66. (1988).

[80] Pomarol-Clotet, E., Oh, TM., Laws, K R and McKenna, PJ. Semantic Priming in Schizophrenia: A Meta-Analysis. *British Journal of Psychiatry,* 192, 92-97. (2008).

[81] Minzenberg M, Ober BA, Vinogradov S. Semantic priming in schizophrenia: a review and synthesis. *J. Int. Neuropsychol. Soc.* 8: 699–720 (2002)

[82] Spitzer, M., Beuckers, J., Maier, S. and Hermle, L. `Contextual Insensitivity in Schizophrenic Patients Is Due to Semantic Network Pathology: Evidence From Pauses in Spontaneous Speech', *Language and Speech* 37: 171-185.(1994).

[83] Spitzer, M., Braun, U., Hermle, L. and Maier, S. Associative semantic network dysfunction in thought disordered schizophrenic patients: direct evidence from indirect semantic priming. *Biological Psychiatry*, 34, 864-877. (1993a).

[84] Kerns, J.K. and Berenbaum, H. Cognitive impairments associated with formal thought disorder in people with schizophrenia. *Journal of Abnormal Psychology*, 111, 211-224 (2002).

[85] Aloia, M.A., Gourovitch, M., Missar, D., Pickar, D., Weinberger, D.R. and Golberg, T.E. Semantic abnormalities in schizophrenia: II. A candidate cognitive mechanism. *American Journal of Psychiatry*, 155, 1677-1684. (1998).

[86] Barch, D.M., Cohen, J.D., Servan-Schreiber, D., Steingard, S., Steinhauer, S.S.A. and Van Kammen, D.P. Semantic priming in schizophrenia: an examination of spreading activation using word pronunciation and multiple SOAs. *Journal of Abnormal Psychology*, 105, 592-601. (1996).

[87] Besche, C., Passerieux, C., Segui, J., Sarfati, Y., Laurent, J. and Hardy-Bayle, M.C.Syntactic and semantic processing in schizophrenic patients evaluated by lexical decision tasks. *Neuropsychology*, 11, 498-505. (1997).

[88] Blum, N. and Freides, D. Investigating thought disorder in schizophrenia with the lexical decision task. *Schizophrenia Research*, 16, 217-224. (1995).

[89] Passerieux, C., Segul, J., Besche, C., Chevalier, J.F., Widlocher, D. and Hardy-Bayle, M.C. Heterogeneity in cognitive functioning of schizophrenic patients evaluated by a lexical decision task. *Psychological Medicine*, 27, 1295-1302. (1997).

[90] Spitzer, M., Braun, U., Hermle, L., and Maier, S. Associative semantic network dysfunction in thought-disordered schizophrenic patients: Direct evidence from indirect semantic priming. *Biological Psychiatry,* 34, 864–877. (1993a).

[91] Spitzer, M., Weisker, I., Winter, M., Maier, S., Hermle, L., and Maher, B. A. Semantic and phonological priming in schizophrenia. *Journal of Abnormal Psychology,* 103, 485–494. (1994).

[92] Weisbrod, M., Maier, S., Harig, S., Himmelsbach, U. and Spitzer, M. Lateralised semantic and indirect semantic priming effects in people with schizophrenia. *British Journal of Psychiatry*, 172, 142-146. (1998).

[93] Spitzer, M., Braun, U., Maier, S., Hermle, L. and Maher, B.A. Indirect semantic priming in schizophrenic patients. *Schizophrenia Research*, 11, 71-80. (1993b).

[94] Chapin, K., McCown, J., Vann, L., Kenney, D. and Youssef, I. Activation and facilitation in the lexicon of schizophrenics. *Schizophrenia Research*, 6, 251-255. (1992).

[95] Ober, B.A., Vinogradov, S. and Shenaut, G.K. Semantic priming of category relations in schizophrenia. *Neuropsychology*, 9, 220-228. (1995).

[96] Henik, A., Priel, B. and Umansky, R. Attention and automaticity in semantic processing of schizophrenic patients. *Neuropsychiatry, Neuropsychology and Behavioural Neurology*, 5, 161-169. (1992).

[97] Warrington EK and Shallice T Semantic access dyslexia, *Brain*, 102, 43-63 (1979).

[98] Rapp B and Caramazza A. On the Distinction between Deficits of Access and Deficits of Storage: a Question of Theory. *Cognitive Neuropsychology*, 10 (2), 113-141 (1993).

[99] Kondel TK, Hirsch SR, and Laws, KR. Name relearning in elderly patients with schizophrenia: episodic and temporary, not semantic and permanent. *Cognitive Neuropsychiatry*, 11, 1-12 (2006).

[100] Laws, K.R., Al-Uzri, M.M., Mortimer, A. M. Lexical Knowledge Degradation in Schizophrenia. *Schizophrenia Research*, 45:123-131. (2000).

[101] Maher B A, Manschreck T C, Redmond D, and Beaudette S Length of illness and the gradient from positive to negative semantic priming in schizophrenic patients. *Schizophrenia Research*, 22, 127-132 (1996).

[102] Laws K R, McKenna P J and Kondel T K. On the Distinction between Access and Store Disorders in Schizophrenia – A Question of Deficit Severity. *Neuropsychologia,* 36(4), 313-21. (1998).
[103] Faglioni P and Botti, C How to differentiate retrieval from storage deficit: a stochastic approach to semantic memory modelling. *Cortex,* **30,** 501–518. (1993).
[104] Spitzer, M. A cognitive neuroscience view of schizophrenic thought disorder. *Schizophrenia Bulletin*, 23, 29-50. (1997).
[105] Goldberg, T.E. and Weinberger, D.R. Thought disorder in schizophrenia: A reappraisal of some older formulations and an overview of some recent studies. *Cognitive Neuropsychiatry*, 5, 1-19 (2000).
[106] Laws KR, Al-Uzri M and Mortimer AM. Lexical Degradation in Schizophrenia. *Schizophrenia Research*, 45, 123-131 (2000).
[107] Zalla, T., Posada, A., Franck, N., Georgieff, N., Sirigu, A., A component analysis of action planning processes in schizophrenia: a comparison with patients with frontal lobe damage. *Cognitive Neuropsychiatry* 6 (4), 271–296. (2001).
[108] Henry, J. D., and Crawford, J. R. A meta-analytic review of verbal fluency performance following focal cortical lesions. *Neuropsychology* 18, 284–295 (2004).
[109] Nathaniel-James, D.A., Brown, R., Ron, M.A., Memory impairment in schizophrenia: its relationship to executive function. *Schizophrenia Research* 21, 85–96. (1996).
[110] Lawrence, V. A., Doughty, O., Al-Mousawi, A., Clegg, F., Done, D. J. Do overinclusion and distorted semantic category boundaries in schizophrenia arise from executive dysfunction? *Schizophrenia Research* 94, 172-179 (2007).
[111] Leeson VC, Simpson, A., McKenna PJ and Laws KR. Executive inhibition and semantic association in schizophrenia. *Schizophrenia Research*, 74, 61-67 (2005).
[112] Spitzer M New frontiers in Schizophrenia Research: Neuroplasticity and Neuromodulation. *Proceedings of Global Medical Conference: Focus on Schizophrenia*, 8-13. (2000).
[113] Westerhausen R, Kompus K, and Hugdhal K Impaired cognitive inhibition in schizophrenia: A meta-analysis of the Stroop. *Schizophrenia Research* (2011).
[114] Waters, F.A.V., Badcock, J.C., Maybery, M.T. and Michie, P.T. Inhibition in schizophrenia: association with auditory hallucinations. *Schizophrenia Research*, 62, 275-280. (2003).
[115] Kvavilashvili, L., Mandler, G. Out of one's mind: A study of involuntary semantic memories. *Cognitive Psychology* 48, 47-94. (2004).
[116] Chan, R.C.K., Huang, J., Guo, L., Cao, X., Hong, X., and Gao, Z. Executive control in schizophrenia in task involving semantic inhibition and working memory. *Psychiatry Research*, 179, 259-266. (2010).
[117] Liddle, P.F., Syndromes of chronic schizophrenia: a re-examination of the positive–negative dichotomy. *British Journal of Psychiatry* 151, 145–151. (1987).
[118] Jensterle, J., Mlakar, J., Vodusek, D.B. and Frith, C.D. Disorganisation in schizophrenia need not result from a failure to inhibit dominant response tendencies. *Cognitive Neuropsychiatry*, 5, 105-121. (2000).
[119] Barch, D.M., Carter, C.S., Perlstein, W., Baird, J., Cohen, J.D. and Schooler, N.Increased Stroop facilitation effects in schizophrenia are not due to increased automatic spreading activation. *Schizophrenia Research*, 39, 51-64. (1999).

[120] Chen, E.Y.H., Wong, A.W.S., Chen, R.Y.L. and Au, J.W.Y. Stroop interference and facilitation effects in first-episode schizophrenic patients. *Schizophrenia Research*, 48, 29-44. (2001).

[121] Taylor, S.F., Kornblum, S. and Tandon, R. Facilitation and interference of selective attention in schizophrenia. *Journal of Psychiatric Research*, 30, 251-259. (1996).

[122] Frith CD. Consciousness, information processing and schizophrenia. *British Journal of Psychiatry*, 134, 225–35(1979).

[123] Peters, E.R., Pickering, A., Kent, A., Glasper, A., Irani, M., David, A., Day, S., Hemsley, DThe relationship between cognitive inhibition and psychotic symptoms. *Journal of Abnormal Psychology* 109 (3), 386– 395.(2000).

[124] Brebion, G., Smith, M., Gorman, J., Malaspina, D., Amador, X. Resistance to interference and positive symptomatology in schizophrenia. *Cognitive Neuropsychiatry* 3, 179–190. (1998).

[125] Soriano, M. F., Jiménez, J. F., Román, P., and Bajo, M. T. Intentional inhibition in memory and hallucinations: Directed forgetting and updating. *Neuropsychology 23*, 61-70 (2009).

[126] Kipp Harnishfeger, K., The development of cognitive inhibition: theories, definitions and research evidence. In: Dempster, F.N., Brainerd, C.J. (Eds.), *Interference and Inhibition in Cognition*. Academic Press, San Diego, pp. 175– 205. Chapter 6. (1995).

[127] Soriano, M. F., Jiménez, J. F., Román, P., and Bajo, M. T. Cognitive substrates in semantic memory of formal thought disorder in schizophrenia. *Journal of Clinical and Experimental Neuropsychology, 30,* 70 – 82. (2008).

[128] Cutting, J. and Murphy, D. Impaired ability of schizophrenic patients, relative to manics or depressives, to appreciate social knowledge about their culture. *British Journal of Psychiatry,* 157: 355-358. (1990).

[129] Mortimer A M, Corridan B, Rudge S, Kho K, Kelly F, Bristow M and Hodges J. Thought, Speech and Language Disorder and Semantic Memory in Schizophrenia. In: Sims A (ed). *Speech and Language Disorders in Psychiatry*, Gaskell, The Royal College of Psychiatrists, 70-80. (1995).

[130] Laws, K.R., McKenna, P.J., and McCarthy, R.A. Delusions about people. *Neurocase*, 1: 349-362. (1995).

In: Psychosis: Causes, Diagnosis and Treatment
Editor: Xenia Anastassiou-Hadjicharalambous
ISBN: 978-1-62081-516-8


*Chapter 8*

# SEMANTIC MEMORY ASSOCIATED WITH NEGATIVE SYMPTOMS IN SCHIZOPHRENIA

***Keith R Laws[1,*] and Mohammed M. Al-Uzri[2,3]***
[1]School of Psychology, University of Hertfordshire, UK
[2]Division of Psychiatry, University of Leicester, UK
[3]Leicestershire Partnership NHS Trust, Leicester, UK

## ABSTRACT

In the chapter, we present a new study examining semantic memory impairment in community-based patients with schizophrenia and its symptoms correlates. We tested 73 community-based patients with schizophrenia and 71 healthy controls for a semantic memory assessment (tests of: category fluency; picture naming; naming-to-description; sorting; and word-picture matching).We used bootstrap ANCOVA (covarying age, NART IQ and education) and bootstrap regression techniques to analyse the data. These relatively well-preserved patients performed within the normal range on some semantic tests (picture naming, picture sorting and word-picture matching), but were impaired on others (category fluency and naming-to-description). Negative symptoms were inversely related to picture sorting, word-picture matching and a composite measure of all five semantic tests. By contrast, positive symptoms correlated positively only with category fluency i.e. better fluency with more positive symptoms. The results indicated that semantic memory deficits in community-based patients were small to moderate and certainly not common across all tasks. Finally, semantic memory impairment was more strongly linked to negative than positive symptomatology.

## INTRODUCTION

In this chapter, we present a study examining a series of issues relating to semantic memory function in people with schizophrenia. We provide a detailed review of the literature relating to semantic memory and schizophrenia in another Chapter in this book [1] and so, will only be briefly outline relevant literature here.

* E-mail: k.laws@herts.ac.uk

Following the pioneering studies of McKenna and colleagues nearly 20 years ago [2,3,4,5], reports have increasingly and consistently documented abnormal semantic memory in schizophrenia across a range of tests, with a recent meta-analysis reporting effects sizes from 91 published studies [6].

Following Cohen's nomenclature (0.2 = small; 0.5 = medium and 0.8 = large), the latter meta-analysis revealed large effect sizes (ESs) for naming ($d$=1.45; $K$=22) and semantic fluency ($d$=1.33; $K$=43); medium ESs for semantic associations ($d$=0.63; $K$=6), word-picture matching ($d$=0.58; $K$=6) and categorisation ($d$=0.49; $K$=20) and a small ES for priming ($d$=0.02; $K$=81).

Interestingly, the number of studies reporting significant differences does not correspond with the reported magnitude of effect sizes – the number of studies reporting significant effects was: naming (59%), semantic fluency (93%), categorisation (80%), word-picture matching (12.5%), associations (50%) and priming (61%). Clearly, mismatches emerge between the effect sizes and the vote count for significant results reported: for example, the largest ES was for naming, but less than 60%of studies reported a significant difference; while for word-picture matching a moderate ES emerges when only 12.5 % of studies actually reported a difference. Conversely, the ES for priming was non-existent but 61% reported a significant effect.

The observation that moderate-large effect sizes emerge despite many nonsignificant individual studies, almost certainly reflects a lack of power in many studies. Meta-analyses may reach positive conclusions despite negative findings from even the overwhelming majority of included studies [e.g. see 7]. By contrast, priming effects were significant in over 60% of studies while the effect size was virtually zero. Examining the funnel plot below (See Figure 1) derived from [20] who also reported a near zero effect size for priming) shows that comparable numbers of studies report increased (positive ES) and reduced priming (negative ES) in schizophrenics.

The importance of studying semantic memory in schizophrenia is highlighted by attempts to link semantic abnormalities with symptomatology [8]. The suggested link stems from the notion that schizophrenics have abnormal *world knowledge* [9,10], which is largely synonymous with semantic memory. In support of this idea, several studies have linked semantic memory impairment in schizophrenia with symptoms such as thought disorder [11,12,13,5] and delusions [14,15,16].

For example, [11] reported that two semantic memory tests (the verbal fluency test and the Peabody Picture Vocabulary test) made significant contribution to predicting the level of thought disorder. In a similar vein, [15] reported findings indicative of illogical semantic connections linked to delusions, showing that responses on a silly sentences task were biased towards the delusional beliefs of patients.

Crucially, in their meta-analysis [6] also looked at the broader relationship between semantic memory and symptomatology. With regard to picture naming, 8 of 11 studies reported no significant correlation between clinical symptoms and naming test performance. For word-picture matching three studies found no significant correlation with symptom severity [17,18,19]. On classification tasks, two studies have investigated the relationship between Formal Thought Disorder and categorisation ability - one found a significant correlation [2] and the other reported no correlation [17].

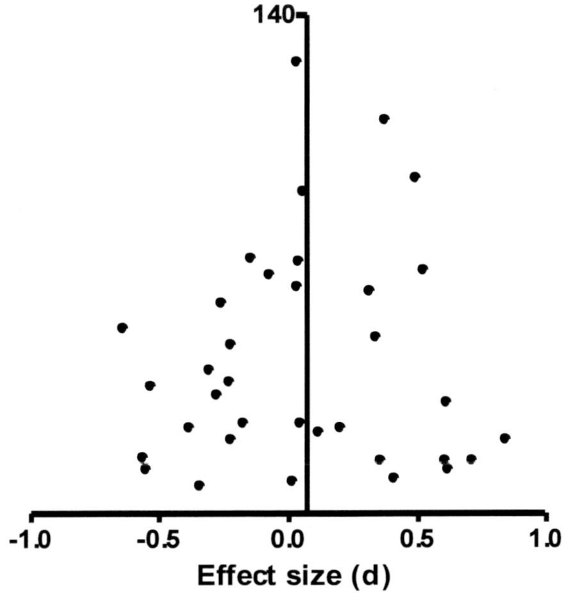


Figure 1. Funnel plot of effect sizes (ESs) for semantic priming in schizophrenia.

In studies of semantic priming (which overall produced a zero effect size), [20] also examined the effect sized in patients with and without thought disorder. The effect size for 14 studies which compared patients without thought disorder with controls yielded an effect size of 0.00, while 18 studies that compared patients thought disordered patients with normal controls was 0.16, indicating significantly increased (albeit small) priming. As can be seen attempts to link semantic memory to symptoms have been quite sporadic, with some emphasis on thought disorder.

Several studies have described the type of the deficit seen in schizophrenia as one of *accessing* semantic information [21, 22, 23], with patients being able to access information intermittently. By contrast, others report an actual loss of semantic knowledge [24, 25, 26] (a so-called store type) that results in a consistent inability to retrieve information. A common denominator that emerges from such studies is that relatively young patients tend to havean access type disorder, while studies of older patients with longer illness duration suggest a picture of a degraded knowledge store [1]. Furthermore, access and storage disorders may well map onto the ability of patients to live and function independently in the community. In the [17] study, which was suggestive of access type disorder, the sample was largely community dwelling and even the inpatients were in community-based rehabilitation units, while in the [26] study, a largely store disorder emerged in more chronically hospitalised patients.

At the extreme end of the illness duration spectrum, [25] examined naming and name relearning in 10 schizophrenics with extremely long illness durations (mean =45.5 years). Compared to 18 Alzheimer patients and 27 healthy elderly controls, the schizophrenics (69% correct) were as anomic as the AD patients (63%) while controls scored near ceiling (96%) at naming 64 simple everyday items (e.g. *chair*, *bike* and *dog*). Moreover, in a second part of the study, Kondel and colleagues attempted to retrain the names of the unnamed items to each patient on a weekly basis for four weeks. While the elderly schizophrenic patients showed some short-term improvement in naming, the gains were not retained when rested one-month after retraining had finished. This study of semantic memory function in this examination of a unique elderly cohort of schizophrenia patients clearly showed that the degree of semantic impairment is comparable to that seen in dementing patients and like, AD patients unresponsive to attempts at relearning. The significance of the access-storage dimension may have important implications for tailoring care profiles and (cognitive) rehabilitation programs to different *types* of patients. It also raises a related issue, which is the possibility that appropriate and speedy intervention in community-dwelling and relatively well patients may impede or halt any potential transition from access to store like disorder.

Indeed, using a case study approach, [12] the extremely thought disordered patient TC who showed a significant semantic memory impairment. On neurocognitive testing, TC's naming (production) was inconsistent across time as was his language comprehension resulting from impaired access to word meaning. They concluded that TC's deficits reflected a disorder of semantic *access* rather than a degradation of the semantic knowledge base itself. Five years later, TC showed a remarkable improvement in his thought disorder symptoms and begun to speak rationally without immediately drifting off into unrelated topics. [27] therefore re-administered the same test battery of tests to TC and his comprehension of language showed a marked and significant improvement with the remitting of his major symptom. Although TC's naming did not improve, he did become more consistent. Together these two studies show that psychotic symptoms and semantic problems may be causally linked. Moreover, *some* aspects of the semantic disorder appear to be state related (to the symptoms),while others may be described better as traits of schizophrenia *per se*.

Two further studies, using a battery based approach, have compared semantic memory function in schizophrenics and patients with Alzheimer's disease. [4] used the *Cambridge Semantic Memory Test Battery* (CSM), which consists of five tests [see 28, developed by 29]: picture naming, picture sorting, word-picture matching, naming to definition and category fluency. They found that, on many of the semantic tests, elderly schizophrenics performed at a level comparable to that of patients with mild to moderate Alzheimer's disease. Two further schizophrenic groups - a mild group who had relapsing and remitting episodes (but were able to live independently) and a core group who were younger (but had unremitting illness) - also showed semantic memory deficits. As expected, the deficits were less severe in the mild group, with the core group displaying impairment intermediate between the elderly and mild groups, thus highlighting the potentially crucial role played by severity and chronicity of illness in the level of semantic memory impairment.

In a further study using the CSM, [30] compared a group of 20 schizophrenia patients with 22 Alzheimer's Dementia (AD).and 15 elderly healthy controls. While the profile of AD patients indicated marked impairment across all tests, the profile for chronic schizophrenics was more uneven. Based on this, and in contrast to [25] and [4], Doughty and colleagues argued that the semantic impairment in schizophrenia patients is unlikely to result from a degraded store. On subordinate sorting and the Camel and Cactus pictures and words[1] test, schizophrenics produced error rates significantly greater that healthy controls and did not differ from the AD group. By contrast, for picture naming, word–picture matching and superordinate category sorting, AD patients made significantly more errors than schizo-

[1] This task is similar to the Pyramids and Palm Trees test – requiring participants to match a target picture or name with one of two distracters e.g. Camel goes with Cactus or Fir Tree

phrenic patients, who performed at a level similar to that of the healthy controls; however, substantial ceiling effects existed on these tests[2]. Doughty and colleagues proposed that the uneven profile in the schizophrenia group does not accord with a degraded semantic store disorder (as per the consistent and widespread impairment in the AD group). Nevertheless, as noted, this conclusion may be somewhat premature given the ceiling effects on several tests preventing the finding of any impairment being revealed some tests. At a general level, the presence of ceiling effects on such tasks stems inevitably from their being primarily devised for use with those who have dementia[3]. Nevertheless, comparisons with controls are invariably required and so, analyses will be detrimentally affected by the ceiling effect (regardless of transforming the data or the use of nonparametric statistics which reduce power and makes the use of covariates complex). One solution, however, is through the use of boostrapping techniques and we will return to these later.

Previous cohort-based studies of semantic memory in schizophrenia have limited their representativeness. Second, as noted, studies have often used single measures of semantic memory functioning (e.g. picture naming), which – if the profile is inconsistent – will produce potentially misleading inferences regarding semantics in schizophrenia. By contrast, semantic batteries provide a more comprehensive view of the components of semantic memory. Third, the performance of controls has often been at or close to ceiling on some semantic memory tasks (e.g. word-picture matching), and therefore represent a challenge to the way the emerging data may be analysed and also likely to produce spuriously large effect sizes because of the small standard deviations. Finally, as suggested above [and see 1] the type of semantic memory impairment can vary across patients with schizophrenia along various dimensions e.g. length of illness. For example, [31] noticed that the type of impairment reported in studies of community-based sample was different to that of chronically hospital based ones [32]. For these reasons, this current study was designed to be population-based, using a robust statistical method and focusing on community-based patients.

# METHODS

## Participants

We identified 190 patients who were potentially eligible for testing (see Figure 1 for flow chart describing recruitment). Of those not eligible, two did not fulfil strict diagnostic criteria for schizophrenia, one died before testing, five had a diagnosis of substance misuse, eight had a history of organic brain disease/head injury, thirty were over age 60 years, and for eleven English was not their first language. Of the 133 eligible patients, 60 declined to take part, leaving 73 (55%) patients who were eligible and volunteered to take part in the study. All patients who took part in the study were stable and living in the community except one who was an inpatient at the time of the study.

[2]Indeed, the authors removed control data from their analyses for this reason; and used a log-linear transform of the patient data

[3]Given that neuropsychologists are typically looking at a performance profile across a range of tests and so, it is crucial to know if the pattern mirrors or deviates from that expected in healthy normal individuals (see Laws 2005 for striking examples)

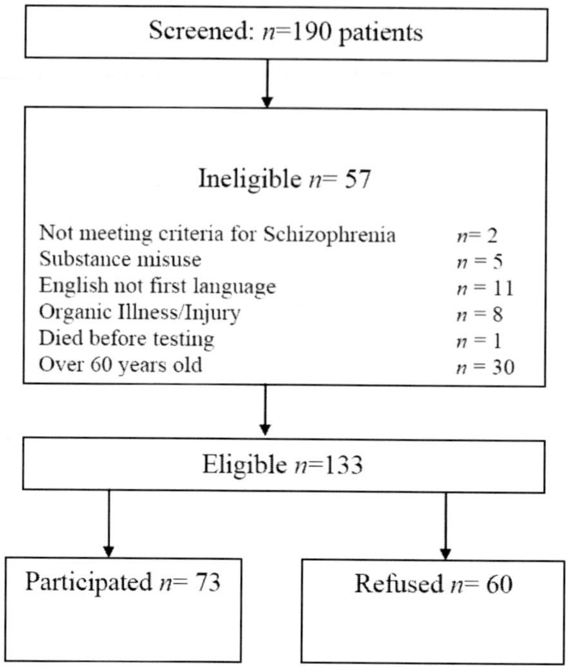


Figure 1.Flow chart of patient selection for the study.

**Table 1. Comparison between Patients who participated or refused to take part in the study**

| | Participants(n=73) | Refused (n=60) | *t-value* | *p* |
|---|---|---|---|---|
| Age | 39.4(11.7) | 40.3 (9.6) | t=-0.50 | *ns* |
| Age illness onset (yrs) | 27.2 (7.9) | 25.7(7.3) | t=1.07 | *ns* |
| Illness duration (yrs) | 669 (545.6) | 752.9(427.5) | t=-.94 | *ns* |
| Inpatient stays (weeks) | 185.7(322.7) | 217.0(208.3) | t=-.61 | *ns* |
| Education | 13.6(2.7) | 12.23(2.5) | t=2.96 | *p*=.004 |
| Gender M:F | 42:31 | 35:25 | 0.01 | *ns* |
| Accommodation* | 17:18:27:10:1 | 21:11:18:7:3 | 4.21 | *ns* |
| Employment** | | | 10.03 | *ns* |
| AnticholinergicsYes:No | 27:46 | 22:37 | 0.25 | *ns* |
| Antipsychotic treatment*** | 37:24:8:4 | 29:22:6:2 | 0.09 | *ns* |

Note. *Accommodation = independent: with partner: with parents: supported: residential
**Employment = Standard Occupational Classification 2000
***Antipsychotic treatment = atypical: typical: mixed: antipsychotic free

We compared the known socio-demographic and clinical characteristics of patients who participated in the study and those who did not take part (see Table 1). Those characteristics included; age, gender, years in education, accommodation, employment status, medication prescribed, age of onset, length of inpatient stay and illness duration. There were no significant differences between the groups apart from the study participants having more years in education.

**Table 2. Demographic details for Schizophrenia Patients and Healthy Controls**

| | Patients (n=73) | Controls (n=71) | |
|---|---|---|---|
| Sex (M:F) | 42:31 | 38:33 | $\chi^2$ = 0.31, ns |
| Age | 39.4 (11.70) | 34.4 (12.40) | t=2.48, p=.014 |
| NART IQ | 112.66 (6.50) | 115.46 (6.47) | t=2.49, p=.014 |
| Education (years) | 13.61 (2.69) | 14.89 (3.52) | t=2.46, p=.015 |
| Illness duration (weeks) | 669.01 (545.65) | | |
| SAPS | 4.10 (3.70) | | |
| SANS | 3.96 (4.58) | | |

Note. SDs in parentheses

The controls lived in the same city and were recruited by adverts in the local hospital, university and supermarkets. They had no history of mental illness and shared the same exclusion criteria as the patients. The demographic information of the patients (n=73) who took part in the study and that of controls (n=71) are summarised in Table 2.

# PROCEDURE

## Semantic Battery

We assessed participants on five tests (picture naming, picture sorting, and word-picture matching tests) from the Cambridge Semantic Memory Battery [29, 30]. The battery assesses input to and output from central representational knowledge about the same group of items through both visual and verbal modalities. Each test contains the same 48 items chosen to represent three categories of animals (land animals, sea creatures and birds; n=24) and three categories of man-made items (household items, vehicles and musical instruments; n= 24). Items were matched on prototypicality within each semantic category: exemplars were chosen to represent the range from highly prototypical (e.g. desk, guitar, lion), to atypical (e.g. rocking chair, French horn, racoon). Participant scores were determined by their correct answers and there was no time limit for responding.

*Category fluency*. Subjects were asked to generate as many items as they could from the category of animals in one minute.

*Picture naming*. Subjects were shown 48 cards of drawings of different items presented in turn, and asked to name them.

*Naming to description*. Subjects were given a description of 24 different living and man made items and were asked to give the name.

*Picture sorting*. Subjects asked to sort the same 48 cards (used in the picture naming task) into: (a) Level one (superordinate) - living (24 items) vs. manmade (24items); (b) Level two (categories) - the living items into land animals, birds, and water creatures, the manmade items into household items, musical instruments and vehicles; and (c) Level three (subordinate) - the land animals into native vs. foreign to Britain, and the household items into electrical vs. non-electrical items.

*Word to picture matching*. The subjects were given the names of each of the 48 items and asked to point to the named item from an array containing the six items in the same category.

## Pre-Morbid Intelligence

The National Adult Reading Test (NART) was used to estimate pre-morbid intelligence [33].

## Clinical Assessment

Patient symptoms were assessed using the *Scales for the Assessment of Negative Symptoms and Positive Symptoms* [34] (SANS and SAPS, respectively). Antipsychotic dosages were converted to the Percentage of Maximum Dose (PMD) according to the British National Formulary [35] in order to investigate associations between dosage and neuropsychological test performance. This method of comparing antipsychotic potency is considered more reliable than using chlorpromazine equivalents [36].

# RESULTS

For the control data, we calculated skewness and kurtosis statistics ($g_1$ and $g_2$ respectively) and also the D'Agostino-Pearson omnibus test for normality [37], which uses both $g_1$ and $g_2$ as input, was calculated to determine if the distributions differed significantly from normality. All distributions (except for category fluency) deviated significantly from normality in controls (see Table 3).

**Table 3. Skew and distribution for healthy controls on semantic measures**

| | Skewness $g_1$ | Kurtosis $g_2$ | D'Agostino- Pearson Omnibus test $K^2$ | $p$ |
|---|---|---|---|---|
| Category Fluency | 0.2 | -0.2 | 0.94 | .62 |
| Picture naming | -1.4 | 2.3 | 23.9 | <.0001 |
| Naming to description | -1.8 | 4.50 | 36.5 | <.0001 |
| Category sorting | -0.8 | -0.01 | 7.8 | .02 |
| Word-Picture matching | -4.6 | 25.3 | 101.8 | <.0001 |

As with all previous studies using this battery, controls perform near ceiling for picture naming, naming-to-description, sorting and comprehension. In this context, the data was analyzed using randomization re-sampling techniques rather than standard parametric analyses. We therefore used bootstrap methods because they require fewer assumptions about the distribution of the responses and represent a useful approach for data that are heavily skewed distributions, have unequal variances across groups, and/or multiple zero errors for controls [see 38]. We ran a series of bootstrap ANCOVA analyses (using education, NART IQ and age as covariates). We created 1000 bootstrap samples, each equal in size to the original sample, by randomly resampling with replacement from the original patient data. For each bootstrap sample, an observation was selected at random to be included in the sample and then made available to be selected again for that same sample. A bootstrap sample may contain several copies of one data point and none for another data point. Then, for each of the 1000 bootstrap samples, the statistic (in this case F for ANCOVA) is recomputed and a distribution of *test statistics* is created. This distribution of results is then compared to the original result and declared significant if it is amongst the most extreme 5%. We ran ANCOVA analyses for each of the semantic memory tests (category fluency, picture naming, naming to definition, picture sorting and word-picture matching). The adjusted means for all comparisons are presented in Table 4. Significant group differences emerged for category fluency and naming-to-description.

**Table 4. Semantic Memory performance for Schizophrenic Patients and Controls**

| Test | Patient (n=73)<br>Mean (95% CI) | Control(n=71)<br>Mean (95% CI) | ANCOVA | *d* |
|---|---|---|---|---|
| Category fluency | 17.81 (16.7 -19.4) | 21.63 (20.2 to 23.1) | $F$=15.3,$p$<.01 | 0.43 |
| Picture naming (n=48) | 45.64 (44.9 to 46.2) | 45.70 (44.4 to 46.4) | $F$=1.7, $p$=.41 | 0.13 |
| Naming to description (n=24) | 20.89 (20.1 to 21.5) | 21.96 (21.3 to 22.4) | $F$=9.4 ,$p$=.03 | 0.37 |
| Picture Sorting (n=120) | 116.16 (114.5 to 117.7) | 116.15 (112.7 to 117.4) | $F$=3.4, $p$=.23 | 0.20 |
| Word-picture matching (n=48) | 47.73 (47.1 to 48.2) | 47.48 (46.0 to 47.9) | $F$=2.9, $p$=.29 | 0.18 |

Note.Adjusted mean (and 95% confidence intervals)

## Regression Analyses and Simple Correlations

We examined the relationship between patient demographic/clinical variables and performance on each of the five semantic memory tests. We also calculated a composite semantic memory score by standardizing (Z-scores) for all five measures within the sample of schizophrenia patients and taking the average of these measures as a proxy for semantic memory function *per se*. We ran the 1000 bootstrap regression analyses for each dependent variable using age, NART IQ, education, SAPS, SANS, percentage maximum dose, length of illness as predictors. Table 5 displays the results of regression analyses. Analysis of the semi-partial correlations within the patient group revealed that neither medication (% of maximum dose) nor age was related to any of the five semantic memory tests. By contrast, NART IQ was related to picture naming and duration of illness was related to category sorting performance. Positive symptoms (SAPS) were positively correlated with category fluency; and negative symptoms (SANS) were negatively related to category fluency, category sorting and word-picture matching i.e. all semantic tasks except those involving naming. For the composite measure of semantic memory, only SANS was a significant predictor, accounting for almost 11% of the variance in test performance. We also performed simple correlations between semantic memory measures and more specific symptom ratings (see Table 6). This revealed that the association with negative symptoms largely reflects the fact that alogia and affective flattening correlated negatively and significantly with every semantic measure.

**Table 5. Semi-partial Correlations and $r^2$ values**

| | Category Fluency | Picture Naming | Name to Des | Category Sorting | W-P Match | Composite Semantic |
|---|---|---|---|---|---|---|
| Age | -.11 | .01 | .19 | .02 | -.21 | -.03 |
| NART | .10 | .34** | .31** | .18 | .17 | .23 |
| Education | .34** | .07 | .05 | .05 | -.06 | .11 |
| Duration of Illness | .02 | -.06 | -.21 | -.25* | -.00 | -.16 |
| Percent max dose | -.06 | .07 | .17 | -.03 | .02 | .00 |
| Positive symptoms | .31** | .05 | -.04 | .08 | .23 | .17 |
| Negative symptoms | -.26* | -.16 | -.15 | -.33** | -.40** | -.33* |
| Multiple $r^2$ | .38 p<0.001 | .23 p=0.05 | .29 p=0.02 | .27 p=0.02 | .28p=0.02 | .42 p=0.01 |

Note. *=p<.05, **=p<.01

**Table 6. Correlations between Patient Symptoms and Semantic Test performance (n=73)**

| | Category Fluency | Picture naming | Naming to des | Picture Sorting | WP match | Composite Semantic |
|---|---|---|---|---|---|---|
| Positive symptoms SAPS | | | | | | |
| Hallucinations | .03 | -.04 | -.09 | .03 | .17 | .03 |
| Delusions | .12 | .04 | -.06 | -.06 | .12 | .03 |
| Bizarre behaviour | .11 | -.15 | -.16 | -.40** | -.02 | -.20 |
| Thought Disorder | .34** | .22 | .20 | .18 | .00 | .25* |
| Negative symptoms SANS | | | | | | |
| Inappropriate affect | .00 | .14 | -.09 | .02 | .10 | .05 |
| Affect flattening | -.26* | -.25* | -.25* | -.48** | -.39** | -.42** |
| Alogia | -.29* | -.28* | -.25* | -.42** | -.36** | -.44** |
| Avolition/apathy | -.18 | -.06 | -.07 | -.22 | -.24 | -.18 |
| Anhedonia/asocialiy | -.10 | -.09 | - .04 | -.22 | -.18 | -.15 |
| Attention | -.21 | -.19 | -.41** | -.37** | -.19 | -.40** |

*Note.* ** <.01; * <.05

## CONCLUSION

As far as we are aware, this is the first study to examine semantic memory in a community-based population of patients with schizophrenia. Our main findings were that community based patients with schizophrenia showed significant impairment on two of the five semantic tasks (category fluency and naming-to-description), but performed within the normal range on tests of picture naming, category sorting and word-picture matching. Additionally, examination of the relationship between symptoms and semantic memory performance revealed a significant role for negative symptoms in semantic memory test performance (for three of the five tasks: category fluency, category sorting and word-picture matching). By contrast, naming ability as measured by picture naming and naming-to-description were better predicted by the premorbid factors of educational attainment and estimated premorbid IQ. Given the catchment-based population approach to recruitment used here, we would suggest that the current study provides a good estimate of semantic memory deficits in community dwelling patients with schizophrenia. The patients who did and did not consent to take part in the study shared almost all demographic and clinical characteristics, although those who participated had significantly more years of education. Therefore, this study can be considered as the closest to a prevalence design when taking various methodological obstacles facing studies of cognitive functions into consideration.

The semantic memory deficits are not attributable to simple differences between patients and controls in terms of age, estimated premorbid IQ or education (all of which were covaried in the analyses). NART IQ was positively correlated with picture naming and naming-to-description inpatients; however, this is quite a normal profile seen in controls and similarly with the positive correlation between education and semantic fluency. We were also able to show that medication (as measured by percentage maximum dose) was not significantly related to semantic memory performance and that duration of illness was modestly correlated with category sorting performance. By contrast, however, negative symptomatology was widely and significantly correlated with semantic memory measures.

In the context of previous studies examining semantic memory function in patients with schizophrenia, the level and range of semantic memory impairment reported here was quite low. Indeed, on three tasks, the patients performed within the normal range; and where patients did perform significantly worse than healthy controls, the differences although significant were small-moderate (as indicated by effect sizes). This contrasts with previous studies (some using the same battery e.g. [4] showing significant impairment on exactly the same tasks, but at a level that was almost indistinguishable from that of patients with Alzheimer's disease. Nonetheless, the patients examined by [4] were chronically hospitalised schizophrenics, while our sample of patients are possibly at the other end of the continuum, living in the community, experiencing low levels of symptoms and with approximately 30% being in employment.

We assessed semantic memory in various ways (production, reception, verbal and visual input) and the resulting dissociations across tasks accords with the idea that some components of semantic memory are more affected than others in schizophrenia. In particular, while category fluency and naming-to-description were significantly impaired, the remaining three tasks (picture naming, picture sorting and word-picture matching) failed to reveal any significant differences. This is consistent with a recent report suggesting that naming-to-description might be an early marker for semantic memory impairment in schizophrenia [32]. Unlike picture naming, naming-to-description requires patients to hold and process information within working memory as well then accessing semantic memory and then derive the name (if stored). Such *online* processing is complex and failure could emanate from a variety of sources between input and output. The fact that naming-to-description was unrelated to positive symptomatology indicates that the possible intrusion and distraction provided by hallucinations or delusions do not account for performance. Rather naming-to-description was significantly related to negative symptomatology including alogia, affective flattening and crucially, attention problems - thus supporting the idea that it may be an input problem i.e. patients may not be able to make the required effort to encode (or retrieve) or cannot hold the information online (in working memory) sufficiently for deriving the name.

Only one measure of semantic memory - category fluency - was related to the global measure of positive symptoms (with increased positive symptomatology leading to *better* fluency), and fluency was also significantly inversely related to negative symptoms [cf. 39]. Studies have often reported significant correlations between negative symptom scores and executive impairment [e.g. 40] and this association is substantiated by a meta-analysis of 40 studies of various fluency measures, which revealed a correlation of -.27 [39].

The correlations between semantic memory and the positive symptoms of delusions and hallucinations were nonsignificant and largely close to zero. The lack of an association between semantics and both delusions and hallucinations is somewhat surprising. Nonetheless, as with previous work, thought disorder was significantly and positively correlated with category fluency [cf. 41]. The small number of functional imaging studies examining formal thought disorder [42] has implicated the temporal lobes and again, this would accord with a semantic problem. Indeed, other lines of evidence reviewed above – primarily from picture naming - suggest that formal thought disorder is associated with an impairment affecting *access* to the semantic knowledge system [e.g. 11, 43, 33, 13, 23].

Finally, the composite measure of semantic memory was significantly related to negative symptomatology and indeed, affective flattening and alogia (i.e. poverty of speech, poverty of content of speech, blocking, and increased latency of response: see [44]) correlated negatively with all five semantic memory measures. This confirms an earlier report of an association between some negative symptoms (alogia) and semantic memory function in schizophrenia [45]. It is also consistent with reports that the semantic memory deficit and negative symptoms may have the same underlying substrate. [22] argued "This discrete association indicates that impaired verbal fluency and alogia reflect a dysfunction of the same cognitive process which is normally involved in gaining access to semantic knowledge and, on the above argument, is possibly mediated by frontostriatal systems." (p.46). As noted in our review [1 this volume] executive functions undoubtedly contribute to the semantic memory problems seen in some schizophrenics (via increased inhibition, the role of executive processes in strategic retrieval, possibly working memory and so on); however, a more *pure* semantic disorder does also exists in some patients. Future research needs to address these varied influences and the relationship with symptomatology.

## REFERENCES

[1] Laws, K.R., Leeson, V.C., Al-Uzri, M.M., and Kondel, T.K (this publication). Semantic memory and symptomatology in schizophrenia: a review.

[2] Chen E, Wilkins A, and McKenna P J. Semantic memory is both impaired and anomalous in Schizophrenia. *Psychological Medicine*, 24(1), 193-202. (1994)

[3] Clare L, McKenna P J, Mortimer A M, and Baddeley A D. Memory in Schizophrenia: what is impaired and what is preserved. *Neuropsychologia* 31(11), 1225-1241 (1993).

[4] McKay, A.P., McKenna, P.J., Bentham, P., Mortimer, A. N., Holbery, A. and Hodges, J.R. Semantic Memory is Impaired in Schizophrenia. *Biological Psychiatry*, 39: 929-37. (1996).

[5] Tamlyn, D., McKenna, P.J., Mortimer, A. N., Lund, C. E., Hammond, S, and Baddeley, A.D. Memory impairment in schizophrenia: It's extent affiliations and neuropsychological character. *Psychological Medicine*, 22:101-115 (1992).

[6] Doughty OJ, and Done DJ. Is semantic memory impaired in schizophrenia? A systematic review and meta-analysis of 91 studies. *Cognitive Neuropsychiatry,* 14, 473 -509 (2009).

[7] Lau, J., Antman, E. M., Jimenez-Silva, J., Kupelnick, B., Mosteller, F., and Chalmers, T. C. Cumulative meta-analysis of therapeutic trials for myocardial infarction. *New England Journal of Medicine,* 327, 248-254 (1992).

[8] McKenna P J, Mortimer A M and Hodges J R. Semantic Memory and Schizophrenia. In: David A S and Cutting J C (eds), *The Neuropsychiatry of Schizophrenia* Lawrence Erlbaum Associates Ltd.163-178 (1994).

[9] Cutting, J. and Murphy, D. Schizophrenic thought disorder: A psychological and organic interpretation. *British Journal of Psychiatry,* 152, 310-319. (1988).

[10] Cutting, J. and Murphy, D. Impaired ability of schizophrenic patients, relative to manics or depressives, to appreciate social knowledge about their culture. *British Journal of Psychiatry,* 157: 355-358 (1990).

[11] Goldberg T E, Aloia M S, Qourovitch M L, Missar D, Pichard D, and Weinberger D R. Cognitive Substrates of Thought Disorder, 1: The Semantic System. *American Journal of Psychiatry*, 155 (12), 1671-1676 (1998).

[12] Laws, K.R., Kondel, T.K., and McKenna, P.J. Receptive and Expressive language Disorders in Schizophrenic Thought Disorder: Impaired Semantic Access and Monitoring. *Cognitive Neuropsychiatry,* 4: 89-106 (1999).

[13] Mortimer A M, Corridan B, Rudge S, Kho K, Kelly F, Bristow M and Hodges J.Thought, Speech and Language Disorder and Semantic Memory in Schizophrenia. In: Sims A (ed). *Speech and Language Disorders in Psychiatry*, Gaskell, The Royal College of Psychiatrists, 70-80 (1995).

[14] Laws, K.R., McKenna, P.J., and McCarthy, R.A. Delusions about people. *Neurocase*, 1: 349-362 (1995).

[15] Rossell, S.L., Shapleske, J., and David, A.S. Sentence verification and delusion: a content specific deficit. *Psychological Medicine*, 28, 1189-98 (1998).

[16] Rossell, S.L., Rabe-Hesketh, S., Shapleske, J., and David, A.S. Is semantic fluency differentially impaired in schizophrenic patients with delusions? *Journal of Clinical and Experimental Neuropsychology,* 21(5), 629-642. (1999).

[17] Al-Uzri MM, Laws KR and Mortimer AM. An early marker for semantic memory impairment in patients with schizophrenia. *Cognitive Neuropsychiatry,* 9(4), 267-279 (2004).

[18] Barrera, A., McKenna, P. J. and Berrios, G. E. Formal thought disorder in schizophrenia: An executive or a semantic deficit? Psychological Medicine, 35(1): 121–132. (2005).

[19] Lawrence, V. A., Doughty, O., Al-Mousawi, A., Clegg, F. and Done, D. J. Do overinclusion and distorted semantic category boundaries in schizophrenia arise from executive dysfunction?. *Schizophrenia Research*, 94(1–3): 172–179 (2007).

[20] Pomarol-Clotet, E., Oh, TM., Laws, K R and McKenna, PJ. Semantic Priming in Schizophrenia: A Meta-Analysis. *British Journal of Psychiatry,* 192, 92-97 (2008).

[21] Allen, H. A., Liddle, P.F., and Frith, C.D. Negative features, retrieval processes and verbal fluency in schizophrenia. *British Journal of Psychiatry,* 163, 769-775. (1993).

[22] Joyce EM, Collinson S L and Crichton P. Verbal Fluency in Schizophrenia: Relationship with Executive Function, Semantic Memory and Clinical Alogia. *Psychological Medicine,* 26(1), 39-49 (1996).

[23] Spitzer, M., Braun, U., Hermle, L. and Maier, S. Associative semantic network dysfunction in thought disordered schizophrenic patients: direct evidence from indirect semantic priming. *Biological Psychiatry*, 34, 864-877. (1993).

[24] Chen, R.Y.L., Chen, E.Y.H., Chan, C.K.Y., Lam, L.C., and Lieh-Mak, F. Verbal fluency in schizophrenia: reduction in semantic store. *Australian and New Zealand Journal of Psychiatry*, 34 (1), 43-48. (2000).

[25] Kondel TK, Hirsch SR, and Laws, KR. Name relearning in elderly patients with schizophrenia: episodic and temporary, not semantic and permanent. *Cognitive Neuropsychiatry*, 11, 1-12. (2006).

[26] Laws, K.R., Al-Uzri, M.M., and Mortimer, A. M. Lexical Knowledge Degradation in Schizophrenia. *Schizophrenia Research*, 45:123-131. (2000).

[27] Leeson VC, McKenna PJ, Murray G, Kondel TK, and Laws KR "What happens to semantic memory when formal thought disorder remits? Revisiting a case study." *Cognitive Neuropsychiatry* 10(1):57-71 (2005)

[28] Adlam AL,Patterson K, Bozeat S, and Hodges JR. The Cambridge semantic memory test battery: detection of semantic deficits in semantic dementia and Alzheimer's disease. *Neurocase* 16, 193–207. (2010)

[29] Hodges J R, Sellman D P and Butters N. Semantic Memory Impairment in Alzheimer's Disease: failure of Access or Degraded Knowledge? *Neuropsychologia*, 30 (4), 301-314. (1992)

[30] Doughty, O.J., Done, D.J., Lawrence, V.A., Al-Mousawi, A., and Ashave, K. Semantic memory impairment in schizophrenia - deficit in storage or access of knowledge? *Schizophrenia Research* 105, 40–48. (2008).

[31] Al-Uzri M. M. Can neuroplasticity improve our understanding of semantic memory deficit in schizophrenia? *History and Philosophy of Psychology*, 6, 1, 48-58. (2004)

[32] Leeson, V.C., McKenna, P.J., and Laws, K.R. Storage and Access Procedures in Schizophrenia: Evidence for a Two Phase Model of Lexical Impairment. *Journal of Clinical and Experimental Neuropsychology*, 27 (6):700-701. (2005)

[33] Nelson, H. E. *National Adult Reading Test (NART).* Windsor :NFER Nelson. (1982)

[34] Andreasen N.C. and Olsen S. Negative v positive schizophrenia. *Archives of General Psychiatry,* 39, 789-794. (1982)

[35] British National Formulary. The British Medical Association. London, U.K. (2004)

[36] Yortson, G., and Pinney A. Chlorpromazine equivalents and percentage of British National Formulary maximum recommended dose in patients receiving high-dose antipsychotics. *Psychiatric Bulletin*, 24, 130–132. (2000).

[37] D'Agostino, R. B., Belanger, A., and D'Agostino, R. B., Jr. A suggestion for using powerful and informative tests for normality. *The American Statistician*, 44, 316–321. (1990).

[38] Delucchi, K.L., and Bostrom, A. Methods for analysis of skewed data distributions in psychiatric clinical studies: working with many zero values. *American Journal of Psychiatry*, 161, 1159-1168. (2004).

[39] Dibben CR, Rice C, Laws K, and McKenna PJ. Is executive impairment associated with schizophrenic syndromes? A meta-analysis. *Psychological Medicine*, 39:381–392. (2009)

[40] Donohoe G, and Robertson IH. Can specific deficits in executive functioning explain the negative symptoms of schizophrenia? A review. *Neurocase* 9 :97–108 (2003)

[41] Bokat C.E., and Goldberg, T.E. Letter and category fluency in schizophrenic patients: a meta-analysis, *Schizophrenia Research,* **64** 73-78. (2003)

[42] Maguire E A, and Mummery CJ. Deferential Modulation of a Common Memory Retrieval Network Revealed by Positron Emission Tomography. *Hippocampus*, 9(1), 54-61. (1999)

[43] Laws K R, McKenna P J and Kondel T K. On the Distinction between Access and Store Disorders in Schizophrenia – A Question of Deficit Severity. *Neuropsychologia,* 36 (4), 313-21. (1998)

[44] Andreasen, N. Negative symptoms in schizophrenia: definition and reliability. *Archives of General Psychiatry* 39, 784-788. (1982)

[45] Sumiyoshi C, Sumiyoshi T, Nohara S, Matsui M, Kurachi M, and Niwa S. Disorganization of semantic memory underlies alogia in schizophrenia: An analysis of verbal fluency performance in Japanese subjects. *Schizophrenia Research*, 74, 91-100 (2005).

In: Psychosis: Causes, Diagnosis and Treatment
Editor: Xenia Anastassiou-Hadjicharalambous
ISBN: 978-1-62081-516-8


*Chapter 9*

# FAMILY WORK FOR FIRST-EPISODE PSYCHOSIS: A SERVICE DELIVERY PROTOCOL

*Nicholas J. K. Breitborde*[1] *and Vinod H. Srihari*[2]
[1]Department of Psychiatry, University of Arizona, Tucson, AZ, US
[2]Department of Psychiatry, Yale University, New Haven, CT, US

## FAMILY WORK FOR FIRST-EPISODE PSYCHOSIS: A SERVICE DELIVERY PROTOCOL

There is growing international support for the benefits of early intervention for psychotic disorders. Clinical services organized around the principal of providing comprehensive phase-specific care and/or reducing the duration between the onset of psychotic symptoms and the receipt of treatment have shown promise with regard to producing better clinical outcomes for individuals with first-episode psychosis [Bertelsen et al., 2008; Melle et al., 2008]. The success of such clinical programs has sparked major health services reform throughout the world, including the development of a national early intervention service network in the UK [Joseph and Birchwood, 2005] and the dedication of 40 million dollars by the US National Institute of Mental Health for the completion of the Recovery After an Initial Schizophrenic Episode (RAISE) initiative [National Institute of Mental Health, 2009].

When providing care to individuals with first-episode psychosis, it is imperative to consider their caregiving relatives. Family members typically provide a plethora of resources and services to facilitate the recovery process of their ill relative (e.g., provision of emotional and/or financial support, assistance with obtaining and maintaining competitive employment, managing psychiatric care visits, etc.). While family members caring for a relative with a chronic illness may experience certain rewards associated with the caregiving process (e.g., feelings of gratification and mastery as well as increased intimacy with their ill relative [Chen and Greenberg, 2004; Heru, 2000]), unfortunately, there are also many negative outcomes commonly associated with the familial caregiving, including feelings of grief and loss [Magliano et al., 1998; Miller, 1996], financial strain [Arno, Levine, and Memmott, 1999; Kuipers, 1993], restrictions in leisure activities [Magliano et al., 1998; Möller-Leimkühler, 2005], and worse physical and mental health outcomes [Breitborde, López, and Kopelowicz,

2010; Gallagher and Mechanic, 1996] including premature mortality [Schulz and Beach, 1999]. Consequently, incorporating family members within the clinical care provided by an early intervention service has several potential benefits. First, given the key role that familial caregivers play in the recovery process from psychotic disorders, assisting them in the completion of their caregiving duties may promote better outcomes among their ill relatives. Moreover, addressing the needs of caregivers within a clinical service for first-episode psychosis may have broader public health implications. Specifically, reducing the strain that often accompanies the caregiving process may result in reductions in morbidity (and potentially mortality) among caregivers themselves.

Within the past thirty years, a number of professionally-led clinical programs have been developed to assist families caring for a relative with a psychotic illness [e.g., Anderson, Reiss, and Hogarty, 1986; Falloon et al., 1985; McFarlane et al., 1995; Mueser and Glynn, 1999]. Typically referenced with the umbrella term "family psychoeducation," these programs provide individuals and caregiving relatives with:

(i) Information with regard to etiology, symptoms, course, and treatment of psychotic disorders;
(ii) Tools to promote better clinical outcomes; and
(iii) Coping strategies to reduce the difficulties associated with living with psychosis or caring for a relative with psychosis [McFarlane, Dixon, Lukens, and Lucksted, 2003].

To date, multiple clinical trials of family psychoeducation have been completed, and it is clear that participation in these interventions is associated with a reduced risk of symptomatic relapse and rehospitalization among individuals with psychosis [Baucom, Shoham, Mueser, Daiuto, and Stickle, 1998; Pilling et al., 2002; Pitschel-Walz, Leucht, Bäuml, Kissling, and Engel, 2001]. Moreover, participation in family psychoeducation is associated with reductions in caregiver burden and distress as well as improvements in overall family functioning and the relationship between the individual with psychosis and their caregiving relative [Cuijpers, 1999].

To date, the majority of studies of family psychoeducation among families caring for a relative with psychosis have focused on individuals with chronic psychotic disorders. This raises the possibility that the effective delivery of these services in the context of a recent onset psychotic disorder in a younger individual may require adaptation of the original models. For instance, although there are many shared concerns among caregiving relatives of individuals with psychotic disorders, recent work by Addington and colleagues [Addington, Addington, Jones, and Ko, 2001; Addington and Burnett, 2004; Addington, Collins, McCleery, and Addington, 2005] has highlighted the unique needs of individuals caring for a relative with first-episode psychosis. As many individuals with first-episode psychosis can achieve symptomatic remission with adequate initial treatment [Lieberman et al., 1993; Perkins et al., 2004], family members of individuals with first-episode psychosis may particularly benefit from guidance and support in fostering responsibility and action on the part of their ill relative in managing her or his own recovery [Addington et al., 2001; Addington and Burnett, 2004]. This is in contrast to family caregivers of individuals with chronic psychotic disorders who often report wanting greater assistance in their personal efforts to manage aspects of their ill relative's care and recovery [Askey, Holmshaw, Gamble, and Gray, 2009; Winefield and Harvey, 1994]. Likewise, caregivers of patients with first-episode psychosis may not benefit from the provision of disorder-specific information [Addington et al., 2001] given the diagnostic ambiguity that is often present early in the course a psychotic disorder [Amin et al., 1999; Schwartz et al., 2000; Whitty et al., 2005]. Rather, it may be best to present these caregivers with information geared specifically toward the specific cluster of symptoms experienced by their ill relative (e.g., auditory hallucinations, depressed mood, etc.) while simultaneously attending to and normalizing any anxiety that these caregivers may experience due to the lack of a definitive diagnosis.

Developing an effective delivery system for family psychoeducation for first-episode psychosis is further complicated by variation among families with regard to both their need for psychoeducation as well as their desire to participate in a family psychoeducation program. A sizeable proportion of families decline or withdraw from formal psychoeducation programs [Glynn, Cohen, and Niv, 2007; Tarrier, 1991]. In an early review of family psychoeducation programs, Smith and Birchwood [1990] found that across studies 13.5% (median) of families refused to participate in the intervention and an additional 11% (median) withdrew from treatment. More recent studies have reported even higher rates (≥ 40%) of refusal and/or non-adherence to family interventions [McCreadie, Phillips, Harvey, Waldron, and et al., 1991; Montero, Asencio, Ruiz, and Hernández, 1999; Szmukler et al., 2003], and there is preliminary evidence that the same may be true for familial caregivers of individuals with first-episode psychosis. For instance, among participants in one of the premier clinical services for first-episode psychosis in the world (i.e., the Calgary Early Psychosis Program: [Addington and Addington, 2001]), 20% of families decline to participate in a family psychoeducation program and 37% of those who do participate drop out of the intervention prior to its completion [Addington et al., 2005]. The inability to successfully engage these families is problematic given that individuals with psychosis whose families decline to participate in family psychoeducation programs may be at greater risk for negative clinical outcomes (e.g., symptomatic relapse [Tarrier, 1991]).

Several recent studies have noted that not all family members caring for a relative with a psychotic disorder may need to participate in formal family psychoeducation programs [Cohen et al., 2008; Mottaghipour and Bickerton, 2005--see also Bickerton, Hense, Benstock, Ward, and Wallance for an example outside of the psychosis literature]. For instance, whereas certain families caring for a relative with a psychotic illness may require participation in a formalized family psychoeducational intervention to relieve their distress, other families may require a less intensive intervention (e.g., a single informational session on psychosis) to achieve the same reduction in distress. Consequently, such studies have devised programs of "family work" in which individuals with psychotic disorders and their caregiving relatives have the option of progressing through increasingly intensive family interventions ranging from brief education on psychosis to participation in formal psychoeducational interventions. This progression is stopped once the family's distress is alleviated, resulting in a clinical delivery system in which not all families would progress to the more intensive interventions (e.g., family psychoeducation). In support of such a model, Cohen and colleagues [2008] draw on the "principle of sufficiency"--a ethical concept most famously outlined by the philosopher Harry Frankfurt [1987; 1997]—arguing that the most appropriate manner in which to distribute a valuable but limited good across individuals (in this case, psychiatric care) is to provide each individual with just enough of that good to prevent the occurrence of a negative outcome. Translated to family work for psychotic disorders, the sufficiency principle suggests that the provision of family services should be guided by the goal of providing each family with the least intensive intervention that will alleviate current distress and reduce the likelihood of future negative outcomes (e.g., continued distress for the caregiver or worsening of symptoms for the individual with psychosis). Applying this ethical construct to the delivery of medical services may reduce the costs by preventing the inappropriate overuse of expensive and intensive services [Shapiro, Lasker, Bindman, and Lee, 1993], and may also be consistent with the goals of caregiving relatives. For instance, familial caregivers of individuals with psychosis have noted that it is problematic both to receive too much or too little information from mental health professionals about psychosis and their ill relative's care [Askey et al., 2009]. This suggests that caregivers, too, prefer family interventions that are only as intensive as needed to address their specific needs.

Thus, the goal of this paper is to outline a service delivery protocol for family work developed over a two year period at the Specialized Treatment Early in Psychosis (STEP) Program. Drawing on past service delivery protocols for psychotic disorders [e.g., Cohen et al., 2008; Mottaghipour and Bickerton, 2005], this service delivery protocol outlines the provision of stepped-care for families specifically caring for a relative with first-episode psychosis. Ultimately, this service delivery system may serve as an example for other clinical services for first-episode psychosis.

## The STEP Program: A Clinical Service for First-Episode Psychosis

The Specialized Treatment Early in Psychosis (STEP) Program is a collaboration between Yale University and the Connecticut Department of Mental Health and Addiction Services [Srihari et al., 2009]. Located in the Connecticut Mental Health Center, STEP is designed to determine the feasibility and cost-effectiveness of a comprehensive early intervention service based in the US public-sector. The components of the complex intervention include medication management, case management, family psychoeducation, and group cognitive-behavioral therapy. Individuals eligible to receive clinical services at the STEP program must be:

(i) Between the ages of 16-45;
(ii) Meet criteria for a psychotic disorder or affective disorder with psychotic features based on the Structured Clinical Interview for the DSM-IV (SCID: First, Spitzer, Gibbon, and Williams, 2002);
(iii) Have had no more than 12 weeks of lifetime treatment with antipsychotic medication; and
(iv) Be willing to receive treatment at the Connecticut Mental Health Center.

Individuals are not eligible to receive clinical services at STEP if they are:

(i) Suffering from a substance-induced psychotic disorder or severe cognitive limitation; or
(ii) Unable to provide informed consent to participate in the research activities associated with the STEP Program.

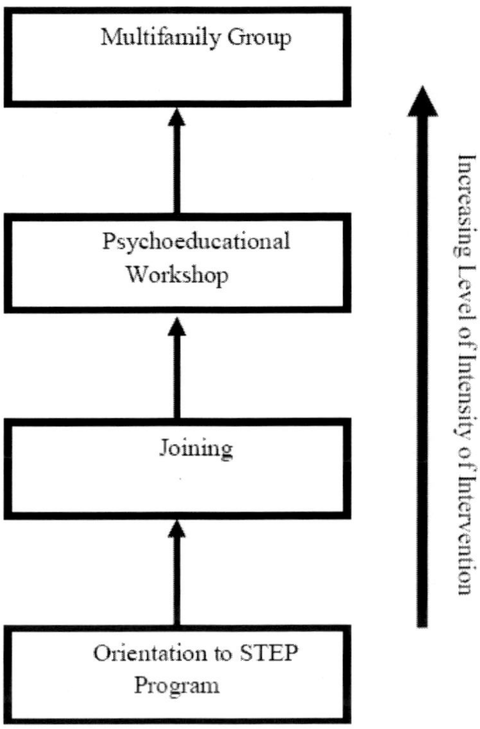


Figure 1. Family Work Model at the Specialized Treatment Early in Psychosis (STEP) Program.

Within the STEP Program, we have developed a program which provides families with the opportunity to personalize their levels of participation in family services based on their needs. The components of this model draw largely from the seminal multifamily group psychoeducation program developed by William McFarlane [McFarlane, 2002; McFarlane et al., 1995] which, in turn, is based on the family psychoeducation programs created by Anderson and colleagues [1986] and Falloon and colleagues [1985]. This decision was informed by past research indicating that this intervention may be particularly beneficial for individuals with first-episode psychosis [McFarlane, 2002] as well as the successful implementation of this family psychoeducation program within exemplary first-episode clinical research programs [Bertelsen et al., 2008; Fjell et al., 2007]. However, as depicted in Figure 1, our model of family work provides families with the opportunity to participate in the STEP program with varying levels of intensity depending on their needs and interests. Moreover, consistent with existing recommendations [Rossberg et al., 2010], we have made a number of modifications to the McFarlane multifamily group model to increase its applicability for families caring for a relative who is early in the course of a psychotic disorder. Below, we outline the components of each level of the model.

## Orientation to the STEP Program

Within the STEP Program, we have designated a specific individual (i.e., the Project Director) to oversee the family work component of the clinical service. The Project Director is responsible for screening all new referrals to the STEP Program and works to ensure that a caregiving relative attends these eligibility screening meetings as well to facilitate early family engagement with the STEP Program. Including family members in the initial eligibility meetings allows for the collection of additional information with regard to the patient's clinical course and symptoms but, more importantly, also facilitates the early establishment of a collaborative relationship between the family members and the clinical staff. The components of the STEP program are explained to both the patient and caregiving relative, and the Project Director answers questions with regard to the treatment, etiology, and course of psychotic disorders as needed.

Patients deemed eligible for the STEP Program are scheduled for a second meeting with the Project Director. For patients, the goal of this second meeting is to complete registration paperwork and the baseline assessment as well as to schedule the first clinical appointments. However, family members are requested to attend this meeting as well to further their engagement with the STEP Program. As caregiving relatives of individuals with a mental illness typically identify increased communication as the area of greatest need of improvement in their relationship with clinical staff [Biegel, Song, and Milligan, 1995], several actions are completed at this meeting to facilitate communication between family caregivers and members of the STEP treatment team. First, written consent is obtained from the patient for bidirectional communication between family members and the treatment staff at this second meeting. To date, some patients have had initial concerns about allowing their family members to talk directly with clinical staff. These clients have each been provided with the opportunity to discuss these concerns confidentially with clinical staff and, during the two years in which this intervention was implemented, no client has refused to allow his or her family members to have bidirectional communication with STEP clinical staff. Second, family members (and the individual with psychosis) are introduced to the various mental health professionals who will be providing care to their relative (i.e., the psychiatrist, primary clinician, and the respective group leaders for the family psychoeducation and cognitive-behavioral therapy interventions). Family members are provided with the opportunity to ask questions to each of these individuals and are provided with each person's contact information should future questions arise. By providing family members with multiple contact points among the STEP clinical staff, we hope to empower family members' active participation in all aspects of the treatment planning and delivery. Finally, family members are also provided with a "Family Information Packet" which includes written information on psychosis and substance abuse, details with regard to the community clinic in which the STEP Program is located, and the common challenges experienced by individuals caring for a relative with psychosis.

Finally, family members are informed about the various additional components of the STEP family work program (i.e., joining sessions, psychoeducational workshop, multifamily group, and family therapy). This discussion includes a description of the additional family work components as well a brief overview of the potential benefits associated with participation in these interventions as demonstrated in the research literature. Family members are informed that their relative with psychosis may still participate in all aspects of the STEP Program regardless of whether the family member chooses to participate in any additional aspect of family work program. Additionally, family members are informed that they may always later choose to participate in any of the more intensive aspects of the STEP family work component even if they initially decline to do so.

## Joining Sessions

Caregiving relatives and clinically stable individuals with first-episode psychosis who desire to participate in additional family services are next invited to participate in three joining sessions with the Project Director. The goals of these sessions are to provide education about psychosis and to strengthen the therapeutic alliance between the family and STEP clinical staff. During these visits, which are modeled on the joining sessions included in McFarlane's multifamily group psychoeducation program [McFarlane, 2002], the Project Director discusses several key topics with the family members, including:

(i) The physiological changes in brain structure and functioning that accompany psychosis;
(ii) The stress-diathesis model of expression of psychotic symptoms;
(iii) Identification of early warning signs that their relative's psychotic symptoms are worsening; and
(iv) Caregivers' explanatory model of their relative's psychotic symptoms.

Given that the McFarlane model was not developed specifically for first-episode psychosis, we discuss two additional key topics with family members at the STEP Program that are specifically related to first-episode psychosis:

(i) The "critical period" hypothesis; and
(ii) Uncertainty with regard to diagnosis and the long-term course of illness in first-episode psychosis.

The order in which these five key topics are presented to family members over the course of the three joining sessions is outlined in Table 1. Typically, two topics are presented during each respective joining session. For example, during joining session one, families are presented with information with regard to brain physiological and psychosis as well as the critical period hypothesis.

The first topic reviewed during the joining session is the physiological changes in brain structure and functioning that accompany psychosis and the link between these changes and the symptoms of psychosis. The goal of this activity is to highlight to family members (i.e., both caregivers and ill relatives) that psychosis is similar to other medical symptoms in that it stems from underlying biological processes. Given the large number of such biological processes that are associated with psychosis, we have found it most useful to provide only a few specific examples of physiological factors that are associated with psychosis [e.g., the loss of grey and white matter that accompanies and may event predate the expression of psychotic symptoms [Glantz and Lewis, 2000; Thompson et al., 2001; Witthaus et al., 2008], disruptions in neurotransmitter systems such as dopamine and glutamate [Davis, Kahn, Ko, and Davidson, 1991; Olney and Farber, 1995], and hypoactivity in the prefrontal cortex [Hill et al., 2004]. These specific examples were selected as they can be communicated easily through visual depictions (e.g., showing slides of the decreased number of dendritic spines on neurons of individuals with psychotic disorders versus individuals without psychotic disorders) and because the hypothesized link between these physiological features and symptoms of psychosis have been relatively well explicated to date [e.g., the link between hypoactivity in the prefrontal cortex and disruptions in working memory [Carter et al., 1998].

Second, caregiving relatives are presented with information with regard to the "critical period" hypothesis for psychotic disorders [Birchwood, 1999; Birchwood and Fiorillo, 2000; Birchwood, Todd, and Jackson, 1998].

**Table 1. Topics Addressed During Joining Sessions**

| |
|---|
| 1. Brain Physiology and Psychosis. |
| 2. The "Critical Period" Hypothesis. |
| 3. The Stress-Diathesis Model of Psychotic Symptoms. |
| 4. Identifying Warning Signs of an Upcoming Symptomatic Exacerbation. |
| 5. Family Members' Explanatory Model of Psychosis. |
| 6. Uncertainty with regard to Relative's Illness. |

Drawing on research suggesting that the majority of functional and clinical deterioration that accompanies psychotic disorders occur early in the course of these illnesses (e.g., within the first 2-5 years [Crumlish et al., 2009; Lieberman et al., 2001; McGlashan, 1998]), the "critical period" hypothesis suggests that targeted intervention provided early in the course of a psychotic illness may have a disproportionately large and positive effective on the long term course of illness. Presenting family members with this information may not only help to increase their motivation to play an active role in the care provided to their ill relative at the STEP Program, but also helps to provide these individuals with a sense of hope with regard to an illness for which it may often be difficult to remain hopeful about [Tuck, du Mont, Evans, and Shupe, 1997].

Third, the Project Director elicits the caregivers' explanatory model of their relative's psychotic symptoms. Such models include perceptions of the causes, course, and appropriate treatment for the ill relative's symptoms [Kleinman, 1980; Kleinman, Eisenberg, and Good, 1978] as well as caregivers' perception of their role in their relative's treatment and recovery [Chesla, 1989]. Understanding caregivers' explanatory models for their relative's psychotic symptoms is important for several reasons. First, this provides an opportunity to highlight ways in which engagement in family interventions is consistent with the caregivers' beliefs with regard to optimal treatment and desired outcomes for their relative with psychosis—a factor which may increase engagement with family work programs for psychosis [Tarrier, 1991]. Second, it allows for the correction of common misunderstandings with regard to psychosis that may lead to the experience of unnecessary distress among caregiving relatives. Examples of such misunderstandings include blaming one's self for the onset of psychosis in a relative, believing that recovery in schizophrenia is impossible, and feeling powerless to help their ill relative in any way.

With regard to the assessment of caregivers' explanatory models of their ill relative's psychosis, we utilize the series of questions identified by Kleinman and colleagues [Kleinman, 1980; Kleinman et al., 1978]:

(i) What do you think is the cause of this symptom?
(ii) What course do you expect this symptom to take;
(iii) How serious is this symptom?
(iv) How does this symptom affect your relative's mind and/or body?
(v) What kind of treatment do you think your relative should receive for this symptom?

(vi) What results do you hope your relative will obtain from this treatment?
(vii) What problems has the symptom caused for you and for your relative?
(viii) What do you fear most about your relative's symptom?
(ix) What do your fear most about the treatment for your relative's symptom?

Fourth, the Project Director reviews the diathesis-stress model of psychosis [Fowles, 1992; Walker and Diforio, 1997] with the caregiving relatives. Specifically, the Project Director explains to family members that due to pre-existing biological vulnerability factors, psychosocial stressors (including substance use) may trigger the onset of future psychotic symptoms in their relative with psychosis. The goal of this discussion is not to encourage family members to remove *all* stressors from their ill relative's life. Doing so would likely be impossible and would potentially prevent their ill relative from participating in positive and meaningful aspects of the recovery process in psychosis which, by their very nature, would include some experience of stress (e.g., participating in educational/vocational activities and forming new friendships or romantic relationships). Rather, the goal of this activity is:

(i) To clarify to the family members that in certain situations the onset of future psychotic symptoms may be outside of their and their ill relative's control; and
(ii) To help families become more proactive in identifying situations in which their ill relative may be exposed to particularly high levels of stress (e.g., during final examination week at school) so that they can be better prepared to provide additional support and care as needed.

Fifth, the Project Director works with family members to identify early warning or "prodromal" signs of a future symptomatic exacerbation. The rationale of this exercise, as explained to the family members, is that the onset of psychotic symptoms is often preceded by the occurrence of non-psychotic psychiatric symptoms and observable changes in behavior on the part of the ill relative (e.g., increased anxiety and depressed mood, sleep difficulties, increased social isolation, etc. [Herz and Melville, 1980; Marder et al., 1991; Subotnik and Nuechterlein, 1988]) and that providing targeted pharmacological and psychological interventions upon the recognition of the presence of these early warning signs (in addition to the continued receipt of maintenance medication) can reduce the likelihood that a relapse of full psychotic symptoms will occur [Birchwood, Spencer, and McGovern, 2000; Clare and Singh, 1994; Hewitt and Birchwood, 2002; Lamberti, 2001]. The importance of preventing future symptomatic relapses is further emphasized to family members by noting findings suggesting that the risk of the development of treatment-resistant and/or residual symptoms increases with each relapse [Lieberman et al., 2001; Shepherd, Watt, Falloon, and Smeeton, 1989; Wiersma, Nienhuis, Sloof, and Giel, 1998]. Available research suggests that the vast majority of familial caregivers (≥90%) can retrospectively identify changes in their ill relative's behavior and emotions shortly before the occurrence of a psychotic relapse [Birchwood et al., 1989; Herz and Melville, 1980], and within the STEP Program, it is our experience that caregivers are typically able to identify several of their relative's idiosyncratic "early warning" signs through recounting the period of time during which they first became concerned about their ill relative's health. Similar results have been reported in other studies of first-episode cohorts [Fjell et al., 2007]. To facilitate this recall, the Project Director reviews with the caregiving relative a list of common early warning signs of an incipient symptomatic exacerbation [see, for example, Tarrier, Barrowclough, and Bamrah, 1991]. However, in some instances in which the family member was not in close contact with their ill relative during the onset of the psychotic symptoms, we have requested that the individual with first-episode psychosis be present for these meetings to provide additional information with regard to the details of the onset of their psychotic symptoms.

The final topic addressed during the joining session is uncertainty experienced by caregivers with regard to their ill relative's illness. Uncertainty among relatives caring for an individual with a chronic illness stems from multiple factors, including inability to predict future outcomes for the ill relative, lack of information or unclear information provided by health providers with regard to their relative's illness, and ambiguity stemming from the presence of unexplained symptoms or the lack of clear rationale for why certain treatments are provided [Mishel, 1983]. Within the context of caring for a relative with first-episode psychosis, there are several factors which commonly contribute to caregivers' sense of uncertainty. For instance, given the diagnostic ambiguity often present early in the course of psychotic disorders, [Amin et al., 1999; Schwartz et al., 2000; Whitty et al., 2005], it is often difficult (if not impossible) to provide caregivers with a definitive diagnosis for their ill relatives. Likewise, as there is considerable heterogeneity in the long term course of psychotic illnesses [Ciompi, 1980; Davidson and McGlashan, 1997; Shepherd et al., 1989; Thara, 2004], mental health practitioners may not always be able to provide caregivers with specific information with regard to their ill relative's prognosis. Finally, although there are several effective pharmacological and psychosocial treatments for psychotic disorders, data to inform the delivery of personalized interventions to individuals with first-episode psychosis based on their unique combination of presenting features (e.g., symptom onset, environmental stressors, treatment motivation, etc.) is lacking [Breitborde, Srihari, Pollard, Addington, and Woods, 2010]. Consequently, determination of what specific interventions will be most effective for a specific individual with first-episode psychosis may often be made based on "trial and error"—a strategy which may increase caregivers' uncertainty with regard to the treatment provided to their ill relative.

Addressing caregivers' uncertainty is a complex task given the varied outcomes that may result from such uncertainty. More specifically, available research has found that uncertainty in the context of chronic illness is associated with both negative and positive outcomes [Babrow, Kasch, and Ford, 1998; Brashers, 2001; Brashers and Babrow, 1996]. Scholars have suggested that these divergent results may stem from individuals' varied appraisal of their uncertainty—uncertainty that is perceived as dangerous may lead to negative outcomes, whereas uncertainty that is perceived as an opportunity may lead to positive outcomes [Babrow et al., 1998; Mishel, 1988, 1990]. For example, studies outside of the schizophrenia literature have demonstrated that uncertainty with regard to whether one's treatment will be effective (uncertainty as danger) is distressing for individuals with a chronic illness and their caregiving relatives, whereas uncertainty with regard to whether one is predestined to experience a negative outcome associated with one's chronic illness (uncertainty as opportunity) may promote hope and optimism among individuals with a chronic illness and their caregiving relatives [Brashers, Goldsmith, and Hsieh, 2002; Brashers et al., 2000; Nelson, 1996; Newton and Mateo, 1994]. Thus, within the STEP clinic, our approach is to inquire into any areas in which caregivers may be feeling uncertain with regard to their ill relative and determine whether this uncertainty is distressing (i.e., uncertainty as danger) or whether this uncertainty is a source of hope for the caregiver (i.e., uncertainty as opportunity).

To assist in this assessment, one could rely on the questions included in the Parents' Perception of Uncertainty in Illness Scale [Mishel, 1983]. If the uncertainty is distressing to the caregiver, the Project Director will use several techniques to assist the caregiver in coping with her or his uncertainty. These techniques, which are drawn from empirically-validated interventions for coping with uncertainty in the context of living with a chronic illness [Hoff et al., 2005; Mishel et al., 2002; Northouse, Kershaw, Mood, and Schafenacker, 2005] as well as Berger and Calabrese's [1975] seminal work on uncertainty reduction, include:

(i) Normalizing the experience of uncertainty associated with caring for a relative with a chronic illness;
(ii) Providing information to the caregiver so as to improve her or his ability to accurately predict the outcome of the uncertain situation (e.g., informing the caregiver that their relative may need to take antipsychotic medication for several weeks before they achieve the full benefit of the medication);
(iii) Teaching the caregivers strategies that they can use to obtain needed information in the future (e.g., providing contact information for all local social service agencies);
(iv) Assisting caregivers in differentiating between behaviors that are under their ill relative's control (e.g., substance use) versus those that are not (e.g., persecutory delusions); and
(v) Instructing caregivers in the use of a structured problem-solving activity that they can use to identify solutions to perplexing problems associated with the caregiving experience (i.e., identify the problem, develop a list of possible solutions, evaluate the advantages and disadvantage of each solution, and enact the solution that provides the best ratio of advantages to disadvantages).

Of note, these techniques are not designed to eliminate all uncertainty associated with the caregiving experience—such a goal is unrealistic [Babrow and Kline, 2000]. Rather, the goal of these activities is to help the caregiver cope with uncertainty in situations in which such uncertainty may be a source of distress and interfere with caregiving.

## Psychoeducational Workshop

Should families express interest in additional services or should family members' distress persist, caregiving relatives and their clinically stable relatives with psychosis are invited to attend a psychoeducation workshop. The goals of this workshop are to:

(i) Review the topics covered during the joining sessions;
(ii) Educate families about the benefits of pharmacological and psychosocial treatments for psychosis with particular attention devoted to reviewing family psychoeducation programs specifically;
(iii) Discuss the format of the family group sessions and review common challenges associated with joining a family group; and
(iv) Identify additional topics that families would like to learn more about during the future family group sessions.

Of note, although a significant portion of the psychoeducational workshop is dedicated to the review of topics that were previously reviewed during the joining sessions, in our experience, family members typically appreciate the recapitulation of these topics.

Following our review of the material covered during the joining session, we next discuss the effects of pharmacological and psychological treatments on the symptoms of psychosis as well as the underlying brain pathology that accompanies this psychiatric symptom. This review includes discussion of the symptomatic reductions and neuroprotective effects of pharmacological and psychosocial treatments for psychosis [e.g., Eack et al., 2010; Thompson et al., 2008]. In highlighting how treatments may influence the physiological processes underlying psychosis, we hope to increase hope among caregivers and ill relatives with regard to the ill relative's course of illness. However, the majority of this time in this section of the workshop is devoted specifically to reviewing the benefits associated with participating in the multifamily group [e.g., lower rates of relapse [McFarlane et al., 1995], reduced negative symptoms [Dyck et al., 2000], and reduced caregiver distress [Hazel et al., 2004]. Per research on health belief theory [Tsang, Fung, and Corrigan, 2006], our goal in providing families with information with regard to the potential benefits of the family group is to increase the likelihood that they will choose to participate in this program. Specifically, health belief theory research has demonstrated that individuals are more likely to participate in a health intervention if they believe that participating in this intervention will allow them to reduce the likelihood of a future negative health outcome (e.g., a psychotic relapse for their relative with first-episode psychosis).

The next topic addressed in the psychoeducation workshop is the format of the family group sessions and common challenges associated with joining a family group. Drawing on Yalom's work [1966; 1975; 1967] suggesting that new members typically experience significant anxiety when entering a therapy group for which the format and expectations are unclear, scholars have hypothesized that providing new group members with pretherapy orientation to the group process and structure may reduce attrition rates [France and Dugo, 1985; Yalom, 1966]. Attrition in group therapy is a significant problem both due to its frequency [i.e., a mean rate of 35% across studies [Bostwick, 1987] as well as its deleterious effects on other group members. More specifically, attrition of group members is often a source of anxiety for both the other group members and the group leader(s) who may fear that such attrition is a precursor of the complete dissolution of the group [Yalom, 1966]. Ultimately, such anxiety may negatively influence the efficacy of the group [Yalom, 1966]. In their review of pretherapy orientation research in the overall psychotherapy literature, Walitzer and colleagues [1999] found that the majority of studies reported results which comport with the hypothesis that pretherapy orientation may reduce client attrition and improve client attendance. As such, we view this orientation as a critical component of the psychoeducation workshop. With regard to group process, we attempt to normalize the anxiety associated with entering an existing group by highlighting that this is a common experience. To further emphasize this, we invite a family member who is already participating in the family group to attend the psychoeducational workshop to talk to the new families about their experience participating in the multifamily group. Additionally, we further attempt to reduce anxiety among the families by providing information about the structure of the multifamily group. A description of this group structure is outlined in subsection below.

The final component of the psychoeducation workshop involves identifying educational topics that family members would like to review during the multifamily group. Including this component in the psychoeducational workshop accomplishes two goals. First, it creates additional incentive for families to attend the multifamily group. Second, identifying these topics during the workshop provides the group leaders with additional time to schedule the required speakers needed to addresses the educational topics requested by the families.

## Multifamily Group

Following the completion of the joining sessions and psychoeducational workshop, family members are invited to join the multifamily group. In situations in which a family member is not interested in participating in the psychoeducation group, the Project Director reviews any concerns that the family member may have with regard to participating in the group. To date, typical concerns have included difficulty with transportation to the group, conflicts between the time of the group and other scheduled activities (e.g., work), and concern about participating in a group program (e.g., concerns about sharing private material in front of other families). When possible, the Project Director works with these individuals to find solutions for these barriers to participation in the family psychoeducation program. For example, family members who were not comfortable participating in a group program are offered the opportunity to participate in meetings with one of the leaders of the family group where they can receive continued individual education about psychosis and support. All family members who choose not to participate in the family group are informed that they can join the group at any future point during their relative's participation in the STEP Program.

During each family group session, families participate in one of two activities. First, certain sessions are dedicated to structured problem-solving activities based on the McFarlane multifamily group model [McFarlane, 2002; McFarlane et al., 1995]. More specifically, through group discussion, the attendees select a specific problem that one family is currently struggling with. Next, the families collectively identify several possible solutions to this problem (e.g., 6-8). The families then collectively review the pros and cons of each suggested solution. Finally, based on this discussion, the specific family that is struggling with the problem addressed during the session identifies the solution(s) that they feel would be most effective in addressing their problem. This family is then expected to attempt to enact these solutions during the two weeks before the next group session. The subsequent session then begins with a review of the problem identified during the previous session and the proposed solution selected by the family. This family provides an update of their attempt to implement this solution. Should this attempt be unsuccessful, the family is asked to identify the factors which prevented the success of this solution and is reminded of the other non-implemented solutions identified during the previous session for this problem. More details with regard to this problem solving activity can be found in McFarlane [2002].

Sessions not devoted to the problem-solving activity are reserved for additional educational activities suggested by the families participating in the group. Typically, these activities involve bringing a speaker to the group to address a topic that falls outside of the range of expertise of the group leaders. To date, educational activities have addressed topics such as estate planning, mental health advocacy, supported housing programs, first-hand accounts of living with mental illness, and strategies to negotiate interactions with law enforcement during behavioral crises. The breadth of such topics is consistent with the conceptualization of recovery in severe mental illness as involving many factors that:

(i) Occur outside of the clinic; and
(ii) Fall outside of the expertise of most mental health providers [Davidson, 2003].

Although many of these topics are identified during the psychoeducational workshop, members of the family group are repeatedly queried over the course of their participation in the group about possible topics for future educational sessions.

With regard to the logistics of the family group, two 90-minute group sessions are scheduled per month. We have relied on a rolling admission policy such that new families may join the family group at anytime. This strategy allows for the development of "veteran" families who can often serve as guides and supports to new families who join the group. Finally, due to the reluctance of many STEP clients to participate in the family group, we allow family members to participate in the group without the concurrent participation of their relative with first-episode psychosis. Given evidence that relapse rates do not vary across family work programs that include caregivers and ill relatives versus programs that include caregivers alone [Leff et al., 1989, 1990], we feel that it is not necessary to require that individuals with first-episode psychosis attend the group with their caregiving relatives.

## Movement through the STEP Family Work Model

Upon enrollment in the STEP Program, families are assessed for their interest in participation in the family work program. Specifically, we seek to obtain an initial assessment of a family's desired level of intensity with regard to participation in the STEP family work model. However, we recognize that families desired level of intensity with regard to participation in the family work model may change over the course of their participation in the STEP Program. For example, following a hospitalization of their ill relative, a family who initially declined to participate in the multifamily group may now desire to join the family group for additional education and support. Consequently, we continuously track negative outcomes among individuals with first-episode psychosis in the STEP program during weekly clinical rounds that the STEP Project Director attends. When such a negative outcome occurs (e.g., hospitalization, relapse of substance use, loss of a job, etc.), the Project Director will offer to schedule a session with the family and to facilitate their participation the educational workshop and/or multifamily group if desired.

**Table 2. Uptake of STEP Family Work Model**

| Level | n/N | Percentage* |
|---|---|---|
| None | 17/42 | 40% |
| Joining | 25/42 | 60% |
| Psychoeducational Workshop | 6/42 | 14% |
| Multifamily Group | 6/42 | 14% |

*Values do not sum to 100% as some families participated in multiple levels of the intervention.

## Uptake of STEP Family Work Model

Families' level of participation in the STEP Family Work Model is summarized in Table 2. Among STEP participants, 40% of families decline to participate in any aspect of the family work model. This figure is consistent with the non-participation rates reported in other studies of family work in first-episode psychosis [e.g., Fjell et al., 2007]. However, among the remaining 60% of families—all of whom would traditionally only have the option of participating in a high intensity family psychoeducation program—only 6 out of 25 (24%) opted to participate in the most intense aspect of the STEP family work program (i.e., the multifamily group). The remaining 76% chose to participate only in the less intense joining sessions. This occurred despite the fact that these families were provided with significant encouragement to participate in the psychoeducational workshop and the multifamily groups. In total, these results are consistent with the available evidence suggesting that not all families desire intensive family interventions [Cohen et al., 2008; Mottaghipour and Bickerton, 2005--see also Bickerton, Hense, Benstock, Ward, and Wallace for an example outside of the psychosis literature]. Rather, many families may prefer to participate only in briefer, less intense family interventions (i.e., individual joining sessions).

# CONCLUSION

Family interventions have a strong empirical basis in the treatment of psychotic disorders [Dixon et al., 2001]. With nearly 25 years of research demonstrating the clear benefits of these interventions, scholars have noted that there is only minimal utility in additional studies of the efficacy of these interventions [Hogarty, 2003]. Thus, what is the future of family work research? We would suggest that important contributions to this field of research can be made by exploring the ways in which existing interventions can be improved and/or adapted for specific populations. These population-specific interventions could be geared to meet the needs of specific clinical populations (e.g., first-episode psychosis), but should likely also consider the varying needs of individual families (i.e., some families may require less intensive interventions that other families). Ultimately, developing more nuanced versions of family work interventions will be an important first step in moving toward a system of care in which families are provided with personalized treatment plans and resources can be deployed more economically.

# REFERENCES

[1] Addington, J., and Addington, D. (2001). Early intervention for psychosis: The Calgary Early Psychosis and Prevention Program. *Canadian Psychiatric Association Bulletin,* 33, 11-16.

[2] Addington, J., Addington, D., Jones, B., and Ko, T. (2001). Family interaction in an early psychosis program. Psychiatric Rehabilitation Skills, 5, 272-286.

[3] Addington, J., and Burnett, P. (2004). Working with families in the early stages of psychosis. In J. F. M. Gleeson and P. D. McGorry (Eds.), Psychological Interventions in Early Psychosis (pp. 99-116). West Sussex, U. K.: John Wiley and Sons.

[4] Addington, J., Collins, A., McCleery, A., and Addington, D. (2005). The role of family work in early psychosis. Schizophrenia Research, 79, 77-83.

[5] Amin, S., Singh, S. P., Brewin, J., Jones, P. B., Medley, I., and Harrison, G. (1999). Diagnostic stability of first-episode psychosis: Comparison of ICD-10 and DSM-III-R systems. British Journal of Psychiatry, 175, 537-543.

[6] Anderson, C. M., Hogarty, G. E., and Reiss, D. (1986). Schizophrenia and the family. New York: Guilford Press.

[7] Anderson, C. M., Reiss, D. J., and Hogarty, G. E. (1986). Schizophrenia and the family: A practitioner's guide to psychoeducation and management. New York: Guilford Press.

[8] Arno, P. S., Levine, C., and Memmott, M. M. (1999). The economic value of informal caregiving. Health Affairs, 18, 182-188.

[9] Askey, R., Holmshaw, J., Gamble, C., and Gray, R. (2009). What do carers of people with psychosis need from mental health services? Exploring the view of carers, service users and professionals. Journal of Family Therapy, 31, 310-331.

[10] Babrow, A. S., Kasch, C. R., and Ford, L. A. (1998). The many meanings of uncertainty in illness: Toward a systematic accounting. Health Communication, 10, 1-23.

[11] Babrow, A. S., and Kline, K. N. (2000). From "reducing" to "coping with" uncertainty: Reconceptualizing the central challenge in breast self-exams. Social Science and Medicine, 51, 1805-1816.

[12] Baucom, D. H., Shoham, V., Mueser, K. T., Daiuto, A. D., and Stickle, T. R. (1998). Empirically supported couple and family interventions for marital distress and adult mental health problems. Journal of Consulting and Clinical Psychology, 66, 53-88.

[13] Berger, C. R., and Calabrese, R. (1975). Some explorations in initial interactions and beyond: Toward a developmental theory of interpersonal communication. Human Communication Research, 1, 99-112.

[14] Bertelsen, M., Jeppesen, P., Petersen, L., Thorup, A., Øhlenschlæger, J., le Quach, P., Christensen, T. O., Krarup, G., Jørgensen, P., and Nordentoft, M. (2008). Five-year follow-up of a randomized multicenter trial of intensive intervention vs standard treatment for patients with a first episode of psychotic illness: The O. P. U. S. study. Archives of General Psychiatry, 65, 762-771.

[15] Bickerton, A., Hense, T., Benstock, A., Ward, J., and Wallace, L. (2007). Safety First: A model of care for working systematically with high risk young people and their families in an acute C. A. M. H. S. service. Australian and New Zealand Journal of Family Therapy, 28, 121-129.

[16] Biegel, D. E., Song, L.-y., and Milligan, S. E. (1995). A comparative analysis of family caregivers' perceived relationships with mental health professionals. Psychiatric Services, 46, 477-482.

[17] Birchwood, M. (1999). Early intervention in psychosis: The critical period. In P. D. McGorry and H. J. Jackson (Eds.), The Recognition and Management of Early Psychosis: A Preventative Approach (pp. 226-264). Port Chester, N. Y.: Cambridge University Press.

[18] Birchwood, M., and Fiorillo, A. (2000). The critical period for early intervention. American Journal of Psychiatric Rehabilitation, 4, 182-198.

[19] Birchwood, M., Smith, J., MacMillan, F., Hogg, B., Prasad, R., Harvey, C., and Bering, S. (1989). Predicting relapse in schizophrenia: The development and implementation of an early signs monitoring system using patients and families as observers, a preliminary investigation. Psychological Medicine, 19, 649-656.

[20] Birchwood, M., Spencer, E., and McGovern, D. (2000). Schizophrenia: Early warning signs. Advances in Psychiatric Treatment, 6, 93-101.

[21] Birchwood, M., Todd, P., and Jackson, C. (1998). Early intervention in psychosis: The critical period hypothesis. British Journal of Psychiatry, 172, 53-59.

[22] Bostwick, G. (1987). "Where's Mary?" A review of the group treatment dropout literature. Social Work with Groups, 10, 117-131.

[23] Brashers, D. E. (2001). Communication and uncertainty management. Journal of Communication, 51, 477-497.

[24] Brashers, D. E., and Babrow, A. S. (1996). Theorizing communication and health. Communication Studies, 47, 243-251.

[25] Brashers, D. E., Goldsmith, D. J., and Hsieh, E. (2002). Information seeking and avoiding in health context. Human Communication Research, 28, 258-271.

[26] Brashers, D. E., Neidig, J. L., Haas, S. M., Dobbs, L. K., Cardillo, L. W., and Russell, J. A. (2000). Communication in the management of uncertainty: The case of persons living with H. I. V. or A. I. D. S. Communication Monographs, 67, 63-84.

[27] Breitborde, N. J. K., López, S. R., and Kopelowicz, A. (2010). Expressed emotion and health outcomes among Mexican-Americans with schizophrenia and their caregiving relatives. Journal of Nervous and Mental Disease, 198, 105-109.

[28] Breitborde, N. J. K., Srihari, V. H., Pollard, J., Addington, D. N., and Woods, S. W. (2010). Mediators and moderators in early intervention research. Early Intervention in Psychiatry, 4, 143-152.

[29] Carter, C. S., Perlstein, W., Ganguli, R., Brar, J., Mintum, M., and Cohen, J. D. (1998). Functional hypofrontality and working memory dysfunction in schizophrenia. American Journal of Psychiatry, 155, 1281-1284.

[30] Chen, F.-p., and Greenberg, J. S. (2004). A positive aspect of caregiving: The influence of social support on caregiving gains for family members of relatives with schizophrenia. Community Mental Health Journal, 40, 423-435.

[31] Chesla, C. A. (1989). Parents' illness models of schizophrenia. Archives of Psychiatric Nursing, 3, 218-225.

[32] Ciompi, L. (1980). The natural history of schizophrenia in the long term. British Journal of Psychiatry, 136, 413-420.

[33] Clare, L., and Singh, K. (1994). Preventing relapse in psychotic illness: A psychological approach to early intervention. Journal of Mental Health, 3, 541-550.

[34] Cohen, A. N., Glynn, S. M., Murray-Swank, A. B., Barrio, C., Fischer, E. P., McCutcheon, S. J., Perlick, D. A., Rotondi, A. J., Sayers, S. L., Sherman, M. D., and Dixon, L. B. (2008). The family forum: Directions for the implementation of family psychoeducation for severe mental illness. Psychiatric Services, 59, 40-48.

[35] Crumlish, N., Whitty, P., Clarke, M., Browne, S., Kamali, M., Gervin, M., McTigue, O., Kinsella, A., Waddington, J. L., Larkin, C., and O'Callaghan, E. (2009). Beyond the critical period: Longitudinal study of 8-year outcome in first-episode non-affective psychosis. British Journal of Psychiatry, 194.

[36] Cuijpers, P. (1999). The effects of family interventions on relatives' burden: A meta-analysis. Journal of Mental Health, 8, 275-285.

[37] Davidson, L. (2003). Living outside mental illness: Qualitative studies of recovery in schizophrenia. New York: New York University Press.

[38] Davidson, L., and McGlashan, T. H. (1997). The varied outcomes of schizophrenia. Canadian Journal of Psychiatry, 42, 34-43.

[39] Davis, K. L., Kahn, R. S., Ko, G., and Davidson, M. (1991). Dopamine in schizophrenia: A review and reconceptualization. American Journal of Psychiatry, 148, 1474-1486.

[40] Dixon, L., McFarlane, W. R., Lefley, H., Lucksted, A., Cohen, M., Falloon, I., Mueser, K., Miklowitz, D., Solomon, P., and Sondheimer, D. (2001). Evidence-based practices for services to families of people with psychiatric disabilities. Psychiatric Services, 52, 903-910.

[41] Dyck, D. G., Short, R. A., Hendryx, M. S., Norell, D., Myers, M., Voss, W. D., and McFarlane, W. R. (2000). Management of negative symptoms among patient with schizophrenia attending multiple-family groups. Psychiatric Services, 51, 513-519.

[42] Eack, S. M., Hogarty, G. E., Cho, R. Y., Prasad, K. M. R., Greenwald, D. P., Hogarty, S. S., and Keshavan, M. S. (2010). Neuroprotective effects of cognitive enhancement therapy against gray matter loss in early schizophrenia. Archives of General Psychiatry, 67,
674-682.

[43] Falloon, I. R. H., Boyd, J. L., McGill, C. W., Williamson, M., Razani, J., Moss, H. B., Gilderman, A. M., and Simpson, G. M. (1985). Family management in the prevention of morbidity of schizophrenia: Clinical outcome of a two-year longitudinal study. Archives of General Psychiatry, 42, 887-896.

[44] First, M. B., Spitzer, R. L., Gibbon, M., and Williams, J. B. W. (2002). Structured Clinical Interview for DSM-IV-TR Axis I Disorders, Research Version, Patient Edition with Psychotic Screen (SCID-I/P W/ PSY SCREEN). New York: Biometrics Research, New York State Psychiatric Institute.

[45] Fjell, A., Thorsen, G. R. B., Friis, S., Johannessen, J. O., Larsen, T. K., Lie, K., Lyse, H.-G., Melle, I., Simonsen, E., Smeby, N. A., Øxnevad, A. L., McFarlane, W. R., Vaglum, P., and McGlashan, T. (2007). Innovations: Psychoeducation: Multifamily group treatment in a program for patients with first-episode psychosis: Experiences for the T. I. P. S. Project. Psychiatric Services, 58, 171-173.

[46] Fowles, D. C. (1992). Schizophrenia: Diathesis-stress revisited. Annual Review of Psychology, 43, 303-336.

[47] France, D. G., and Dugo, J. M. (1985). Pretherapy orientation as preparation for open psychotherapy groups. Psychotherapy, 22, 256-261.

[48] Frankfurt, H. (1987). Equality as a moral ideal. Ethics, 98, 21-43.

[49] Frankfurt, H. (1997). Equality and respect. Social Research, 64, 3-15.

[50] Gallagher, S. K., and Mechanic, D. (1996). Living with the mentally ill: Effects on the health and functioning of other household members. Social Science and Medicine, 42, 1691-1701.

[51] Glantz, L. A., and Lewis, D. A. (2000). Decreased dendritic spine density on prefrontal cortical pyramidal neurons in schizophrenia. Archives of General Psychiatry, 57, 65-73.

[52] Glynn, S. M., Cohen, A. N., and Niv, N. (2007). New challenges in family intervention for schizophrenia. Expert Review of Neurotherapeutics, 7, 33-43.

[53] Hazel, N. A., McDonell, M. G., Short, R. A., Berry, C. M., Voss, W. D., Rodgers, M. L., and Dyck, D. G. (2004). Impact of multiple-family groups for outpatients with schizophrenia on caregivers' distress and resources. Psychiatric Services, 55, 35-41.

[54] Herz, M. I., and Melville, C. (1980). Relapse in schizophrenia. American Journal of Psychiatry, 137, 801-805.

[55] Hewitt, L., and Birchwood, M. (2002). Preventing relapse of psychotic illness: Role of self-monitoring of prodromal symptoms. Disease Management and Health Outcomes, 10, 395-407.

[56] Hill, K., Mann, L., Laws, K. R., Stephenson, C. M., Nimmo-smith, I., and McKenna, P. J. (2004). Hypofrontality in schizophrenia: A meta-analysis of functional imaging studies. Acta Psychiatrica Scandinavica, 110, 243-256.

[57] Hoff, A. L., Mullins, L. L., Gillaspy, S. R., Page, M., C., Van Pelt, J. C., and Chaney, J. M. (2005). An intervention to decrease uncertainty and distress among parents of children newly diagnoses with diabetes: A pilot study. Families, Systems, and Health, 23, 329-342.

[58] Hogarty, G. E. (2003). Does family psychoeducation have a future? World Psychiatry, 2, 29-30.

[59] Joseph, R., and Birchwood, M. (2005). The national policy reforms for mental health services and the story of early intervention services in the United Kingdom. Journal of Psychiatry and Neuroscience, 30, 362-365.

[60] Kleinman, A. (1980). Patients and healers in the context of culture: An exploration of the borderland between anthropology, medicine, and psychiatry. Berkeley: University of California Press.

[61] Kleinman, A., Eisenberg, L., and Good, B. (1978). Culture, illness, and care: Clinical lessions from anthropologic and cross-cultural research. Annals of Internal Medicine, 88, 251-258.

[62] Kuipers, L. (1993). Family burden in schizophrenia: implications for services. Social Psychiatry and Psychiatric Epidemiology, 28, 207-210.

[63] Lamberti, J. S. (2001). Seven keys to relapse prevention in schizophrenia. Journal of Psychiatric Practice, 7, 253-259.

[64] Leff, J., Berkowitz, R., Shavit, N., Strachan, A., Glass, I., and Vaughn, C. (1989). A trial of family therapy v. a relatives group for schizophrenia. British Journal of Psychiatry, 154, 58-66.

[65] Leff, J., Berkowitz, R., Shavit, N., Strachan, A., Glass, I., and Vaughn, C. (1990). A trial of family therapy versus a relatives' group for schizophrenia: Two-year follow-up. British Journal of Psychiatry, 157, 571-577.

[66] Lieberman, J. A., Jody, D., Geisler, S., Alvir, J., Loebel, A., Szymanski, S., Woerner, M., and Borenstein, M. (1993). Time course and biologic correlates of treatment response in
first-episode schizophrenia. Archives of General Psychiatry, 50, 369-376.

[67] Lieberman, J. A., Perkins, D., Belger, A., Chakos, M., Jarskog, F., Boteva, K., and Gilmore, J. (2001). The early stages of schizophrenia: Speculations on pathogenesis, pathophysiology, and therapeutic approaches. Biological Psychiatry, 50, 884-897.

[68] Magliano, L., Fadden, G., Madianos, M., Caldas de Almeida, J. M., Held, T., Guarneri, M., Marasco, C., Tosini, P., and Maj, M. (1998). Burden on the families of patients with schizophrenic results of the BIOMED I study. Social Psychiatry and Psychiatric Epidemiology, 33, 405-412.

[69] Marder, S. R., Mintz, J., Van Putten, T., Lebell, M., Wirshing, W. C., and Johnston-Cronk, K. (1991). Early prediction of relapse in schizophrenia: An application of receiver operating characteristic (R. O. C.) methods. Psychopharmacology Bulletin, 27, 79-82.

[70] McCreadie, R. G., Phillips, K., Harvey, J. A., Waldron, G., and et al. (1991). The Nithsdale schizophrenia surveys: VIII. Do relatives want family intervention--and does it help? British Journal of Psychiatry, 158, 110-113.

[71] McFarlane, W. R. (2002). Multifamily groups in the treatment of severe psychiatric disorders. New York: Guilford Press.

[72] McFarlane, W. R., Dixon, L., Lukens, E., and Lucksted, A. (2003). Family psychoeducation and schizophrenia: A review of the literature. Journal of Marital and Family Therapy, 29, 223-245.

[73] McFarlane, W. R., Lukens, E., Link, B., Dushay, R., Deakins, S. A., Newmark, M., Dunne, E. J., Horen, B., and Toran, J. (1995). Multiple-family groups and psychoeducation in the treatment of schizophrenia. Archives of General Psychiatry, 52, 679-687.

[74] McGlashan, T. H. (1998). A selective review of recent North American follow-up studies on schizophrenia. Schizophrenia Bulletin, 14, 515-542.

[75] Melle, I., Larsen, T. K., Haahr, U., Friis, S., Johannessen, J. O., Opjordsmoen, S., Rund, B. R., Simonsen, E., Vaglum, P., and McGlashan, T. (2008). Prevention of negative symptom psychopathologies in first-episode schizophrenia: Two year effects of reducing the duration of untreated psychosis. Archives of General Psychiatry, 65, 634-640.

[76] Miller, F. E. (1996). Grief therapy for relatives of persons with serious mental illness. Psychiatric Services, 47, 633-637.

[77] Mishel, M. H. (1983). Parents' perception of uncertainty concerning their hospitalized child. Nursing Research, 32, 324-330.

[78] Mishel, M. H. (1988). Uncertainty in illness. Image: Journal of Nursing Research, 20, 225-232.

[79] Mishel, M. H. (1990). Reconceptualization of the uncertainty in illness theory. Image: Journal of Nursing Scholarship, 22, 256-262.

[80] Mishel, M. H., Belyea, M., Germino, B. B., Stewart, J. L., Bailey, D. E. J., Robertson, C., and Mohler, J. (2002). Helping patients with localized prostate carcinoma manage uncertainty and treatment side effects: Nurse-delivered psychoeducational intervention over the telephone. Cancer, 94, 1854-1866.

[81] Möller-Leimkühler, A. M. (2005). Burden of relatives and predictors of burden. Baseline results from the Munich 5-year-follow-up study on relatives of first hospitalized patients with schizophrenia or depression. European Archives of Psychiatry and Clinical Neuroscience, 255, 223-231.

[82] Montero, I., Asencio, A. P., Ruiz, I., and Hernández, I. (1999). Family interventions in schizophrenia: An analysis of non-adherence. Acta Psychiatrica Scandinavica, 100, 136-141.

[83] Mottaghipour, Y., and Bickerton, A. (2005). The pyramid of family care: A framework for family involvement with adult mental health services. Australian e-Journal for the Advancement of Mental Health, 4, 1-8.

[84] Mueser, K. T., and Glynn, S. M. (1999). Behavioral family therapy for psychiatric disorders. Oakland, C. A.: New Harbinger.

[85] National Institute of Mental Health. (2009). Major N. I. M. H. research project to test approaches to altering the course of schizophrenia: Recovery act funds will support first phase of project. Retrieved January 28, 2010, from the World Wide Web: http://www.nimh.nih.gov/science-news/2009/major-nimh-research-project-to-test-approaches-to-altering-the-course-of-schizophrenia.shtml.

[86] Nelson, J. P. (1996). Struggling to gain meaning: Living with the uncertainty of breast cancer. Advances in Nursing Science, 18, 59-76.

[87] Newton, C., and Mateo, M. A. (1994). Uncertainty: Strategies for patients with brain tumor and their families. Cancer Nursing, 17, 137-140.

[88] Northouse, L., Kershaw, T., Mood, D., and Schafenacker, A. (2005). Effects of a family intervention on the quality of life of women with recurrent breast cancer and their family caregivers. Psycho-Oncology, 14, 478-491.

[89] Olney, J. W., and Farber, N. B. (1995). Glutamate receptor dysfunction and schizophrenia. Archives of General Psychiatry, 52, 998-1007.

[90] Perkins, D. O., Lieberman, J. A., Gu, H., Tohen, M., McEvoy, J., Green, A. I., Zipursky, R. B., Strakowski, S. M., Sharma, T., Kahn, R. S., Gur, R., and Tollefson, G. (2004). Predictors of antipsychotic treatment responses in patients with first-episode schizophrenia, schizoaffective and schizophreniform disorders. British Journal of Psychiatry, 185, 18-24.

[91] Pilling, S., Bebbington, P., Kuipers, E., Garety, P., Geddes, J., Orbach, G., and Morgan, C. (2002). Psychological treatments in schizophrenia: I. Meta-analysis of family intervention and cognitive behaviour therapy. Psychological Medicine, 32, 763-782.

[92] Pitschel-Walz, G., Leucht, S., Bäuml, J., Kissling, W., and Engel, R. R. (2001). The effect of family interventions on relapse and rehospitalization in schizophrenia--A meta-analysis. Schizophrenia Bulletin, 27, 73-92.

[93] Rossberg, J. I., Johannessen, J. O., Klungsoyr, O., Opjordsmoen, S., Evensen, J., Fjell, A., Haahr, U., Joa, I., Langeveld, J., Larsen, T. K., Melle, I., Rund, B. R., Simonsen, E., ten Velden, W., Vaglum, P., Friis, S., and McGlashan, T. (2010). Are multi family groups appropriate for patients with first episode psychosis? A 5-year naturalistic follow-up study. Acta Psychiatrica Scandinavica, 122, 384-394.

[94] Schulz, R., and Beach, S. R. (1999). Caregiving as a risk factor for mortality. J. A. M. A., 282, 2215-2219.

[95] Schwartz, J. E., Fenning, S., Tanenberg-Karant, M., Carlson, G., Craig, T., Galambos, N., Lavelle, J., and Bromet, E. J. (2000). Congruence of diagnoses 2 years after a first-admission diagnosis of psychosis. Archives of General Psychiatry, 57.

[96] Shapiro, D. W., Lasker, R. D., Bindman, A. B., and Lee, P. R. (1993). Containing cost while improving quality of care: The role of profiling and practice guidelines. Annual Review of Public Health, 14, 219-241.

[97] Shepherd, M., Watt, D., Falloon, I., and Smeeton, N. (1989). The natural history of schizophrenia: A five year follow-up study of outcome and prediction in a representative sample of schizophrenics. Psychological Medicine, 19 (Monograph Supplement 15), 1-46.

[98] Smith, J., and Birchwood, M. (1990). Relatives and patients as partners in the management of schizophrenia: The development of a service model. British Journal of Psychiatry, 156, 654-660.

[99] Srihari, V. H., Breitborde, N. J. K., Pollard, J., Tek, C., Hyman, L., Frisman, L. K., McGlashan, T. H., Jacobs, S., and Woods, S. W. (2009). Public-academic partnership: Early intervention for psychotic disorders in a community mental health center. Psychiatric Services, 60, 1426-1428.

[100] Subotnik, K. L., and Nuechterlein, K. H. (1988). Prodromal signs and symptoms of schizophrenic relapse. Journal of Abnormal Psychology, 97, 405-412.

[101] Szmukler, G., Kuipers, E., Joyce, J., Harris, T., Leese, M., Maphosa, W., and Staples, E. (2003). An exploratory randomised controlled trial of a support programme for carers of patients with a psychosis. Social Psychiatry and Psychiatric Epidemiology, 38, 411-418.

[102] Tarrier, N. (1991). Some aspects of family interventions in schizophrenia: I. Adherence to intervention programmes. British Journal of Psychiatry, 159, 475-480.

[103] Tarrier, N., Barrowclough, C., and Bamrah, J. S. (1991). Prodromal signs of relapse in schizophrenia. Social Psychiatry and Psychiatric Epidemiology, 26, 157-161.

[104] Thara, R. (2004). Twenty-year course of schizophrenia: The Madras longitudinal study. Canadian Journal of Psychiatry, 49, 564-569.

[105] Thompson, P. M., Bartzokis, G., Hayashi, K. M., Klunder, A. D., Lu, P. H., Edwards, N., Hong, M. S., Yu, M., Geaga, J. A., Toga, A. W., Charles, C., Perkins, D. O., McEvoy, J., Hamer, R. M., Tohen, M., Tollefson, G. D., Lieberman, J. A., and the H. G. D. H. Study Group. (2008). Time-lapse mapping of cortical changes in schizophrenia with difference treatments. Cerebral Cortex, 19, 1107-1123.

[106] Thompson, P. M., Vidal, C. N., Giedd, J. N., Gochman, P., Blumenthal, J., Nicolson, R., Toga, A. W., and Rapoport, J. L. (2001). Mapping adolescent brain change reveals dynamic wave of accelerated grey matter loss in very early-onset schizophrenia. Proceedings of the National Academy of Sciences of the United States of America, 98, 11650-11655.

[107] Tsang, H. W. H., Fung, K. M. T., and Corrigan, P. W. (2006). Psychosocial treatment compliance scale for people with psychotic disorders. Australian and New Zealand Journal of Psychiatry, 40, 561-569.

[108] Tuck, I., du Mont, P., Evans, G., and Shupe, J. (1997). The experience of caring for an adult child with schizophrenia. Archives of Psychiatric Nursing, 11, 118-125.

[109] Walitzer, K. S., Derman, K. H., and Connors, G. J. (1999). Strategies for preparing clients for treatment: A review. Behavior Modification, 23, 129-151.

[110] Walker, E. F., and Diforio, D. (1997). Schizophrenia: A neural diathesis-stress model. Psychological Review, 104, 667-685.

[111] Whitty, P., Clarke, M., McTigue, O., Browne, S., Kamali, M., Larkin, C., and O'Callaghan, E. (2005). Diagnostic stability four years after a first episode of psychosis. Psychiatric Services, 56, 1084-1088.

[112] Wiersma, D., Nienhuis, F. J., Sloof, C., and Giel, R. (1998). Natural course of schizophrenic disorders: A 15 year follow-up of a Dutch incidence cohort. Schizophrenia Bulletin, 24, 78-85.

[113] Winefield, H. R., and Harvey, E. J. (1994). Needs of family caregivers in chronic schizophrenia. Schizophrenia Bulletin, 20, 557-566.

[114] Witthaus, H., Brüne, M., Kaufmann, C., Bohner, G., Özgürdal, S., Gudlowski, Y., Heinz, A., Klingebiel, R., and Juckel, G. (2008). White matter abnormalities in subjects at ultra high-risk for schizophrenia and first-episode schizophrenic patients. Schizophrenia Research, 102, 141-149.

[115] Yalom, I. D. (1966). A study of group therapy dropouts. Archives of General Psychiatry, 14, 393-414.

[116] Yalom, I. D. (1975). The Theory and Practice of Group Psychotherapy. New York: Basic Books.

[117] Yalom, I. D., Houts, P. S., Newell, G., and Rand, K. H. (1967). Preparation of patients for group therapy: A controlled study. Archives of General Psychiatry, 17, 416-427.

In: Psychosis: Causes, Diagnosis and Treatment
Editor: Xenia Anastassiou-Hadjicharalambous

ISBN: 978-1-62081-516-8


*Chapter 10*

# FAMILY INTERVENTIONS: FUNDAMENTAL CONSIDERATIONS WHEN DEVELOPING ROUTINE AND FORMAL FAMILY INTERVENTIONS SERVICES

***Frank R. Burbach****

Somerset Partnership NHS Foundation Trust, United Kingdom

## ABSTRACT

Family interventions (FI) have been recognised as an important part of the biopyschosocial treatment package for people with schizophrenia and other psychoses. The addition of family interventions to routine care, including medication, results in significantly superior clinical outcomes for people with psychosis.

The needs of caregivers is discussed and the rationale for working with families is presented. The substantial evidence-base for formal family interventions (structured goal-orientated sessions) with individual families and with multi-family groups is briefly reviewed. This well-known research was largely conducted with chronic populations, but the subsequent development of FI has been significantly influenced by the more recent focus on people experiencing their first episode of psychosis. This contemporary literature, and its implications for service delivery, is discussed.

Research into some of the underlying constructs regarding family stress levels and a model which integrates the findings regarding family emotional climate, attributions and interactions is presented.

It will be argued that although the 'critical ingredients' of a successful family intervention have not yet been established, the creation of a collaborative relationship between the family, patient and services probably contributes significantly to the positive clinical outcomes identified in research studies. The constituents of a 'collaborative engagement with families' as well as 'formal family interventions' will be clearly delineated and the implications for service delivery will be explored.

* E-mail: frank.burbach@sompar.nhs.uk

This chapter is intended to help clinicians and service managers to successfully develop FI in real-world clinical settings, by clarifying what is required, considering FI service models and the implications for staff training, as well as suggesting how best to overcome the commonly reported barriers to the implementation of FI.

## INTRODUCTION

With the onset of community-based care for people with psychosis, the crucial role of the family in providing care and support has been increasingly recognised. It is clear that an effective bio-psycho-social treatment package depends on the collaborative engagement of the service user (patient) as well as their key supporters/ caregivers.

Although many people with chronic mental health problems lose contact with family members, most young people experiencing a first episode of psychosis (FEP) are in close contact with their families [1] and mental health services thus have an ideal opportunity to forge treatment partnerships with family members from this early stage.

Following the realization that medication alone does not 'cure' schizophrenia and other psychoses, there has been a burgeoning interest in psychological treatments, beginning in the 1980s when the early family intervention studies clearly demonstrated improved outcomes. This was followed by the subsequent development of individual psychotherapeutic interventions for psychosis such as Cognitive Behavioural Therapy [2] as well as a renewed emphasis on social interventions, including evidence-based employment support programmes [3, 4]. This chapter will focus on family interventions (FI) for psychosis, and aims to provide an overview of the field as well as a guide to the implementation of FI.

## RATIONALE FOR WORKING WITH FAMILIES

When someone has a severe mental health problem such as psychosis there are numerous benefits to working collaboratively with families and other significant members of the social support network (e.g. landladies; members of the local church or college tutors) and numerous rigorous research studies have shown that formal family interventions (FI) result in significantly superior clinical outcomes for people with psychosis [5]. Family members are crucial to optimal recovery of the person with psychosis, as they are often the ones who initiate and maintain contact with the specialist services, and physically provide the bulk of the care.

Medical and psychosocial interventions often require ongoing encouragement, support and reinforcement, and the family is a valuable resource in this regard. When the lives of people with psychosis are chaotic and they are poorly engaged with services, working with family members is sometimes the best way to maintain therapeutic input. In addition, research [6] has shown that family members experience a significant amount of stress in caring for someone in the early stages of a psychotic disorder, and that this may develop into unhelpful, critical or over intrusive behaviours [7, 8, 9] which, in turn, may contribute to subsequent relapse [10]. The extensive research literature examining the family emotional climate associated with relapse and the associated theoretical debates will be explored later in this chapter.

## FAMILY NEEDS

Although aspects of caregiving can be perceived as positive, many caregivers find that caregiving is time-consuming and stressful. They often have difficulty in accessing services and are forced to cope with challenging situations and high-risk behaviour, without adequate support and guidance. Many caregivers have to deal with numerous crises, sometimes involving contact with the police, ambulance and other services. It can become difficult to maintain employment and carers can suffer financially. In addition, many carers find that they cannot continue their previous leisure activities and their social networks shrink. The stigma associated with severe mental health problems in many communities often contributes to caregivers becoming socially isolated. Many caregivers also experience a complicated grief reaction as they struggle to come to terms with their relative's ongoing difficulties and many experience depression as a result of hopelessness and loss. Athough caregivers commonly experience stress, exhaustion and distress, mental health services have traditionally focused on treating the patient's symptoms. More recently, it is encouraging to note increased acknowledgement both of the fact that carers need support in their own right, to maintain their physical and mental wellbeing, and that family members need to be enabled to provide care, in order to optimise recovery of their relative. Additionally, it is now being recognized that the meeting of carers' needs may require an appreciation of the factors pertaining to their particular situation - an individually tailored approach to supporting carers. Family caregivers may be parents, partners, siblings or even children; they will have a range of understandings about the situation they find themselves in; they will have a range of resources and coping strategies available to them; and they will have had a range of 'premorbid relationships' with the person experiencing psychosis. There is therefore no simple formula that can be applied to determine the needs of family caregivers. The needs of particular family members will also change over time.

A helpful heuristic may be to consider families' needs in terms of a hierarchy [11], although it must be emphasised again that families' needs will not necessarily present in single categories and will not necessarily develop in a step-wise manner. When first involved with services, families tend to require information (about mental health issues, treatment options, how services work etc.) and the opportunity to talk about their traumatic experiences. This commonly includes a need to discuss their experiences in relation to the development of psychosis; difficulties in accessing appropriate help and feelings of fear, anger, loss and grief. Many will also welcome further help with solving problems (for example about roles, chores or achieving goals) and improving communication (eg. when misattributions result in patterns consisting of criticism and withdrawal), and some will seek more in-depth exploration of issues.

In our experience, some families engage more with psychoeducational interventions, while others are more interested in reflecting on family relationships and interactions in the context of family history and cultural issues. It is not just a tiny minority of families that are interested in having more multi-facetted family discussions and thus our Family Needs diagram (Figure 1 below) has a trapezoid rather than pyramidal shape. This conceptualization of family needs also differs from service-related models in that families referred to in the top sections of the diagram are not viewed as more challenging or needing greater input.

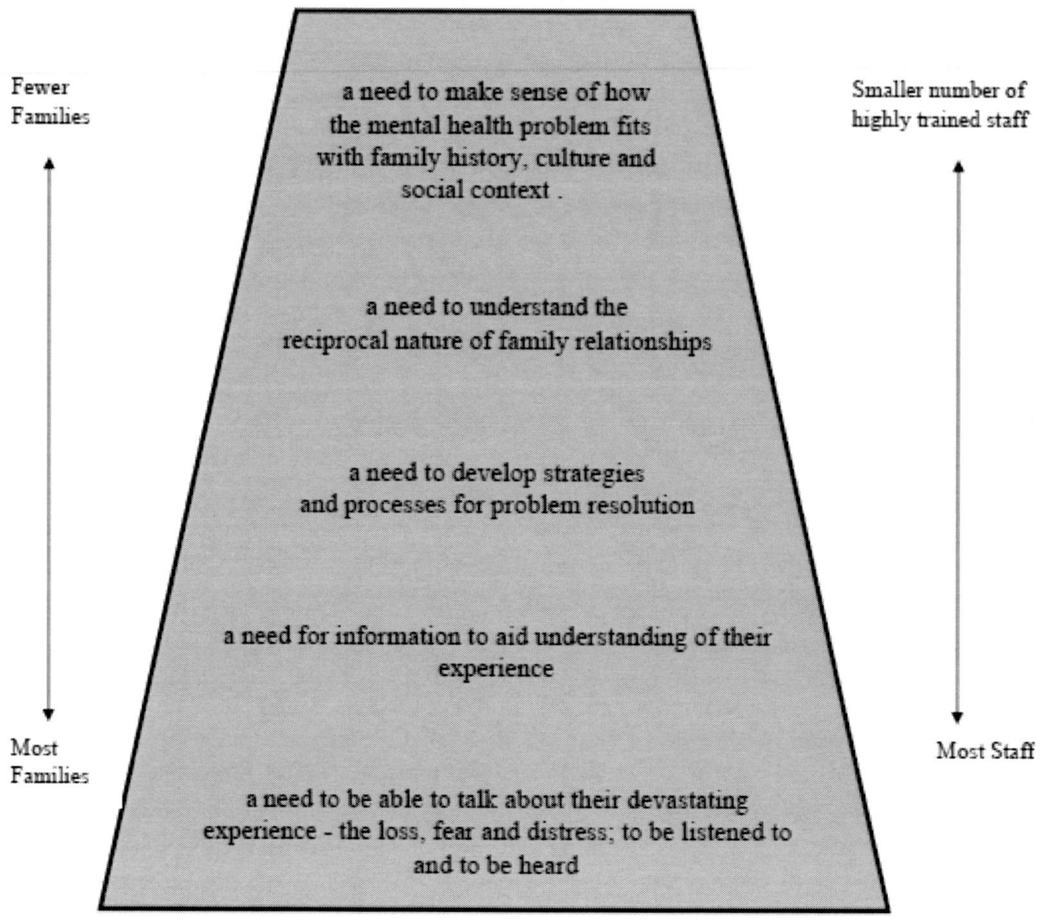


Figure 1. A hierarchy of family needs.

In services where staff have more extensive training in working with families (eg. Somerset [12, 13], or Western Lapland in Finland [14]) it is often possible to have family sessions in which multi-facetted, systemic issues are addressed in a relatively brief but comprehensive manner. It remains to be shown whether such approaches confer additional benefits over the psychoeducational interventions in terms of outcome for the person with psychosis or the other family members, but the evidence is encouraging [15]. We have found our trapezoid model helpful as it also reflects the relationship between the number of families with particular needs and the training needs of staff. The relationship between family needs, staff training and service provision is also addressed in Mottaghipour and Bickerton's (2005) 'pyramid of family care' model [16]. This model proposes a minimum level of care to meet families' basic needs for information regarding illness and orientation to the mental health service, and, in a hierarchical fashion, builds more specialist interventions to meet more complex family needs. They conclude that all staff will need to possess an ability to form supportive therapeutic relationships with families, be able to provide relevant information in a manner which takes into account the families' current knowledge and beliefs, and have some ability to enable families to reduce stress levels by improving communications and developing coping strategies and problem-solving skills.

However, in some circumstances, families may require more complex psychotherapeutic intervention, for example where pre-existing relationship problems are impacting on the person with a first-episode psychosis or in situations of pre-existing trauma or abuse. The traumatising effect of the onset of psychosis, and the guilt, denial, anger or hopelessness that frequently accompany this would probably require the more skilled input of an experienced therapist.

## EVIDENCE BASE

Numerous randomised controlled trials (RCT's) have shown that the inclusion of Family Intervention (FI) with standard care, including medication, significantly reduces relapse rates, improves social functioning, reduces 'family burden' and reduces overall treatment costs for schizophrenia [17, 18, 19]. In addition, a systematic review has recently confirmed that FI reduces relapse and hospital admission rates for young people with FEP [20].

Arguably the most scientifically rigorous of these reviews was the 2009-10 updated Cochran Collaboration meta-analysis of 53 carefully selected RCT's [5]. They calculated the relative risk (RR) and its 95% confidence interval (CI) based on the fixed-effect model. They reported reductions in relapse rates (RR 0.55) and readmission to hospital (RR 0.78), increased medication compliance (RR 0.6), and general improvements in social impairment and in the levels of 'expressed emotion' in the family. They also calculated the number needed to treat (NNT) to prevent a relapse and concluded "family intervention significantly reduces hospital admission at one year, with one patient out of every eight treated with family intervention prevented from hospitalization compared with standard care" (p23). Although the Cochrane review recognises methodological limitations in many of the included studies, it is encouraging that their robust meta-analytic approach continues to conclude that family intervention is worth the time and effort, especially if families could be clearly shown to also benefit from this approach as well as patients (to date relatively few studies have investigated the benefits for family members).

The original research studies established that the addition of FI to routine care, including medication, dramatically reduced the relapse rates. At 9 months to 1 year the relapse rates ranged from 6–12%, whereas in routine treatment controlled groups' relapse rates ranged from 41–53%. At 2-year follow-up the advantages of FI over controls were maintained, although the relapse rates had increased (17–40% versus 66–83%). Once the original research studies had established that the addition of FI to routine care more than halved relapse rates, a second generation of studies established that psychoeducational family interventions could be replicated across cultures and in routine clinical settings [21]. Comparative FI studies [22] appear to indicate that a range of psychoeducational approaches are effective and that no one model or "brand" of FI is superior. However, Multiple Family Groups (MFGs) appear to offer a slight advantage over individual family interventions, particularly for families having to cope with significant ongoing symptomatology [23, 24]. Unfortunately MFGs also have a higher drop-out rate and are not acceptable to some families. Thus it can only be concluded that MFGs should be one of a number of options available, rather than viewing them as the family treatment of choice. A detailed treatment manual for MFGs is now available [25]. Although the 'critical ingredients' of a successful FI have not yet been established, the creation of a collaborative relationship between the family, client and services probably contributes significantly to the positive clinical outcomes identified in research studies. However, specific therapeutic techniques are required with particular families to have an impact on the emotional climate and the family members' ability to cope with the often-extreme stress of the advent of a psychotic episode.

## CONTENT OF FAMILY INTERVENTIONS

The clinical approaches developed for the family intervention research studies conducted in the 1980s and 1990s incorporated a range of behavioural, cognitive and systemic techniques but had a similar philosophical basis and a common emphasis on psychoeducation. These approaches were based on a stress-vulnerability model of schizophrenia [26] and had been developed largely as a result of the research findings that relapse rates were higher when families were rated as high in 'expressed emotion' (viz. criticism, hostility or over involvement) [27, 28]. The psychoeducational approaches commonly included an educational component regarding etiology, symptoms, prognosis and medication adherence; formal or informal problem solving, and addressed issues of communication (often through behavioural skills training). A number of treatment manuals describing the approaches used in the early studies have been published [29, 30, 31, 32]. Although they have much in common, family interventions also differ in a number of respects and it is therefore impossible to draw definitive conclusions about the 'critical ingredients'. Variations include whether the patient is involved in the family sessions, the extent to which formal skills training is used, the differing combinations of individual or group family sessions, the intensity of contact and the length of the interventions.

In addition, studies examining the hypothesized mediating variables (e.g. problem solving or communication skills) have been inconclusive and a forum of family intervention experts concluded that key confounding factors (e.g. easier access to the treatment team or use of relapse prevention plans) had not been sufficiently controlled for [33]. With the development of first episode psychosis (FEP) services family interventions have undergone further development. There is a consensus in the early intervention treatment guides that FI for people with FEP requires a different approach to the first generation research models originally developed for people with longstanding psychotic symptoms/chronic disability [34, 1, 35].

Besides embracing diagnostic uncertainty and providing information about psychosis rather than schizophrenia, the main difference in early FI is a focus on helping the family to cope with the trauma of having a family member who develops psychosis. Rather than primarily engaging families by providing information, early FI is more flexible and crisis – oriented, with an initial focus on the family members' emotional needs. The Open Dialogue (OD) family and network approach developed in Finnish Western Lapland [14, 15] appears to demonstrate the benefits of continuity of care and the active mobilization of the wider support network eg. employers and fellow employees, in addition to the focus on the development of coping skills, which is the main focus of most psychoeducational approaches. This community-based crisis intervention approach puts the family and social network at the center of the treatment, with the team aiming to establish contact within 24 hours of a crisis and subsequently involving them in all treatment discussions and decisions. The same team takes responsibility for the entire treatment process, whether the patient is in hospital or the community, and adopts the family's language and concepts in order to create a dialogue that increases their sense of agency.

In a descriptive study the OD approach appears to result in better functional outcomes for people with first episode psychosis than those achieved by other approaches. Although the 5-year relapse rates [15] did not differ significantly between the comparison approaches, the evidence appears to show that the OD group recovered more quickly, had fewer days in hospital, was more likely to have returned to education or employment and had used less antipsychotic medication. Although the OD approach differs in it's philosophical basis to psychoeducational approaches, the superior outcomes may be due to the quality of the family-based intervention- a highly skilled treatment team is able to respond flexibly and creatively to the needs of the family, uses medication sparingly in a carefully targeted way, focuses on functional outcomes, and brokers acceptance in the wider social network. Although it may be unattainable in many current service settings, the comprehensive service provided in this area of Finland illustrates the principles that an optimum service might aspire to.

Although there is considerable variation in the FI approaches developed to date, it is suggested that the common factors underpinning them deserve more recognition. A particularly important aspect of FI sessions is that they provide a safe forum for family members to express their emotions, to reach a more helpful shared understanding of what has happened, and to receive emotional and practical support to deal with the treatment services and their relative's symptoms and behaviour. However, these positive outcomes can be enabled through a variety of contacts with families, not only in formally constituted family sessions but also during the impromptu discussions with families that can occur as part of routine psychiatric care. It is for this reason that the engagement of families in a collaborative working relationship from their first contact with mental health services should be a priority. Relatively brief contact with families can facilitate the sharing of information, and the provision of emotional support and guidance/skills to cope with their relative's distress and symptoms. This is sometimes sufficient to prevent the development of unhelpful attitudes and interactional patterns, and can thus contribute to a reduction in relapse and the minimization of family members' distress. In order to create appropriate services to meet the varied needs of family members we have found it helpful to delineate what constitutes 'formal family interventions' and 'collaborative engagement with families'. This has enabled the planning of workforce training initiatives [36] and the evaluation and audit of different types of family work [37].

## Collaborative Engagement of Families/ Carers

It is likely that much of the improvement in relapse/hospital admission rates in the early FI studies was due to the development of a treatment partnership between the professionals and the family. Families have traditionally experienced difficulties in getting appropriate professional help for the young person with an emerging psychosis and have felt excluded from their relative's care at the first and subsequent episodes. Involving families in a collaborative partnership [38] from the beginning can create a very different long-term relationship with services.

**Table 1. Routine Family Interventions**

| Collaborative engagement of families in the delivery of care |
|---|
| • Provision of clear messages about the advantages of working together in a 3-way partnership (client, family/carers, clinicians) |
| • Routine involvement of family/carers in the assessment process |
| • Routine involvement of family/carers in treatment planning and reviews |
| • Family/carer involvement in Early Warning Signs monitoring and the agreement of a robust Relapse Prevention Plan (this ensures that families/carers know whom to contact in a crisis) |
| • Exploration of relatives' distress and provision of emotional support |
| • Ongoing clarification with the client regarding the sharing of information and the limits of confidentiality |
| • Provision of information and guidance to help the family/carers to maintain hope and optimize their coping |
| • Provision of information on self-help support groups |
| • Offering a Carer's Assessment and referral to carer support services or family intervention services as appropriate |
| • Consider the welfare of dependent children, siblings and vulnerable adults and carers' physical, social and mental health needs |

Such a two-way partnership would ideally contain the following: an open exchange of information, involvement in the ongoing review and planning of their relative's care, involvement in the setting of realistic recovery goals, the monitoring of stress levels and the emergence of symptoms, and a robust plan to ensure that they could get appropriate help in a crisis. This could be described as 'routine family interventions' (see Table 1). Relatively straightforward information, support and guidance can encourage medication concordance and can enable the family to develop coping strategies, which result in an environment that promotes recovery.

All services should therefore strive to involve family members in routine care wherever possible and appropriate. This will require sensitive ongoing negotiation about the extent of information-sharing, in the context of a clear policy regarding client confidentiality [39, 40].

Routine early engagement with families as part of the assessment process will also enable the gathering of invaluable information about the young person who has developed their FEP as well as enabling the low-key assessment of family members' needs. In the UK this may lead to a more formal Carer's Assessment and referral to mental health or carers' support services.

## FORMAL FAMILY INTERVENTIONS

In addition to routine family involvement in care, a range of formal goal oriented family interventions are required to meet the needs of a significant proportion of families. In recent years there has been a growing consensus amongst clinicians about the content of FI (see Table 2), as well as an appreciation that the interventions should be provided flexibly, tailored to the particular needs of each family.

Family psycho-education initiatives with individual families [30, 31, 32] or in multi-family groups [25] are helpful for most families. Such approaches are based on the stress-vulnerability model [26] and usually focus on helping families to develop their problem-solving skills and to communicate in a calm and consistent manner.

Whilst families are helped to maintain a low stress environment for the client, they are also encouraged to set appropriate goals for their relative, tailored to the client's stage of recovery [35]. Working together to identify the early warning signs of relapse and the prior agreement of an intervention plan should this occur, is another important aspect of such family work. These (cognitive) behaviourally- oriented approaches are often usefully augmented with a focus on systemic issues such as the unhelpful patterns of belief and behaviour in which families members have become trapped [41, 42]. In addition, a smaller number of families may require more in-depth psychotherapeutic input to help them negotiate more complex and longstanding conflicts, more entrenched negative interaction patterns, or more intense and destructive feelings, attitudes and behaviours; or to address significant pre-existing or recently developed risk factors (e.g. abuse or violence).

**Table 2. Formal Family Interventions**

| Structured, goal oriented family sessions |
|---|
| • Validating and normalising the family's emotional reactions and helping them to maintain hope<br>• Discussing with the family/carers their appraisal of the situation<br>• Developing a more helpful shared understanding about what has happened<br>• Information sharing about psychosis, stress and vulnerability, medication, psychosocial interventions, services etc.<br>• Support in accessing and getting the best out of services<br>• Counselling about grief, loss and adjustment to changed expectations<br>• Goal setting and encouragement of realistic steps towards recovery<br>• Encouragement of 'low EE' behaviours (non-critical encouragement; support without being over-intrusive or fostering dependence)<br>• Practicing clear, direct, positive communication<br>• Identifying and changing unhelpful interactions<br>• Problem-solving about everyday issues<br>• Enhancing family members' skills for dealing with crises and challenging symptoms<br>• Early warning signs monitoring and relapse prevention planning<br>• Stress management and encouraging all family members/ carers to look after their own needs, including referral to mental health/ carer support services when required<br>• Helping family members/carers to make contact with others in similar situations to reduce feelings of isolation, stigma and powerlessness<br>• Addressing pre-existing or newly developed risk issues<br>• Different types of family input at different points in time; meeting different combinations of family members/ significant others as appropriate |

## Service Models

A number of service models, for example [16, 43] and Breitborde and Srihari this volume, provide helpful frameworks for matching family needs to different types of family interventions. These are based on the increasing recognition that it is not necessary (or feasible) to offer in-depth interventions to all families. Such 'stepped care' models reflect the 'sufficiency principle' – by providing a range of family-based services the needs of clients and family members can be met with the least intensive intervention [33]. There are a number of examples in the literature which are briefly summarized below:

A group of American experts [33] recommended a model which contained a number of steps consisting of very brief interventions which are designed to meet the needs of a large number of families: 1 Family-friendly agencies and the non-judgmental exchange of information; 2 Brief education; 3 Intermittent family consultation (1-5 sessions) to resolve specific issues; and 4 Intensive family psycho-education (a 9-12 month course of skills training).

The model developed in Sydney, Australia [16] may reflect a greater availability of trained staff and recommends 5 steps, with psycho-education seen as the middle step: 1 Connection and assessment; 2 General education; 3 Psycho-education; 4 Consultation; and 5 Family Therapy. They propose that all families be offered a minimum level of care (steps 1 and 2) before being assessed and referred to higher level interventions.

A model developed in India [43], where there are fewer mental health professionals, conceptualizes the hierarchy of family-based services quite differently: 1 Baseline interventions – provision of information and support; 2 Interventions designed to impact on client-family interactions – learning to manage symptoms, improving communication and problem-solving; and 3 Interventions that foster self-help (e.g. encouraging participation in self-help groups and the establishment of work co-operatives).

Unlike the other 2 models, this is not based on the idea that meeting more complex family needs requires more complex, higher-level interventions provided by more highly skilled clinicians. The Indian model views the professionals as responsible for the baseline interventions, conceptualizes Level 2 interventions as a partnership between families and professionals, and pre-supposes the family as pre-eminent (and professionals as secondary, or catalysts) in Level 3.

In the more established mental health services, the 'pyramid of care' service model has been proposed as an effective way of matching family needs with intensity of service provision and staff skill mix. The basic needs of most families can be met by existing mental health service staff with minimal additional training, but some highly trained staff are required to meet the needs of a smaller number of families with complex needs. Using these principles, it is possible to create a composite stepped care model (see Figure 2).

### *Role of Assessment*

Although the American and Australian models emphasise assessment at each stage, to determine whether the family should progress to the next level of intervention, a service able to offer this range of interventions could also be organized on the basis of assessed needs. A thorough initial assessment, as part of the minimum level of family engagement, could trigger immediate referral to the most appropriate level of intervention, rather than requiring the family to progress through the steps. One way of achieving this is to initially involve a more highly-trained member of staff in the lower-level family intervention with particular families (eg. those with longstanding, complex presentations or high risk issues) so that the family can be offered a more intensive intervention seamlessly. In an ideal mental health service, the principles of 'assessed care' as well as 'stepped care' would be implemented on a flexible, case-by-case basis.

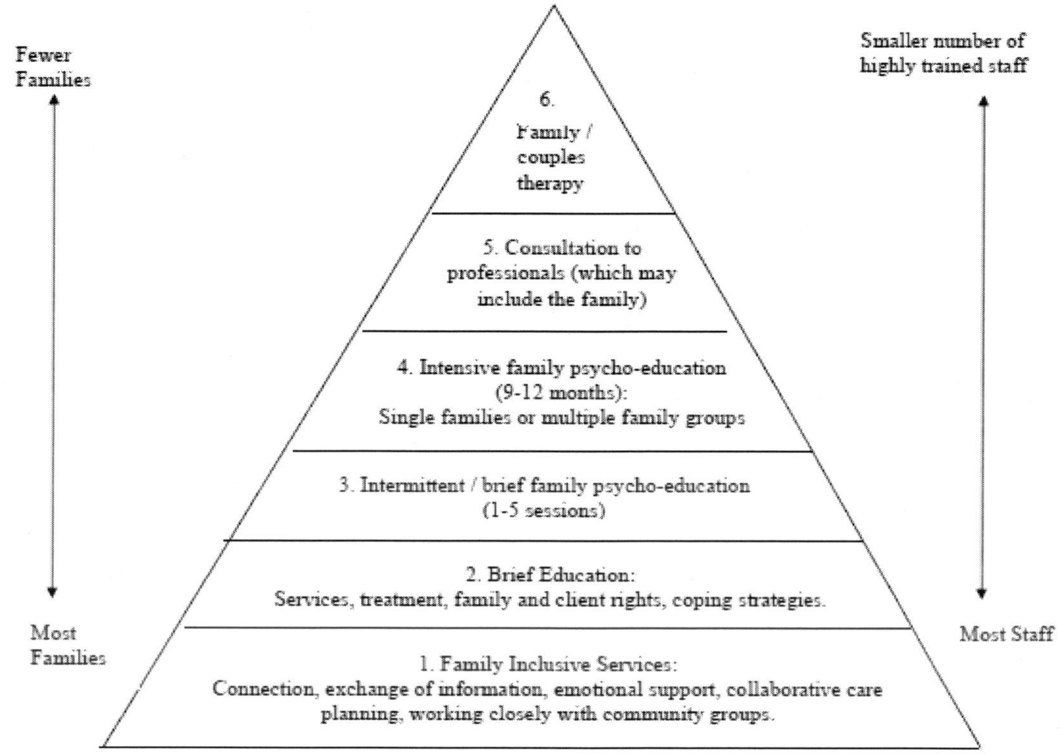


Figure 2. An aggregated stepped-care family interventions model.

## THEORETICAL DEBATES REGARDING MODELS OF FAMILY INTERVENTIONS

The original Family Intervention studies were based on earlier research into the family emotional atmosphere and relapse conducted by George Brown and colleagues. [44, 27]. They had developed the Expressed Emotion (EE) rating scales, which were subsequently used in a large number of studies. Although this contributed to the widespread recognition of the benefits of working with relatives of people with psychosis, the focus of the research effort on relapse has led to a widespread, over-simplified perception of expressed emotion (EE) as a unidirectional, binary concept. In this section we will briefly examine the considerable debate about the theoretical concepts underpinning research in this area, the clinical implications, and consider possible future directions.

Brown and colleagues conducted three research projects in the 1950's and 60's investigating family relationships associated with relapse [44]. The first study appeared to show that patients with schizophrenia were more likely to relapse if they returned to live with parents or wives, whereas those with other disorders appeared to do better on their return to live with the family. The second study found that ratings based on the relatives' attributions and beliefs effectively predicted deterioration in the patient's clinical state in the follow-up period, while ratings based on the patient did not. They also found that low face-to-face contact could be protective for those returning to "highly emotionally-involved" homes.

In the third study, a structured interview schedule, the Camberwell Family Interview (CFI) was used with parents while patients were still hospitalised, and was repeated 9 months after discharge; when 35 out of 101 people had relapsed. The audiotape of this interview was rated on five subscales (criticism, hostility, emotional over-involvement (EOI), warmth and positive comments), taking into account both the content and tone of the comments. In order to simplify the analysis, the three scales most clearly related to relapse (criticism, hostility, EOI) were combined into a single index of EE and relatives assigned to either a High-EE or Low-EE group. This combined index of EE gave a better prediction of relapse than any individual component: 58% of patients returning to High-EE relatives relapsed, compared with 16% discharged to Low-EE homes.

Warmth was also related to relapse, but had complex interrelationships with the other scales. Those rated low in warmth also tended to be highly critical, whereas those high in warmth tended to be associated with over-involvement. However, if relatives showed considerable warmth without criticism or over-involvement, patients did very well (9% relapse rate).

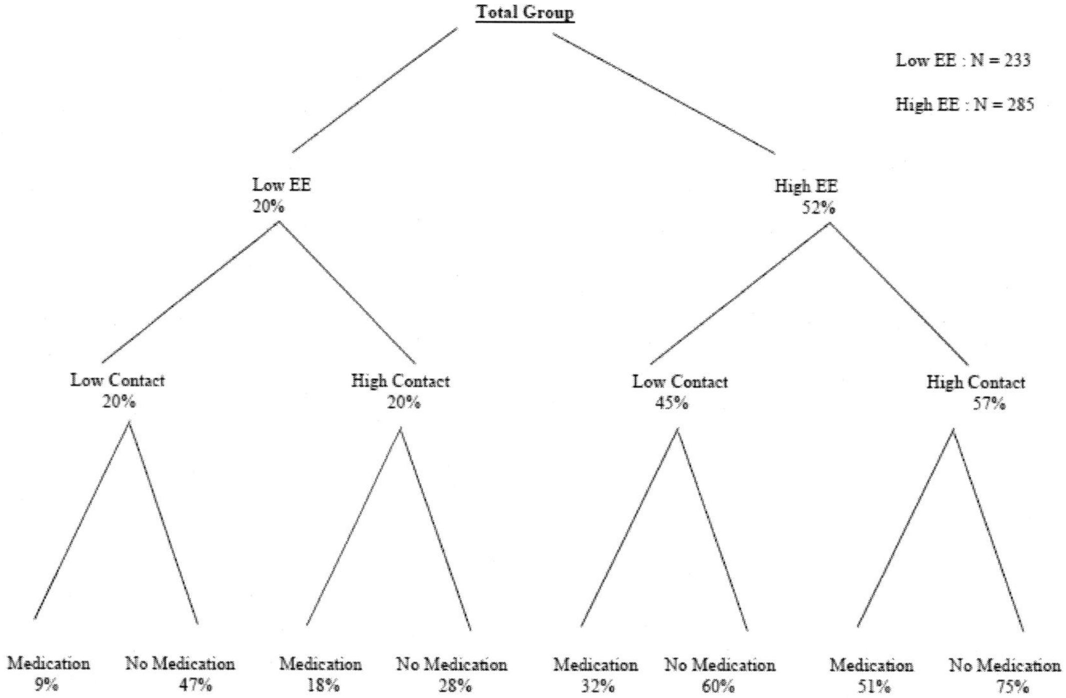


Figure 3. Percentage Relapse according to EE, Contact and Medication status from Bebbington and Kuipers' (1994) aggregate analysis.

The findings of an independent, small-scale replication study [28] were remarkably consistent with the original study [27], which allowed the results to be combined to explore the interaction between medication, the family environment, contact with relatives and relapse rates. While these findings suggested that either low face-to-face contact or regular maintenance on medication gives a measure of protection in a High-EE environment, the role of medication in Low-EE environments was unclear. However, an aggregate analysis of data from 25 studies [45] indicated that medication reduces the relapse rate for those living with High- or Low-EE relatives (see Fig.3). This study also confirmed that high contact with a High-EE relative increased the risk of relapse but indicated that high contact with Low-EE families might be protective.

The predictive validity of the expressed emotion index in a range of settings has been confirmed by numerous studies, with few negative results. Following their meta-analysis of 26 studies, Butzlaff and Hooley [46] concluded that EE was now established as a robust predictor of schizophrenic relapse (High-EE relapse rate = 65%; Low-EE = 35%) and suggested that further replication studies were no longer required. Research has also confirmed that EE is significantly associated with relapse in depression and a range of other psychiatric and medical conditions [47].

Although there are a number of useful reviews [46, 47, 48] the casual browsing of the current EE literature can quickly lead to confusion due to the range of research studies attempting to explore different facets of EE, and their relationship to other concepts. EE has also been critiqued from a number of angles. One of the originators of the field, Julian Leff [49], has acknowledged that it was "unfortunate that the general term Expressed Emotion was applied to (the) index" (p135) as it has led to assumptions that any emotional expression by a relative is harmful to the person with psychosis.

If the 'warmth' scale had not been excluded from the EE index, or other positive scales such as 'compassion' or 'tolerance' had been included, then the research effort could have had an equal emphasis on resilience or recovery. As it was the development of the index resulted in numerous studies of relatives' attitudes negatively impacting on the person with psychosis.

Many clinicians in the field are also unaware of the more recent research studies concerning EE. The most important developments in this field involve the exploration of appraisals [50, 51], coping styles [52, 53, 54, 55] and the interactional nature of the unhelpful emotions and behaviours identified by the unidirectional EE index [56, 57]. It is interesting that EE is increasingly recognised as reflecting interactions between the person with psychosis and their relative/care-giver, but relatively little use has been made of systemic theory to guide research in this area.

However, some therapists have overcome problems inherent in the earlier linear psycho-educational approaches by integrating systemic family therapy and psycho-educational family management [41, 42, 58], and have made particular use of Circular Questioning – therapeutic questions which reveal relationships between members of a family.

Many contemporary systemic therapists also adopt constructivist or social constructionist approaches [59, 60, 61], exploring how people use language in a way that shapes and defines appraisals. There is a particular interest in the way in which family members both construe one another, and behave in a way that is coherent with that construction; and how the actions of each validate or invalidate the other's construction of their relationship. These elegant approaches are therapeutically useful and appear to be compatible with the emerging literature on appraisals, interactions and family emotional atmosphere.

Although Barrowclough and Tarrier's classic 1997 cognitive-behavioural family interventions text [30] has not been updated, Barrowclough and Lobban [62] recently presented a format for the formulation of problem behaviours in the context of family interactions, reflecting the more recent research on appraisals and interactions. They describe their approach as a 'basic family CBT model' of 'linked vicious circles' with behaviours of one person triggering thoughts/beliefs, feelings and behaviours of another. Their joint formulation diagram mirrors the earlier work of Harry Procter [63, 64] who integrated George Kelly's personal construct therapy and systemic therapy (see also Dallos [65]).

Procter's bow-tie diagram and interview format link "the individual processes of meaning making to the delicate social ecology of intimate personal relationships that sustain them" and is "particularly useful as a means of clarifying complex interactive sequences in conflicted couples and families, and in suggesting a road map for intervention" (Neimeyer, p.41) [66].

A simplification of this diagram is used in the 'cognitive - interactive approach' [67] developed in the Family Interventions Service in Somerset (for an example see Fig. 4). We use such 'cognitive-interactional' diagrams clinically with families to explore unhelpful patterns of interaction, thereby enabling reconsideration of attributions and desired behavioural change [42].

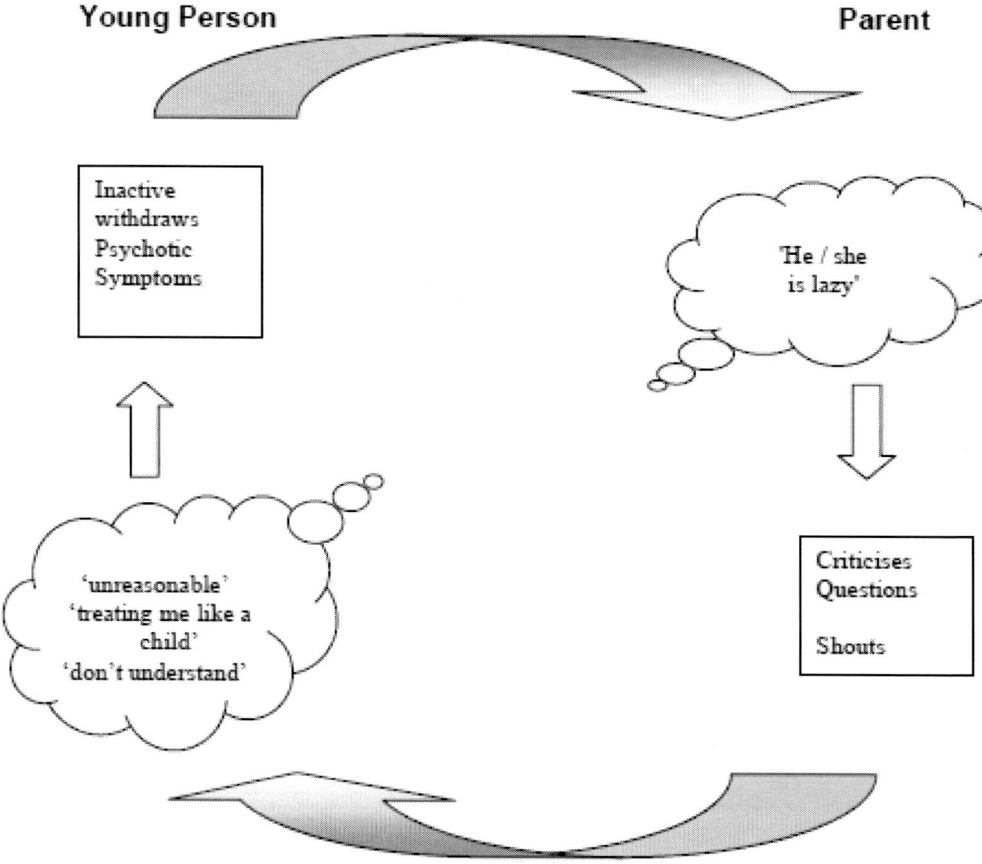


Figure 4. A cognitive interactional diagram of a pursuit – withdrawal cycle.

The diagram illustrates a complementary pattern of interaction which is likely to become increasingly entrenched over time: The more frustrated, critical or intrusive the parent becomes, the more the young person feels overwhelmed and hopeless, consequently doing less and withdrawing.

Sustained or increasing inactivity and withdrawal strengthens the parents' belief that their child is lazy and results in increased attempts to control their behaviour through criticism or intrusiveness.

In behavioural terms, these processes can be described as intermittent reinforcement of the parents' behaviour (e.g. the young person sometimes complies with demands) and negative reinforcement of the young person's behaviour (e.g. withdrawal reduces exposure to parental criticism). In systemic terms, the family members could be described as being caught up in a pursuit – withdrawal cycle.

Further detailed research will be required to clarify the common interactional patterns underlying family emotional atmosphere and their relationship to outcome after psychosis, but the UCLA (University of California Los Angeles) group has clearly described how High-EE (critical) relatives tend to become locked into chains of negative interactions with their offspring with schizophrenia [68].

Critical relatives display more negative verbal and non-verbal behaviour, and less positive verbal and non-verbal behaviour. The patients in these interactions are themselves more critical of their parents, use more justifications for their behaviour, express more disagreements and display more negative non-verbal behaviour.

In contrast, Low-EE relatives were able to break negative chains of interaction sooner and to adopt a more neutral, non-critical, facilitative stance. This was associated with more frequent use of autonomous statements by the young person with schizophrenia and enabled more effective problem solving by the family.

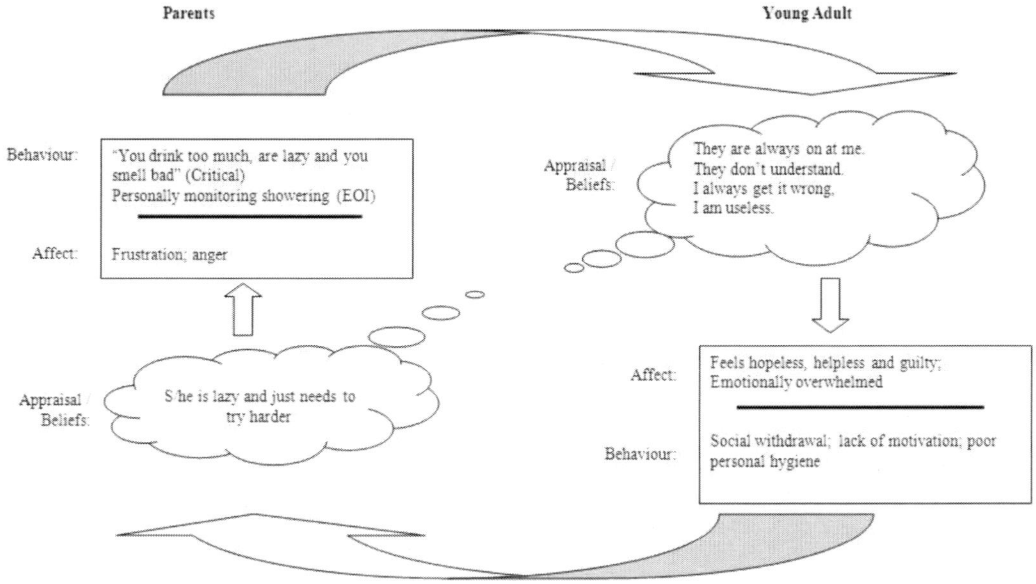


Figure 5. A cognitive – interactional diagram of a complementary transactional pattern.

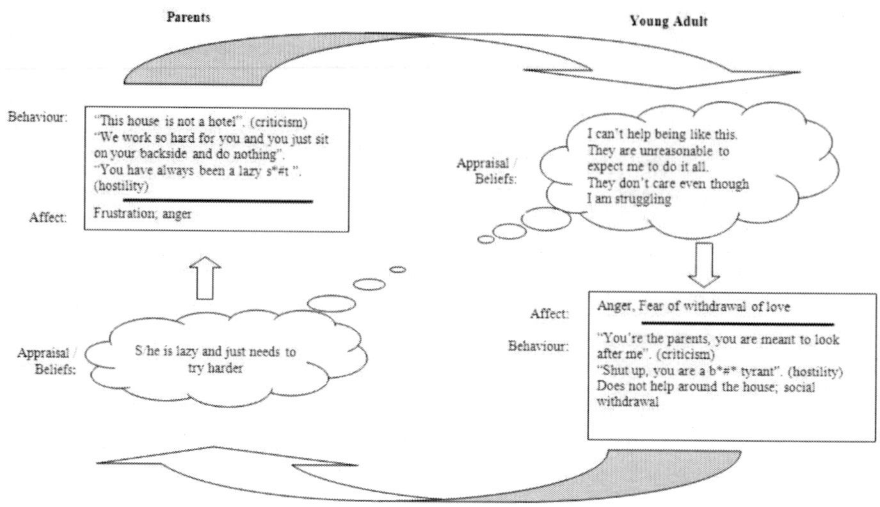


Figure 6. A cognitive – interactional diagram of symmetrical counter – criticism.

Miklowitz and colleagues [69] found that High-EE-critical families became locked either into symmetrical critical interactions or complementary interactions. Figure 5 illustrates the complementary pattern, in which the young person with schizophrenia is self-denigrating and appears to have internalised the criticism. A symmetrical pattern of mutual criticism is illustrated in Figure 6. These interactional cycles are all illustrating simple dyadic relationships. However, young people with psychosis commonly receive different messages because various family members perceive them differently. A common example is illustrated in Figure 7. Clinicians will find formulations of this kind a 'better-fit' than the oversimplified ideas based on the earlier EE research. They will also find that they enable conversations that are non-blaming and therefore more therapeutic [70].

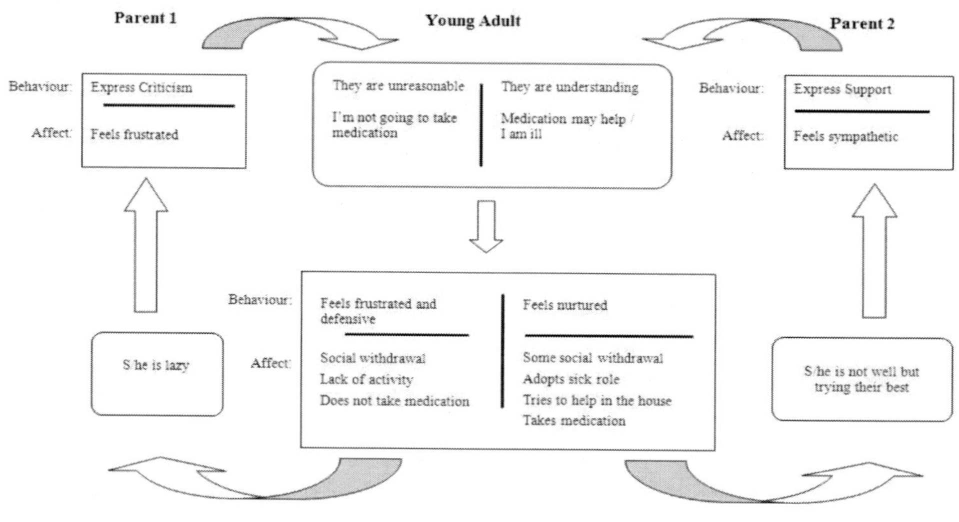


Figure 7. A Cognitive interactional diagram illustrating mixed messages and resultant confusion.

## SERVICE DELIVERY

Developing appropriate services for families coping with early psychosis may seem a daunting prospect, but it is clear that a range of services will be required to meet the range of family needs. Different families require different services, and the same families will require different services at different times. The ideal solution to this would be to have a 'menu' of help available for families to choose from (see Table 3). This concept may also be helpful to teams as it means that the menu of services can be developed incrementally, as resources allow. Similarly, the World Health Organization Early Psychosis Consensus Statement [71] recognizes that mental health services are at different stages of development and therefore translates the principles of good practice contained therein into realistic, context- specific goals taking into account local capacities and cultural diversity. Aspirations regarding family involvement range from self-help psychosocial support in settings with low levels of resources to the routine availability of formal family interventions in countries with high levels of resources. In many less industrialized countries there is greater community solidarity and the Consensus Statement focuses on the facilitation of practical psychosocial support via family, friends and community organizations which may be achieved through minimal funding of self-help groups and other initiatives. In countries with high levels of resources the Consensus Statement sets the aspirational standard that 'families and key supporters will receive effective services appropriate to their needs'. Services are challenged to systematically demonstrate effectiveness in terms of early engagement of families and significant others, and in terms of whether families feel valued as partners in care.

So where should mental health services begin? The evidence suggests that all Psychosis Services should aim to provide 'routine' as well as 'formal' family interventions.

**Table 3. A Menu of Family Interventions**

| | |
|---|---|
| 1. | Provision of written information |
| 2. | Educational groups (provision of information by professionals or other Carers) |
| 3. | Psycho-educational groups (staff-led groups which focus on tailoring information to the particular families' needs and problem solving) |
| 4. | Routine FI (involving families as partners in the care of their relative, enhancement of coping strategies, and promoting recovery through balancing stress reduction and encouragement of appropriate activity) |
| 5. | Formal FI (structured, goal-oriented family work with individual families) |
| 6. | Multi-family groups (ongoing structured FI with a group of families) |
| 7. | Carer support groups including sibling groups (providing tailored information and support) |
| 8. | Carer-to-carer counselling support |
| 9. | Involvement of carers in the development of services, lobbying or public awareness raising |

In addition, the provision of written information and a programme of educational or psychoeducational groups is often achievable. Multi-family groups are particularly helpful for the provision of ongoing peer support, and groups with siblings have also been found to be extremely valuable. Carers organizations (eg. Rethink in the UK or NAMI in the USA) are often a valuable resource, providing information and support either in the form of educational programmes, self-help support groups or in the form of trained carer-to-carer counselling support programmes [72]. In addition, involvement of family members in political lobbying, public awareness raising/anti-stigma campaigns, and in the shaping of local mental health services as carer consultants or as carer representatives, on steering groups or committees, can often be empowering and help family members to find meaning in their new caring role. Many services reach the point where they recognize family members' needs, are willing to develop family interventions, and recognize the need to provide additional training for key groups of staff. However, they often adopt a short-term, 'tick-box' approach rather than a comprehensive and strategic method of service development. The Somerset model [36, 73] of developing both specialist FI as well as routine family inclusive services provides an example of a more systematic approach that may be a useful guide to other services willing to develop a range of services for families. The Meriden Programmeme in the West Midlands region of the UK provides another model for the systematic development of FI services [74]. Those wishing to develop FI services may also wish to take note of the research into the implementation of FI training initiatives. There is now considerable evidence that training in FI does not, in itself, lead to the delivery of FI in routine care [75, 76, 77]. Clinicians often report that they find it difficult to integrate FI with the other demands on their time, and also cite insufficient clinical supervision and a lack of management support for FI as reasons for not practicing post-training in FI. Some newly trained clinicians also appear to lack the confidence to apply their newly developed skills in a sufficiently family needs-led manner, find it difficult to engage families and may lack the basic therapeutic skills which FI training courses take for granted.

**Table 4. Recommendations to Maximise Implementation of Family Interventions Post Training**

- Ensure support for the programme of training and service development at all levels of the organisation, including the highest level of management and lead professionals
- Agree a service development strategy to ensure an appropriate service context and the availability of sufficient resources to enable practice post training (protected time; smaller caseloads; practical support for clinicians)
- Establish robust supervision structures to ensure post-training expert clinical supervision is available
- Use a team training approach or ensure that there is a local 'critical mass' of trained practitioners who can support one another
- Involve families/carers in the training programme and in the design and governance of the service
- Appoint local service leads/champions who are responsible for the development and maintenance of the service

However, a number of factors have now been identified which can facilitate successful implementation of family work post training (see Table 4). In particular, it is crucial that the

FI training initiative is part of a service development strategy that has clear support throughout the organization. This may be a considerable challenge in many organizations and may depend on the successful forging of alliances between family members, key professionals and managers. Besides ensuring that staff undertake effective training, subsequent organizational support and encouragement of family work will be required. Encouraging FI clinicians to support each other, ongoing clinical supervision and further 'top-up' training are all essential if the new FI services are to survive and develop. It may be useful to consult a recent guidebook on the implementation of family work [78] for a detailed consideration of many of these issues and numerous examples of successful development of family services.

## CONCLUSION

Family Interventions are underpinned by a substantial and convincing evidence-base, although there are still many questions remaining unanswered. Better clinical outcomes appear to be associated with comprehensive family-oriented approaches, but there is also an increasing recognition of the diversity of family needs, the fact that it may be more effective and efficient to offer the majority of families briefer initial interventions, and the potential role of factors which are common to a range of FI models. The constructs underlying the bulk of the research in the field are currently also undergoing considerable development.

The challenge for mental health services is to translate this into a range of family based interventions, some of which should be offered on a routine basis to all and others should be available as needed. The delineation of formal and routine family interventions, and the description of pyramidal or trapezoid models integrating family needs, levels of care and staffing (numbers and levels of training), will hopefully prove useful in the design of services for families. Although the ideal scenario may be for all staff to be sufficiently well trained to respond flexibly to the full range of family needs, in reality, these more complex needs are often best met either by having some staff on the team who have received more specialist training and therefore have a more developed level of therapeutic skill, or through co-work with a more experienced family therapist, or referral to specialist psychotherapeutic services.

Readers are urged to work closely with families using their services and existing family organisations/ groups, in order to develop a range of services for families supporting someone with psychosis. The key to better outcomes for many, however, is likely to lie with the practice of routine collaborative family engagement and the establishment of a co-operative working partnership between the patient, family and treatment team.

## REFERENCES


[1] J. Addington and P. Burnett, in *Psychological Interventions in Early Psychosis: a Treatment Handbook* J. F. M. Gleeson, P. D. McGorry, Eds. (John Wiley and Sons, Chichester, UK, 2004) pp.99-116.

[2] T. Wykes, C. Steel, B. Everitt and N. Tarrier, *Schiz.Bull.* 34, 523-537 (2008).

[3] R. E. Drake, G. J. McHugo, R. R. Bebout, D. R. Becker, M. Harris, G. R. Bond and E. Quimby, *Arch. Gen. Psychiatry 56,* 627-633 (1999).

[4] T. Burns, J. Catty, T. Becker, R. E. Drake, A. Fioritti, M. Knapp, C. Lauber, W. Rössler, T. Tomov, J. van Busschbach, S. White and D. Wiersma, *The Lancet* 370, 1146-1152 (2007).

[5] F. M. Pharoah, J. J. Mari, J. Rathbone and W. Wong Family intervention for schizophrenia (update) (Cochrane review), in *The Cochrane Library* 11 (John Wiley and Sons, Chichester, UK, 2010).

[6] D. Raune, E. Kuipers and P. E. Bebbington, *Br. J. Psychiatry* 184, 321–326 (2004).

[7] W. R. McFarlane and W. L. Cook, *Fam. Process* 46, 185–197 (2007).

[8] P. Patterson, M. Birchwood and R. Cochrane, *Br. J. Psychiatry,* 187, 59–64 (2005).

[9] J. Stirling, D. Tantam, P. Thomas, D. Newby, L. Montague, N. Ring and S. Rowe, *Psychol. Med.* 23, 771–778 (1993).

[10] R. L. Butzlaff and J. M. Hooley, *Arch. Gen. Psychiatry* 55, 547–552 (1998).

[11] D. Pearson, F. R. Burbach and R. I. Stanbridge, *Context* 93, 9-12 (2007).

[12] R. Bailey, F. R. Burbach and S. Lea, *J. Ment. Health* 12, 131-141 (2003).

[13] J. Allen, F. R. Burbach and J. Reibstein, *Psychology and Psychotherapy: Theo, Res, Pra. doi: 10.1111/j.2044-8341.2011.02057.x* (2012).

[14] J. Seikkula, B. Alakare and J. Aaltonen, *J. Constructivist Psychol.* 14, 247-265 (2001).

[15] J. Seikkula, J. Aaltonen, B. Alakare, K. Haarakangas, J. Keränen and K. Lehtinen *Psychoth. Res.* 16, 214-228 (2006).

[16] Y. Mottaghipour and A. Bickerton, *Aust. e-J. Advance. Ment. Health* 4, 1-8 (2005).

[17] D. L. Penn, E. J. Waldheter, D. O. Perkins, K. T. Mueser and J. A. Lieberman, *Am. J. Psychiatry*, 162, 2220-2232 (2005).

[18] S. Pilling, P. Bebbington, E. Kuipers, P. Garety, J. Geddes, G. Orbach and C. Morgan, *Psychol. Med.* 32, 763-782 (2002).

[19] G. Pitschel-Walz, S. Leucht, J. Bäuml, W. Kissling and R. R. Engel, *Schizophr. Bull.* 27, 73-92 (2001).

[20] V. Bird, P. Premkumar, T. Kendall, C. Whittington, J. Mitchell and E. Kuipers, *Br. J. Psychiatry* 197, 350–356 (2010).

[21] G. Fadden, *J. Fam. Ther.* 31, 293-309 (1998).

[22] N. R. Schooler, S. J. Keith, J. B. Severe, S. M. Matthews, A. S. Bellack, I. D. Glick, W. A. Hargreaves, J. M. Kane, P. T. Ninan, A. Frances, M. Jacobs, J. A. Lieberman, R. Mance, G. M. Simpson, M. G. Woerner, *Arch. Gen. Psychiatry* 54, 453-463 (1997).

[23] W. R. McFarlane, E. Lukens, B. Link, R. Dushay, S. A. Deakins, M. Newmark, E. J. Dunne, B. Horen and J. Toran, *Arch. Gen. Psychiatry* 52, 679-687 (1995).

[24] W. R. McFarlane, B. Link, R. Dushay, J. Marshall and J. Crilly, *Fam. Process* 34, 127-144 (1995).

[25] W. R. McFarlane, *Multifamily groups in the treatment of severe psychiatric disorders,* Guilford Press, New York (2002).

[26] J. Zubin and B. Spring, *J. Abnorm. Psychol.*, 86, 103-126 (1997).

[27] G. W. Brown, J. L. T. Birley and J. K. Wing, *Br. J. Psychiatry* 121, 241–258 (1972).

[28] C. E. Vaughn and J. P. Leff, *Br. J. Soc. Clin. Psychol.* 15: 157–165 (1976).

[29] C. M. Anderson, D. J. Reiss and G. E. Hogarty, *Schizophrenia and the family: A practitioner's guide to psychoeducation and management,* Guilford Press, New York (1986).

[30] C. Barrowclough and N. Tarrier, *Families of schizophrenic patients: Cognitive behavioural intervention,* Chapman and Hall, London (1992).

[31] I. R. H. Falloon, K. Mueser, S. Gingerich, S. Rappaport, C. McGill, V. Graham-Hole, G. Fadden and F. Gair, *Family Work Manual,* Meriden Family Programmeme, Birmingham, UK (2004).

[32] L. Kuipers, J. Leff and D. Lam, *Family Work for Schizophrenia: A Practical Guide (2nd Edition)* Gaskell, London (2002).

[33] A. N. Cohen, S. M. Glynn, A. B. Murray-Swank, C. Barrio, E. P. Fischer, S. J. McCutcheon, D. A. Perlick, A. J. Rotondi, S. L. Sayers, M. D. Sherman and L. B. Dixon, *Psychiatr. Serv.* 59, 40-48 (2008).

[34] F. R. Burbach, G. Fadden and J. Smith, in *Promoting Recovery in Early Psychosis* P. French, M. Read, J. Smith, M. Rayne, D. Shiers, Eds. (Wiley-Blackwell, Chichester, UK, 2010) pp.210-225.

[35] J. Gleeson, H. J. Jackson, H. Stavely and P. Burnett, in *The Recognition and Management of Early Psychosis: A Preventive Approach* P.D McGorry, H.J. Jackson, Eds. (Cambridge University press, Cambridge, UK, 1999) pp.376-406.

[36] F. R. Burbach and R. I. Stanbridge, R.I. (2008) *J. Ment. Health Training, Ed. Practice* 3, 23- 31 (2008).

[37] F. R. Burbach, D. J. Grinter and S. E. A. Bues, *Early Interv. Psychiatry,* 3, 231-235 (2009).

[38] A. Worthington and P. Rooney, *The Triangle of Care. Carers included: A guide to best practice in acute mental health care.* National Mental Health Development Unit and The Princess Royal Trust for Carers www.carers.org (2010).

[39] M. Slade, V. Pinfold, J. Rapaport, S. Bellringer, S. Banerjee, E. Kuipers and P. Huxley, *Br. J. Psychiatry* 190, 148-155 (2007).

[40] M. Furlong and M. Leggatt, *Aust. N. Z. J. Psychiatry* 30, 614-622 (1996).

[41] F. R. Burbach and R. I. Stanbridge, *J. Fam. Ther.* 20, 311-325 (1998).

[42] F. R. Burbach and R. I. Stanbridge, *J. Fam. Ther.* 28, 39-57 (2006).

[43] R. Shankar and M. S. Menon, *Psychosoc. Rehabil.* J. 16, 75-91 (1993).

[44] G. W. Brown, in *Expressed Emotion in Families* J. P. Leff, C. Vaughn, Eds (Guildford Press, New York, 1985) pp 7-25.

[45] P. Bebbington and L Kuipers, *Psychol. Med.* 24, 707–718 (1994).

[46] R. L. Butzlaff and J. M. Hooley, *Arch. Gen. Psychiatry* 55, 547–552 (1998).

[47] A. J. Wearden, N. Tarrier, C. Barrowclough, T. R. Zastowny, and A. A. Rahill, *Clin. Psychol. Rev.* 20, 633–666 (2006).

[48] L. Kuipers and P. Bebbington, *Psychol. Med.* 18, 893–909 (1988).

[49] J. Leff, *Int. J. Soc. Psychiatry,* 35, 133–145 (1989).

[50] C. Barrowclough and J. M. Hooley, *Clin. Psychol. Rev.* 23, 849–880 (2003).

[51] M. Scazufca and E. Kuipers, *Br. J. Psychiatry* 168, 580-587 (1996).

[52] M. Birchwood and R. Cochrane, *Psychol. Med.* 2, 857-865 (1990).

[53] L. Magliano, G. Fadden, M. Madianos, J. M. Caldas de Almeida, T. Held, M. Guarneri, C. Marasco, P. Tosini and M. Maj, *Soc. Psychiatry Psychiatr. Epidemiol.* 33, 405-412 (1998).

[54] M. Scazufca and E. Kuipers, *Br. J. Psychiatry* 174,154-158 (1999).

[55] E. Kuipers, P. Bebbington, G. Dunn, D. Fowler, D. Freeman, P. Watson, A. Hardy and P. Garety , *Br. J. Psychiatry* 188, 173-179 (2006).

[56] F. Lobban, C. Barrowclough and S. Jones, *Soc. Psychiatry Psychiatr. Epidemiol.* 41, 50–55 (2006).

[57] M. P. O'Brien, J. L. Gordon, C. E. Bearden, S. R. Lopez, A. Kopelowicz and T. D. Cannon, *Schizophr. Res.* 81, 269-275 (2006).

[58] S. Meddings, I. Gordon and D. Owen, in *Reaching Out – the Psychology of Assertive Outreach* C. Cupitt, Ed. (Routledge, Hove, East Sussex, UK, 2010) pp163-185.

[59] P. Bertrando, *The Dialogical Therapist*, Karnac, London (2007).

[60] H. Anderson, *Conversation, Language and Possibilities: A Postmodern Approach to Therapy*, Basic Books, New York (1997).

[61] S. McNamee and K. J. Gergen, *Therapy as Social Construction*, Sage, London (1992).

[62] C. Barrowclough and F. Lobban, "Family Intervention in Psychosis: Using an illness cognition framework", Workshop presented at British Association for Behavioural and Cognitive Psychotherapies (BABCP) Conference, 15 July 2009 (Exeter, UK).

[63] H. G. Procter, in *Personal Construct Theory and Mental Health* E. Button, Ed. (Croom Helm, Beckenham, Kent, UK, 1985) pp.327-350.

[64] H. G. Procter, in *Personal Construct Therapy Casebook* R. A. Neimeyer, G. J. Neimeyer, Eds. (Springer, New York, 1987) pp. 153-171.

[65] R. Dallos, *Family Belief Systems, Therapy and Change*, Open University Press, Buckingham, UK (1991).

[66] R. A. Neimeyer, *Constructivist Psychotherapy: distinctive features*, Routledge, Hove, UK (2009).

[67] F. R. Burbach, "Combining psychoeducational family work and systemic approaches", Paper presented at Working with Families: Making it a Reality Conference, 21 March 2000 (Stratford-upon-Avon, UK).

[68] K. Hahlweg, M. J. Goldstein, K. H. Nuechterlein, J. A. Doane, D. J. Miklowitz and K. S. Snyder, *J. Consulting Clin. Psychol.* 57, 11-18 (1989).

[69] D. J. Miklowitz, M. J. Goldstein, J. A. Doane, K. H. Nuechterlein, A. M. Strachan, K. S. Snyder and A. Magana-Amato, *Fam. Process* 28, 153-167 (1989).

[70] F. R. Burbach, in *Psychosis and Emotion: The role of emotions in understanding psychosis, therapy and recovery,* A. Gumley, A. Gilham, Eds. Brunner-Routledge, in press (2012).

[71] J. Bertolote and P. McGorry, *Br. J. Psychiatry* 187 (suppl.48), s116-s119 (2005).

[72] M. Leggatt, *Med. J. Aust.* 187, s61-s63 (2007).

[73] F. R. Burbach and R. I. Stanbridge, in *A casebook of family interventions for psychosis* F. Lobban and C. Barrowclough, Eds. (Wiley-Blackwell, Chichester, UK, 2009).

[74] G. Fadden, J. *Fam. Ther.* 28, 23-38 (2006).

[75] C. Brooker and A. Brabban *Measured Success: A scooping review of evaluated psychosocial interventions training for work with people with serious mental health problems.* NIMHE/Trent WDC (2004).

[76] C. Brooker, C. Saul, J. Robinson, J. King and M. Dudley, *Int. J. Nursing Studies* 40, 731-747 (2003).

[77] G. Fadden, *J. Ment. Health* 6, 599-612 (1997).

[78] D. Froggatt, G. Fadden, D. L. Johnson, M. Leggatt and R. Shankar, *Families as partners in care: A Guidebook for Implementing Family Work*, Worldwide Fellowship for Schizophrenia and Allied Disorders, Toronto, Canada (2007).

In: Psychosis: Causes, Diagnosis and Treatment
Editor: Xenia Anastassiou-Hadjicharalambous
ISBN: 978-1-62081-516-8


*Chapter 11*

# COERCED TREATMENT IN PSYCHOSIS: IMPLICATIONS OF INSIGHT, DURATION OF UNTREATED PSYCHOSIS AND STIGMA

***Constantin Tranulis****
McGill University, Montreal, Canada

## ABSTRACT

Coerced treatment is a topic of intense debate and current practice in psychiatry. Three recent developments make it is particularly timely for contemporary discussions of early intervention in psychosis. Firstly, highly publicized violent acts of persons suffering from psychosis are awakening stigmatizing stereotypes and calls for social exclusion through re-institutionalization. Secondly, the first episode psychosis movement argues that intervening early in the course of a psychotic disorder has beneficial effects, raising moral arguments for early involuntary treatment. Finally, the neurocognitive research in the clinical phenomenon of lack of insight suggests that its neurological base renders the persons suffering from psychosis unfit to make treatment decisions by themselves.

In this chapter we are analyzing these recent developments around coerced treatment through a selective review of the literature and by presenting pertinent illness narratives collected from first episode psychosis patients and their family members.

This critical analysis suggests that coercion into treatment is a profoundly moral and social decision and should thus be based on moral values and human rights principles. The disempowering effects of biogenetic and neurocognitive models of schizophrenia had deeply stigmatizing effects in the past. Thus, increased coercion in psychosis is a manifestation of the stigma of psychosis rather than a sign of progress in psychiatric care.

* E-mail: constantin.tranulis@gmail.com

## Introduction

E. Fuller Torrey is one the most vocal advocates for increasing involuntary treatment in psychiatry. In his book "The insanity offence" [1], he argues that violence by mentally ill persons is growing ever since the deinstutionalisation movement: "The news clippings of this tragedy [a person suffering from paranoid schizophrenia killing somebody else] become the first entry in my "*preventable tragedies*" file, which was to grow over the years to fill entire file drawers." (pp xi-xii, our emphasis). Manifesto-like titles ("The consequences of unconstrained civil liberties: violent and homicidal" chapter 9), detailed repetitive descriptions of tragic violence and selective citation of scientific data bring him to conclude that the US mental health care system is "a disaster". He proposes a 4-step solution: modification of the laws, identification of the target population, provision and enforcement of treatment and, finally, assessment and research (pp 177-196). His "successful" law modifications examples are all aiming at broader powers to coerce persons into hospitals and treatment. The identification of target populations of potentially violent mentally ill persons is based on a list of attributes, among which lack of insight and non-adherence to treatment and the proposal of an identification method similar to the ones employed in the anti-terrorist policies (e.g. centralized lists). "There are many methods for ensuring that people with severe psychiatric disorders take medication, and almost all of them are effective" (p188) is followed by a long list of informal and formal coercive methods to enforce treatment (in case the reader was in doubt about content: "the treatment of severe mental illnesses involve, first and foremost, the use of antipsychotic medication" pp185). Our aim here will not be to criticize this position as this was done previously by others, but to reveal some of its key discursive arguments as they have great relevance for understanding the authoritarian trends of contemporary psychiatry.

A first discourse concerns the dominant view of mental illness (and of humans in general) as essentially biologically-determined. This view not only puts emphasis on the biological treatment of psychosis through antipsychotic medication, but undermines a key argument against forced psychiatric treatment by the biologization of insight and its relabeling as anosognosia. Secondly, Fuller Torrey emphasizes the importance of untreated mental illness as a risk factor for violent acts. Thus, he offers a simple answer to the security concerns raised by his text: eradicate the *untreated* psychotic periods and the society is going to be safe. This concept of untreated psychosis is also central to the emerging early intervention movement. These threads will be developed in more detail later.

Thirdly, the overarching discourse is centrally concerned with the links between mental illness and violence. This is done in a specific manner, namely in a very graphic and explicit, quasi-journalistic style: the numerous individual cases of violence are often filled with horrific details, the material is essentially retrieved from newspapers and the legal implications have precedence over other dimensions (e.g. socio-economic or cultural determinants are virtually absent). The perpetrators are described in the absence of a humanizing context, their acts seem meaningless and random. Such descriptions foster sentiments of terror and tap on societal fears exacerbated by the 9/11 events. The discourse on fighting terror gains thus applicability to mentally ill persons, the new insider "terrorists" of Unites States. Identification, surveillance, targeting and neutralization of the threat of untreated psychosis become the principal tasks to be solved by psychiatric care, with the help and assistance of law enforcement agencies. The civil rights discourse is the main argument against this approach and, as in the case of the war on terror, it gets dismissed as misguided idealism and dangerous denial of the gravity of the situation (or illness in this case). Indeed, in a society that enshrines security as the most important value, it is difficult to argue for alternative views based on abstract concepts such as liberty, personal freedom, choice or human dignity.

# I. VIOLENCE AND PSYCHOSIS IN THE POST 9/11 ERA

As convincingly argued by Michel Foucault [2], societal responses to madness varied widely throughout history and geography. When the lepers, the Middle Age excluded group, began to disappear in Europe, he noticed the development of an exclusion movement of the "mad", initially by sending them away from cities on boats ("stultifera naves"). Then, in the 17$^{th}$ century, a movement of exclusion through confinement in asylums of the "unreasonables" developped - the "Great Confinement". He traced the evolving definitions of these « unreasonables » from an amorphous group of feeble minded, sexually deviant, homeless and mad persons to a medicalized group of « mentally ill ». Social order and the preservation of morality were arguments for confinement in asylums. Violence per se was not a crucial dimension for these social processes. The founders of modern psychiatric nosology, Kraepelin and Bleuler, did not focus on violence neither in their detailed descriptions of the mentally ill. Interbellum German psychiatry was dominated by concerns of genetic purification and encouraged "cleaning the gene pool" and purifying the race through forced sterilization and, later, annihilation of the mentally ill [3]. A historian of XXth century American psychiatry argues that the notion of violent psychotics gained traction during the period of social unrest following the second World War [4]. Tapping in social anxieties raised by social unrest, namely by African American requests for equal rights, Metzl argues that political protest was translated into psychosis and that psychosis was racialized as a "Black disease". Thus, the contemporary concern over psychosis and violence is neither a universal characteristic of mental illness, nor a timeless link.

Why this societal obsession with violence in psychosis? Tentative answers to this question may be separated in two groups. Firstly, the 9/11 and previous terrorist attacks raised societal anxieties and concerns over risk of violence. Given the medicalization trends in Western cultures, a huge body of scientific literature was developed on the psychological dimensions of terrorism [5, 6]. It is enlightening that both proponents and critics of antiterrorist measures may pathologize terrorists as mentally ill, with the end result of excluding them from politics and subjecting them to coercive measures in the name of order, security and liberty [7]. The explanation of violence by psychosis can thus be understood as a particular example of the broader cultural trend of medicalization of social suffering [8]. Secondly, the new biogenetic understandings of psychosis can increase perceived links to violence. In the last decades, destigmatizing efforts involved disseminating a biogenetic model of mental illness in the general population ("mental illness is an illness like any other" – i.e. biologically-based). There is significant data showing that this strategy, while diminishing blame, has the unforeseen effect of increasing perceived unpredictability and dangerousness [9] and overall stigma [10].

This section described some factors allowing a discourse linking violence and psychosis to become pervasive both in the general public and clinical discourses. This discourse developed in spite of *lack* of strong evidence for an increase in violent acts by persons suffering from psychosis and the fact that the attributable risk of violence to mental illness is actually small [11, 12]. And, of course, the facts that mentally ill persons suffer from institutional violence and are at increased risk of being victimized themselves [13] are mostly ignored by this discourse.

In the next section, we will explore how the recent emphasis on early intervention and on diminishing untreated psychosis periods favors involuntary treatment tendencies.

## II. The Sooner, the Better: the Costs of Early Intervention in Psychosis

"If you are concerned that you or a person you know is at risk for, or may be developing psychosis or schizophrenia we recommend you *call today* the clinic closest to you, to schedule an appointment. *The sooner a person gets diagnosis and treatment, the better the outcome.* » *(http://www. schizophrenia.com/earlypsychosis.htm, accessed February 10, 2010, original emphasis).*

As one can see from this excerpt from a popular and respectable website, the contemporary view of what is at stake for persons suffering from psychosis or schizophrenia is a race against time for early diagnosis and treatment. Indeed, the last two decades gave birth to a radically new way of defining and treating persons suffering from schizophrenia, so much so that the very term for defining the problem becomes "episode of psychosis" instead of the century-old diagnosis of "schizophrenia". The movement of early intervention for persons diagnosed with a first episode of psychosis (FEP) led this major shift.

The FEP movement has the core premise that treating early and using best practices will improve the life of persons suffering from psychosis. The diagnosis of *schizophrenia* cannot be made before having been ill for at least 6 months, so the field chose to use *psychosis* (which has no minimal duration) as the principal diagnostic category.

Through early intervention, the FEP movement aimed at moving clinical practice away from traditional hospital-based approaches to community-based services, proposing to articulate evidence-based medicine with a person-centered philosophy of care.

In contrast to an initial goal of changing the "natural" course of schizophrenia [14], the FEP clinics observed very early the negative effects of stigma on help seeking delays, the difficult access to services, the treatment drop-out and medication non-adherence rates [15, 16]. Instead, the FEP movement aimed to change the "social" and "clinical" courses of psychosis, proposing interventions rooted in recovery principles and an optimistic discourse about the illness [17]. These therapeutic principles are very close to what could be considered destigmatizing interventions. In fact, reducing stigma and offering treatment in the least coercive settings were explicit core objectives in FEP interventions [18].

As elsewhere in medicine, boundaries of disease and health are continually defined and shaped by science, cultural factors and social actors [19-21] and these nosological and clinical definitions have profound everyday consequences [22]. The redefinition of schizophrenia/ psychosis also has profound implications.

The FEP movement raised ethical concerns and intense debates regarding the proposal of treatment for pre-morbid prodromal states, the aggressive efforts to bring persons into treatment as early as possible and the implications of broadening the diagnostic criteria as the lifetime prevalence of psychosis in the general population is 3% as compared to around 1% for schizophrenia [23].

While these ethical risks were deemed acceptable in research contexts [24], as early intervention becomes widely accepted and mainstreamed in psychiatry and in service organization, it becomes imperative to revise and study its clinical and social implications. We will focus here on some unforeseen developments in FEP interventions as related to coercion into treatment.

Issues of coercion arise as the FEP movement is mainstreamed into "standard" psychiatric care. In the initial, research-based, small FEP clinic, clinicians' enthusiasm and their efforts to make the clinical care acceptable and desirable were empowering the patient, thus contributing to lower stigma. *Diminishing* coercion was one of the principal objectives and a criterion for judging the success of the early intervention [25]. However, the global recognition of the FEP movement gives more power to the clinicians, who can now argue that given the proven benefits of early intervention and the treatment non-adherence rates, they should receive more powers to constrain patients into treatment. This logic results in statements like: "...long-acting injectable formulations such as Risperdal(R) Consta(R) should be considered as first line therapy for people experiencing a first episode of psychosis and may improve the long term outcomes for those patients." (Emsley cited in (Today 2006)).

The periods of untreated diagnosable psychosis (or even "at risk" states) are deemed to be neurotoxic [26], or at least socially toxic [27] as they were repeatedly related to worse prognosis [28].

We described elsewhere the illness narratives of a woman who delayed seeking help for psychosis for five years [29]. The patient was describing her choice in the following terms: "It was totally a strange experience for me, and it had been there for such a long time. At no time did it occur to me that it was an illness, something which I haven't heard of, and something like this. I didn't even realize this was an illness, I just thought this was something with my life, and things going, happening naturally ». Through a careful analysis of illness narratives by the patient and her husband, we unveiled the development of a literal and figurative space within which they were able to share, explore and make sense of psychotic experiences : the patient and her husband would meet daily in a coffee shop before going back home and she would share her daily experiences (« the stories » as they called them). They would discuss them, building together meaning around them and finding concrete ways of dealing with them (e.g. he would counsel her not to pay attention at what her colleagues might say). This was a space where the abnormality of her experiences was not relabeled as psychiatric pathology (husband : « I focused mostly on her upbringing, family habits, all that, but never gave emphasis to what illness that she had''). This ''safe space,'' where she would be able to tell the 'stories' of her psychotic experiences without risking pathologization (which was highly stigmatizing and a threat to the marriage because of the cultural background of the couple) had also positive dimensions, promoting spousal connection and sharing (husband : « Sometimes I am now bored, that I do not hear all the stories that she comes and tells me in the evenings, all these strange stories. In the evening that I come, she would take me to the Starbucks and tell all these strange stories, and I'd been accustomed to the stories now for what, five years, and now I, you know, a part of me says when I go home, ''What happened to all these stories? »). We concluded by questioning the value of a hypothetical early intervention in this case, as the data was giving a more nuanced answer to the fundamental question of whether the five years of ''untreated psychosis'' were a ''delay'' or just plainly part of the subjects' life.

But the related concepts of early intervention and duration of untreated psychosis tend to evacuate such rich meanings by considering these periods as merely "untreated psychosis" – an unwanted medical entity. A clinical case will exemplify how this may translate into coercion into treatment. This clinical case is part of an ongoing ethnography of the First Episode Psychosis movement. As part of a First Episode Psychosis clinic treating about 450 persons suffering from psychosis, I was the treating psychiatrist of a 45-year-old female of Haitian origin, brought to the Emergency room by the police because of a complaint from a neighbor. Her conflict with the neighbor was based on paranoid delusions and olfactory hallucinations (odors coming from his apartment). She was calm and cooperative on the psychiatric unit, but refused vehemently the possibility of having a mental illness. She denied any desire to become aggressive or violent against her neighbor and asked to be discharged. The multidisciplinary evaluation revealed a chronic low socio-economic situation because of isolation (immigrant with no close family), loss of employment (the textile jobs she used to do disappeared as manufacturing was outsourced in Asian countries) and cultural barriers (including limited schooling and language barriers). In spite of the recent psychotic symptoms and the long-term low-grade paranoia, she was managing to have a stable life, visiting a gym regularly and not creating frictions in her social interactions. After a team discussion and a careful assessment of risk, we concluded that we did not have enough arguments to keep her against her will in the hospital. She signed a discharge against medical advice and refused follow-up. A year later, she was brought again to the Emergency Room. This time, her conflict with the neighbor deteriorated to the point that she was evicted from her subsidized apartment – a major loss given her situation – and she was technically homeless. She was also angrier, more rigid in her thinking and clearly suffering. The treating team reacted strongly to this deterioration of her condition, expressing sorrow and grief. The team discussion evolved around concerns that not enforcing treatment at the first hospitalization was potentially not ethical and morally wrong given her deterioration. The final conclusion of the clinical team was to consider coercion in the treatment earlier in such situations. An alternate attitude would have been to empathize with the deep stigma resented by the patient and understand her refusal to accept a diagnosis and psychiatric care, eventually acknowledging the limits of resolving such conflicts deeply engrained in socio-cultural backgrounds. In a qualitative inquiry into how persons learned the importance of adherence to antipsychotic treatment, learning through personal experiences of stopping medication was an essential step in most cases (95% of subjects stopped their medication at least once during their psychiatric career) [30]. In clear contrast, this ethnographic data highlights the process of potential increase in coercion when periods of untreated psychosis are considered simply negative and toxic for the patient.

A new expert consensus on the use of long-acting injectable (LAI) antipsychotics reveals the practical implications of this view of untreated psychosis [31]. The LAIs are long-term intramuscular versions of oral antipsychotic medications. Their therapeutic action lasts for 1 to 4 weeks and adherence is ensured upon reception of the injection. Most newer antipsychotics became available in long-acting injectable formulations and they are actively promoted by the pharmaceutical companies as they offer better profit margins (patents often expired for oral formulations). In this Canadian expert consensus, LAIs are proposed as a first-line treatment for first episode psychosis. The treatment algorithm suggests proposing LAIs in adherent patients. For non-adherent patients (data shows that at least 50% of patients stop their antipsychotic medication in the first year of treatment [32]) or for those « at risk of non-adherence » (i.e. clinicians could argue that this represents the vast majority of treatment-naive patients), the algorithm suggests starting a LAI antipsychotic. Not only the LAI treatment of this algorithm represents a form of coercion as it is specifically designed for cases of non-adherence, but most patients will probably react negatively to this treatment plan, in which case the algorithm suggests either the use of oral medication surveillance (either through electronic pill dispensers, or therapeutic interventions) or coercion into treatment through legal measures. Given the present knowledge of adherence behaviors in the first year of treatment for psychosis, it is most likely that a significant proportion of patients (up to 50%) will end up under formal legal requirement to take LAIs if this algorithm is followed.

Here, the person-centered, non-coercive goals of early intervention in psychosis are transformed into exactly the opposite: an epidemic of coercion from the earliest phases of treatment for psychosis.

## III. Insight in Psychosis and Coercion

Insight ('a correct attitude to a morbid change in oneself' [33, 34]) and especially its lack in psychosis, are long-debated topics. Insight is usually measured on a uni-dimensional scale (item G12 of PANSS [35]) and sometimes as a tri-dimensional construct (awareness of mental disorder, awareness of benefit from medication and awareness of social consequences of the disorder [36]).

While insight is considered a desirable attribute in North America, it has not always been the case. For example, lobotomy was performed with the express desire to suppress awareness – this was not an adverse effect, but part of the intended consequences of the operation so that persons will suffer less from the overcrowded and depressing everyday life in an asylum [37]. Until recently, diagnoses of schizophrenia were told with great reluctance in France and not at all in the majority of cases in Japan [38]. It is widely accepted that insight in psychosis correlates with increased suicidality [39]. Moreover, the concept of insight was repeatedly criticized as having limited validity [40], being a sociocultural process [41] and rather representing the level of agreement and compliance with the clinicians' views [42, 43].

Regardless of the moral valence of having insight, lack of insight was shown to be one of the most common symptoms in schizophrenia [44] and psychoeducational interventions showed little capacity to change it [45]. In the last decades, a significant body of research explored the neurocognitive correlates of insight – bringing to the forefront a conceptualization of insight as a neurocognitive deficit similar to anosognosia [46, 47].

Legal responsibility and competency to make informed choices are based on the prerequisite of being aware of the situation and of the moral and practical consequences of one's acts (for a detailed and more nuanced analysis, see [48]). If a neurological process such as anosognosia impairs these capacities, the person suffering from psychosis looses competency and the right to make clinical decisions on one's own. This line of arguments is put forward by some ethicists and clinicians [49, 50] in order to amend the laws to broaden coercive powers even in the absence of dangerousness and, consequently, to promote earlier coercion into treatment for persons suffering from psychosis.

The socio-cultural and psychological contexts of care are glossed over in this legalistic debate. Refusal of treatment is related to access to treatment, to acceptability of interventions and to the costs of being identified as a patient (i.e. stigma and discrimination). Collapsing all these dimensions into a neurobiological discourse on anosognosia is reductive and limits the capacity to develop appropriate responses such as better and more acceptable clinical interventions.

## Conclusion: Ominous Trends

These new discourses on violence, untreated psychosis and insight have tremendous and synergistic effects on how society will react and treat persons suffering from psychosis. They might explain the increased coercion proposed in the clinical care for psychosis.

In this critical analysis we tried to advance the position that coerced treatment is a profoundly moral and social decision and should thus be decided based on moral values and human rights principles. It is not a scientific or a technical decision, nor a purely clinical issue, to be sorted through randomized clinical trials.

The disempowering effects of biogenetic and neurocognitive models of psychosis had deeply stigmatizing effects in the past. Coercion might be interpreted as a manifestation of the stigma of psychosis. The recent increase in coercion signals thus a return of troubled times for those suffering from psychosis rather than a progress in clinical care. If our treatments were that good, how come people are still voting with their feet against them?

In conclusion, in spite of societal pressures, let's hope that psychiatry will reject the perverse postulate that coercion is psychiatric treatment. Doing the contrary will only validate Thomas Szasz' critique [51] and it will impose additional suffering on persons who are already struggling with serious mental health problems.

## Acknowledgments

This work was supported by a Fonds de Recherche en Sante du Quebec grant. Data was collected as part of a CIHR grant. I would like to thank Robert Whitley for his helpful comments on an earlier draft of the manuscript.

## References:

[1] Torrey, E.F., The insanity offense: how America's failure to treat the seriously mentally ill endangers its citizens. 2008: W.W. Norton.

[2] Foucault, M., Histoire de la folie à l'âge classique, ed. Gallimard. 1972: Gallimard. 688.

[3] Seeman, M.V., Psychiatry in the Nazi era. *Can. J. Psychiatry*, 2005. 50(4): p. 218-25.

[4] Metzl, J., The protest psychosis: how schizophrenia became a Black disease. 2010: Beacon Press.

[5] Horgan, J., *The psychology of terrorism*. 2005: Frank Cass.

[6] Victoroff, J., The mind of the terrorist. *Journal of Conflict resolution*, 2005. 49(1): p. 3.

[7] Howell, A., Victims or Madmen? The Diagnostic Competition over ìTerroristî Detainees at Guant·namo Bay. *International Political Sociology*, 2007. 1(1): p. 29-47.

[8] Kleinman, A., V. Das, and M.M. Lock, Social suffering. 1997, Berkeley: University of California Press. xxvii, 404 p.

[9] Read, J., et al., Prejudice and schizophrenia: a review of the 'mental illness is an illness like any other' approach. Acta Psychiatrica Scandinavica, 2006. 114(5 %R doi:10.1111/j.1600-0447.2006.00824.x): p. 303-318.

[10] Pescosolido, B.A., et al., " A Disease Like Any Other"? A Decade of Change in Public Reactions to Schizophrenia, Depression, and Alcohol Dependence. *American Journal of Psychiatry*, 2010. 167(11): p. 1321.

[11] Angermeyer, M.C., Schizophrenia and violence. *Acta Psychiatrica Scandinavica Supplementum,* 2000. 407: p. 63-67.

[12] Van Dorn, R., J. Volavka, and N. Johnson, Mental disorder and violence: is there a relationship beyond substance use? *Social Psychiatry and Psychiatric Epidemiology*, 2011: p. 1-17.

[13] Maniglio, R., Severe mental illness and criminal victimization: a systematic review. *Acta Psychiatrica Scandinavica*, 2009. 119(3): p. 180-191.

[14] McGlashan, T.H. and J.O. Johannessen, Early detection and intervention with schizophrenia: rationale. *Schizophr Bull*, 1996. 22(2): p. 201-22.

[15] Aitchison, K.J., K. Meehan, and R. Murray, First episode psychosis. 1999, London, Malden, Mass.: Martin Dunitz; Distributed in the United States by Blackwell Science. 138 p.

[16] Edwards, J. and P.D. McGorry, Implementing early intervention in psychosis : a guide to establishing early psychosis services. 2002, London, Florence, KY, USA: Martin Dunitz ; Distributed in USA by Fulfilment Center Taylor and Francis. xv, 186 p.

[17] Zipursky, R.B. and S.C. Schulz, The early stages of schizophrenia. 1st ed. 2002, Washington, D.C.: American Psychiatric Pub. xx, 259 p.

[18] NICE, N.C.C.f.M.H.-. Schizophrenia Core interventions in the treatment and management of schizophrenia in primary and secondary care Clinical Guideline. 2002 8 February 2010]; Available from: http://www.schizophreniaguidelines. .uk/schizophrenia/index2.php?ln_id=8.

[19] Canguilhem, G., The Normal and the Pathological. 1989/1966, New York: Zone Books.

[20] Miller, F.A., et al., Redefining disease? The nosologic implications of molecular genetic knowledge. *Perspect Biol. Med*, 2006. 49(1): p. 99-114.

[21] Bayer, R., Homosexuality and American psychiatry : the politics of diagnosis. Princeton paperbacks. 1987, Princeton, N.J.: Princeton University Press. viii, 242 p.

[22] Bowker, G.C. and S.L. Star, Sorting things out : classification and its consequences. Inside technology and indexes. 1999, Cambridge, Mass.: MIT Press. xii, 377 p.

[23] Perala, J., et al., Lifetime Prevalence of Psychotic and Bipolar I Disorders in a General Population. *Arch. Gen. Psychiatry*, 2007. 64(1): p. 19-28.

[24] McGorry, P.D., A. Yung, and L. Phillips, Ethics and early intervention in psychosis: keeping up the pace and staying in step. *Schizophrenia Research*, 2001. 51(1): p. 17-29.

[25] Bertolote, J. and P. McGorry, Early intervention and recovery for young people with early psychosis: consensus statement. *The British Journal of Psychiatry*, 2005. 187(48): p. s116-s119.

[26] Lieberman, J.A., B.B. Sheitman, and B.J. Kinon, Neurochemical sensitization in the pathophysiology of schizophrenia: deficits and dysfunction in neuronal regulation and plasticity. *Neuropsychopharmacology*, 1997. 17(4): p. 205-229.

[27] Norman, R.M.G., A.K. Malla, and R. Manchanda, Is untreated psychosis socially toxic? *Early Intervention in Psychiatry*, 2007. 1(3): p. 267-270.

[28] Perkins, D.O., et al., Relationship between duration of untreated psychosis and outcome in first-episode schizophrenia: a critical review and meta-analysis. *American Journal of Psychiatry*, 2005. 162(10): p. 1785.

[29] Tranulis, C., et al., Early Intervention in Psychosis: A Case Study on Normal and Pathological. *Cult Med. Psychiatry*, 2009. 33(4): p. 608-622.

[30] Tranulis, C., et al., Becoming Adherent to Antipsychotics: A Qualitative Study of Treatment-Experienced Schizophrenia Patients. *Psychiatric Services*, 2011. 62(8): p. 888.

[31] STIP, E., et al., Les antipsychotiques injectables ‡ action prolongÈe: avis d'experts de l'Association des mÈdecins psychiatres du QuÈbec. *Canadian journal of psychiatry*, 2011. 56(6): p. 367-376.

[32] Coldham, E.L., J. Addington, and D. Addington, Medication adherence of individuals with a first episode of psychosis. *Acta Psychiatr. Scand*, 2002. 106(4): p. 286-90.

[33] David, A.S., "To see oursels as others see us". Aubrey Lewis's insight. *Br. J. Psychiatry*, 1999. 175: p. 210-6.

[34] Lewis, A.J., The psychopathology of insight. *British Journal of medical Psychology*, 1934. 14: p. 332-48.

[35] Kay, S.R., A. Fiszbein, and L.A. Opler, The positive and negative syndrome scale (PANSS) for schizophrenia. *Schizophrenia Bulletin*, 1987. 13(2): p. 261-76.

[36] Amador, X.F., et al., Assessment of insight in psychosis. *American Journal of Psychiatry*, 1993. 150(6): p. 873-9.

[37] Braslow, J.T., History and evidence-based medicine: lessons from the history of somatic treatments from the 1900s to the 1950s. *Ment Health Serv Res*, 1999. 1(4): p. 231-40.

[38] Kim, Y. and G.E. Berrios, Impact of the term schizophrenia on the culture of ideograph: the Japanese experience. *Schizophr Bull*, 2001. 27(2): p. 181-5.

[39] Kim, C.H., K. Jayathilake, and H.Y. Meltzer, Hopelessness, neurocognitive function, and insight in schizophrenia: relationship to suicidal behavior. *Schizophrenia Research*, 2003. 60(1): p. 71-80.

[40] Anonymous, Real insight. *The Lancet*, 1990. 336(8712): p. 408.

[41] Kirmayer, L. and E. Corin, Inside knowledge : cultural constructions of insight in psychosis., in Insight and psychosis : awareness of illness in schizophrenia and related disorders., X.F. Amador and A.S. David, Editors. 2004, Oxford University Press, 2004: New York. p. 197-230.

[42] Koren, D., et al., The course and nature of insight change in patients with recent-onset schizophrenia: from unawareness to disagreement. Schizophrenia Research Supplement - 5th International Conference on early Psychosis, Birmingham, UK, 2006. 86(October): p. S106.

[43] Tranulis, C.S., O. Freudenreich, and L. Park, Narrative insight: rethinking insight in psychosis. *International Journal of Culture and Mental Health*, 2009. 2(1): p. 16 - 28.

[44] WHO, Report of the International Pilot Study of Schizophrenia. 1973, Geneva, Switzerland: World Health Organization Press.

[45] Pekkala, E. and L. Merinder, Psychoeducation for schizophrenia. *Cochrane Database Syst Rev*, 2002(2): p. CD002831.

[46] Amador, X.F. and A.S. David, Insight and psychosis : awareness of illness in schizophrenia and related disorders. 2nd ed, ed. X.F. Amador and A.S. David. 2004, New York: Oxford University Press, 2004. 402.

[47] Amador, X.F. and A.L. Johanson, I am not sick, I don't need help!: helping the seriously mentally ill accept treatment : a practical guide for families and therapists. 2000: Vida Press.

[48] Kress, K.J., Why lack of insight should have a central place in mental health law, in Insight and Psychosis, X.F. Amador and A. David, Editors. 2004, Oxford University Press: Oxford, UK. p. 257-279.

[49] Large, M., et al., Mental health laws that require dangerousness for involuntary admission may delay the initial treatment of schizophrenia. *Social Psychiatry and Psychiatric Epidemiology*, 2008. 43(3): p. 251-256.

[50] Dawson, J. and R. Mullen, Insight and use of community treatment orders. *Journal of Mental Health*, 2008. 17(3): p. 269-280.

[51] Szasz, T.S., Coercion as cure : a critical history of psychiatry. 2007, New Brunswick, N.J.: Transaction Publishers. xv, 278 p.

In: Psychosis: Causes, Diagnosis and Treatment
Editor: Xenia Anastassiou-Hadjicharalambous
ISBN: 978-1-62081-516-8


*Chapter 12*

# PSYCHOSIS IN SYSTEMIC LUPUS ERYTHEMATOSUS

***Aline Tamires Lapa,[1] Mariana Postal[2], Fernando Augusto Peres,[2] Caio Rodrigues Guirau[2] and Simone Appenzeller[2,*]***

[1]Pediatrics Department/ State University of Campinas, Brazil
[2]Department of Medicine-State University of Campinas, Brazil

## ABSTRACT

Systemic lupus erythematosus (SLE) is an autoimmune disorder that affects 0.1% of the world population. The disorder is characterized by systemic inflammation, auto-antibody production, and immune dysregulation, and it may lead to significant neurologicaland psychiatric morbidities. Both adults and children are diagnosed according to a set of clinical and laboratory criteria with a high sensitivity and specificity. A diagnosis of SLE in any age-group depends on excluding systemic infections or malignancies and the presence of at least 4 of 11 American College of Rheumatology (ACR) diagnostic criteria. Nephritis (leading to hypertension and renal dysfunction) and nervous system involvement are two of the more ominous manifestations in all age-groups. There are 19 case-based peripheral and central nervous syndromes that are postulated to be associated with SLE. Syndromes requiring prompt neurological evaluation include seizures, cerebrovascular accidents, demyelination, movement disorders, and peripheral neuropathies. Manifestations that may prompt psychiatric consultation include acute confusional state (delirium), affective disorders (anxiety and depression), cognitive impairment, and psychosis. Neuropsychiatric presentations may be caused by hypercoagulability in cerebral vessels (vasculopathy), proinflammatory cytokines, auto-antibody effects on neuronalstructures or receptors, and blood–brain barrier disruption. Alteration in the regulation of neurotransmitters such as dopamine and serotonin appear to play a role in behavioral changes seen in lupus-prone mice.

Psychiatric manifestations in all age-groups may also be influenced by significant disease-related psychosocial stressors and by medication. Psychotic manifestations in adult patients are associated with early and severe clinical presentations and are described in up to 11% of patients in retrospective reviews of adult cohorts.

We will review the prevalence, etiology and clinical presentation of psychosis in SLE. In addition we will discuss treatment protocol for this serious manifestation in SLE.

* E-mail: appenzellersimone@yahoo.com, FAX: +55 19 3289-1818

## INTRODUCTION

Systemic lupus erythematosus (SLE) is an autoimmune disease of unknown etiology which affects different organs, such as the skin, kidney, and the brain. A large fraction of patients with SLE demonstrate organic psychiatric and neurological disorders, indicating central nervous system (CNS) involvement [1-4]. Neuropsychiatric (NP) manifestations occur in up to 75% of the patients and may include major manifestations (i.e., stroke syndromes, severe organic brain syndrome, seizures, psychotic episodes, etc.) or minor abnormalities, including mood disorders and less severe cognitive deficits [5, 6]. The frequency of these manifestations in SLE studies varies widely, depending on the type of manifestations included and the method used for evaluation [7-11]. The involvement is heterogeneous and may vary from subtle signs such as headache and mood disorders to severe, and life threatening conditions, such as stroke, myelopathy and acute confusional state [6]. Any part of the peripheral or CNS may be affected by the disease [12]. The diagnosis of primary NP involvement by SLE is often difficult, as both focal and diffuse manifestations may occur and a gold standard for diagnosis is still absent [2, 13, 14]. Psychiatric syndromes associated with SLE are diverse in etiology and presentation [15,16]. These manifestations can be the presenting manifestation of SLE or occur at any time during the disease [15].

Controversy exists concerning the pathophysiology of psychiatric manifestations in SLE [17], since in addition to inflammation and antibody-mediated etiology, iatrogenic effects of corticosteroids [18], and psychosocial stressors related to chronic disease may influence its occurrence [12]. Psychiatric manifestations in adult SLE patients are associated with early and severe clinical presentations and are described in up to 11% of patients in retrospective reviews of adult cohorts [13, 14, 17, 19- 27] (Table 1). Psychiatric manifestations occur in all age-groups may also be influenced by significant disease-related psychosocial stressors and by medication.

We will review the prevalence, etiology and clinical presentation of psychosis in SLE. In addition we will discuss treatment protocol for this serious manifestation in SLE.

## CLASSIFICATION CRITERIA

The large number of papers published about NP manifestations in SLE evidence more manifestations attributable to SLE than seizures and psychosis described in the original classification criteria by Tan et al. [28]. In addition, the several distinct pathologic mechanisms of NP damage in SLE predispose to different central and peripheral presentations, including focal and diffuse disease. The lack of definitions of individual manifestations and the absence of standardization for investigation were reflected in the prevalence and frequency of NP manifestations in different reports, varying from 24-74% of SLE patients [7, 9, 13, 17, 29, 30-37].

## Table 1. SLE: Classification criteria of neuropsychiatric manifestations: analysis of CNS

| Authors/ year | No of patients | Prevalence NP (%) | Headache (%) | Seizure disorder (%) | Anxiety disorder (%) | Mood disorder (%) | Movement disorder (%) | Cognitive dysfunction (%) | Cerebrovascular disease (%) | Acute confusion (%) | Asepitc meningitis (%) | Myelopathy (%) | Psychosis (%) | Demyelinating syndrome (%) |
|---|---|---|---|---|---|---|---|---|---|---|---|---|---|---|
| Ainiala et al., 2001 (33) | 46 | 91 | 54 | 9 | 13 | 44 | 2 | 80 | 15 | 7 | 2 | 0 | 0 | 2 |
| Mok et al., 2001 (27) | 518 | 19 | 4 | 28 | 1,5 | 6 | 2 | NR | 19 | 14 | 1 | 8 | 11 | 1,5 |
| Brey et al, 2002 (17) | 128 | 80 | 57 | 16 | 24 | 23,0 | 1 | 79 | 2 | 0 | 0 | 5,0 | 6,5 | 0 |
| Alfreta et al., 2003 (20) | 61 | 72 | 21 | 11 | 6 | 27 | 0 | 52 | 24 | 0 | 0 | 0 | 0 | 3 |
| Sanna et al., 2003 (26) | 323 | 57,3 | 24 | 8,3 | 7,4 | 16,7 | 1,2 | 10,8 | 17,6 | 3,7 | 0 | 1,2 | 7,7 | 0,9 |
| Mikdashi et al.,2004 (29) | 130 | 56,9 | NR | 7,6 | 0 | NR | 0 | 27,3 | 25,7 | 0 | 0 | 6,1 | 15,1 | 0 |
| Appenzeller et al., 2005 (24) | 72 | NR | 30 | 11,3 | NR | 10,5 | 0,8 | 27,1 | NR | 7,5 | 0,8 | 2,3 | 4,5 | NR |
| Hanly et al., 2005 (12) | 53 | 31 | 9,4 | 0 | | 0 | 0 | 1,9 | 0 | 3,8 | 0 | 0 | 0 | 1,9 |
| Shimojima et al., 2005 (31) | 25 | 100 | 12 | 36 | 0 | 0 | 0 | 12 | 24 | 0 | 0 | 4 | 32 | 0 |
| Robert et al., 2006 (30) | 50 | 78 | 55,6 | 20,5 | 0 | 0 | 23,1 | 18 | 16,2 | 16,2 | 0 | 0 | 16,2 | 0 |
| Hanly J et al., 2009 (27) | 209 | NR | 32,1 | 6,7 | 8 | 23,4 | 0,3 | 8,4 | 5,7 | 3,7 | 0,3 | 0,3 | 1,7 | 2 |

In 1999, the American College of Rheumatology developed case definitions that included appropriate terminology, classification criteria and complementary examinations for 19 NP syndromes (Table 2) [38].

**Table 2. Central nervous system manifestation following ACR case definitions. Adapted from [38]**

| Central nervous system manifestations | Peripheral nervous system manifestations |
|---|---|
| Aseptic meningitis | Acute Inflammatory Demyelinating Polyradiculoneuropathy |
| Acute Confusional State | Autonomic Disorders |
| Anxiety Disorder | Cranial Neuropathy |
| Cerebrovascular Disease | Mononeuropathy |
| Cognitive Dysfunction | Myasthenia Gravis |
| Demyelinating Syndrome | Plexopathy |
| Headache | Polyneuropathy |
| Movement Disorder | |
| Mood Disorders | |
| Myelopathy | |
| Psychosis | |
| Seizures | |

**Table 3. Suggested preliminary diagnostic criteria for classification of lupus psychosis. Adapted from [41]**

| |
|---|
| I. Fulfill the 1982 (revised in 1999) ACR criteria for the classification of SLE |
| II. Show at least one of the following psychiatric manifestations defined in the 1999 ACR nomenclature |
| Acute confusional state<br>Cognitive dysfunction<br>Psychosis<br>Anxiety disorder<br>Mood disorder (depression) |
| III. Elevation of CSF IL-6 (more than 4.3 pg/ml |
| IV. Exclusion |
| 1. Cerebrovascular disease of a new onset |
| 2. Infectious meningoencephalitis |

I + II + III + IV lupus psychosis

These criteria were a result of a consensus meeting of experts of several subspecialties (rheumatology, neurology, immunology, and psychiatry). Furthermore, in 2001, these criteria have been validated in a cross-sectional study with a specificity of 46% [39]. Several studies have used these classification criteria in order to determine frequency and prevalence of CNS involvement in SLE population [17, 29, 30-37]. Although these studies show a substantial variability between the frequency of CNS manifestations, suggesting differences between cohorts or bias in data acquisition, this classification allows us to compare the results across cohorts [6, 13, 14].

In this classification, psychosis was defined according In the DSM-IV, and refers to delusions or prominent hallucinations, without insight into their pathological nature [40]. Recently specific diagnostic criteria for lupus psychosis have been suggested and are shown in Table 3. [41].

Patients with psychosis have to be carefully evaluated, in order to differentiate primary psychotic disorders unrelated to SLE, substance or drug-induced psychotic disorders and psychologically mediated reactions to SLE as a major stressor. In all patients with psychosis, other causes such as infection, metabolic disturbance and structural lesions have to be excluded by clinical, laboratory and MRI when indicated [14].

Corticosteroid-induced psychiatric disturbances is defined as a new symptoms that appears temporally within 8 weeks of institution or augmentation of steroids and resolves completely after reduction of steroid dosage without additional immunosuppressive agents [14].

## Clinical Relevance

The clinical relevance of NP manifestations in SLE has been intensively studied [6, 13, 34-36, 42, 43].

Using mortality as indicative for poor outcome in NP manifestations, there are studies suggesting that patients with NP have increased mortality when compared to SLE patients without these manifestations [44-47]. Although some studies did not find an increased mortality among patients with CNS manifestations when compared to SLE patients without CNS manifestations and controls [42, 48-51], the presence of CNS manifestations, independently of its etiology, seems to have a negative impact in quality of life [52], overall damage scores [34, 35, 42], higher fatigue scores [34, 43] and unemployment [42, 43, 53].

The association of lower quality of life with NP events over time, independent of progression in cumulative organ damage, emphasizes the persistent negative effect of NP events in the lives of patients with SLE [52].

The ACR damage score (ACR/SLICC-DI) has been developed to determine irreversible damage in SLE patients, irrespectively if attributed to disease itself or secondary to comorbidities or medications [6]. In the ACR/SLICC-DI seizures, psychosis, mood disorders, cerebrovascular disease, neuropathy, mononeuritis multiplex, acute confusional state and myelopathy are scored in addition to several other clinical manifestations in order to determine the global damage score. Using the items of NP in order to create a NP damage score, the strongest risk factors for the development of significant NP damage was the presence of greater disease activity at the time of CNS involvement onset and the presence of antiphospholipide antibodies [35]. Cumulative organ damage was higher in patients with NP disease because they were more likely to have received corticosteroids or immunosuppressive drugs [34]. Fatigue is also an important aspect of life in SLE patients. A recent study shows the main reasons for being unemployed were fatigue, hours of work missed, pain, and cognitive impairment [43]. Another study in the same area proved that patients with NP disease reported more fatigue and had significantly lower scores on 7 of 8 subscales of the SF-36 (Short form 36 health survey questionnaire) [34]. Working disability has been studied in NP in several studies [42, 43, 53]. The number of cognitive spheres, and especially attention, memory, and executive functions, were important factors associated with unemployment in patients with SLE [43]. The association between memory function and employment status in patients with SLE underscores the need for judicious assessment of cognitive function and for the development of appropriate strategies that will either reverse cognitive impairment or help patients overcome obstacles they may face in daily life. Pertaining to employment, persons with cognitive impairment may benefit from specific training programs [53]. In conclusion, the presence of CNS manifestations does not seem to influence mortality, but it does seem to have a negative impact in quality of life [42, 52], overall damage scores [34, 35, 42], higher fatigue scores [34, 42] and unemployment [43, 53].

## PSYCHOSIS IN SLE

A challenging problem in the diagnosis and management of SLE is psychiatric disorder [14]. Abnormal behavior was first described in SLE by Hebra and Kaposi [54], followed by Osler [55]. Many psychiatric symptoms can be observed in SLE patients, such as depression, anxiety, mood disorders, but psychosis was considered as one of the most important and included in the classification criteria for SLE in 1982, despite the widely diverse clinical manifestations [56] and varying degree of severity [57, 58].

Psychosis may be a primary event of CNS manifestation of SLE or associated with a, such as corticosteroids and antimalarics [17] (Figure1).

Adverse psychiatric effects, including mild euphoria, emotional lability, alteration of behavior, panic attacks, psychosis and delirium, are seen in 3–10% of all patients receiving corticosteroids and are unpredictable from the regimens of corticosteroids used [59, 60-62].

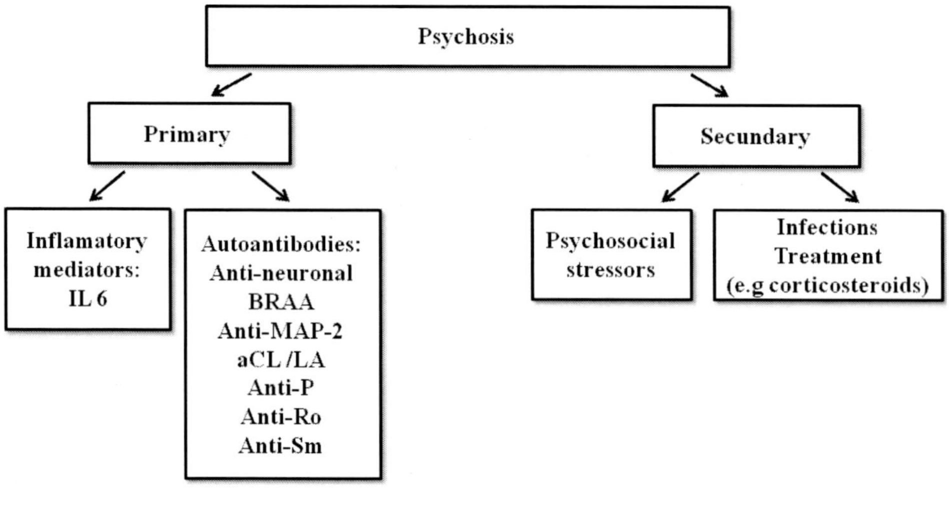


Figure 1. Psychosis may be a primary event, with variety of drugs and infections.

Psychosis is defined as a severe disturbance in the perception of reality characterized by delusions and/or hallucinations, in the absence of delirium, causing clinical distress or impairment in social, occupational or other relevant areas of functioning. This is not a common feature in SLE [14].

There are very few studies specifically exploring the characteristics of this psychiatric complication of SLE published after the ACR standardized definitions were developed and prevalence of psychosis varies from 11-18% [13, 14].

We observed that acute psychosis secondary to SLE at disease onset was more frequently associated with disease activity, whereas cutaneous manifestations were less frequently seen [14]. This may be one of the reasons why these patients are usually first seen by psychiatrist [14, 63]. In patients who had acute psychosis during the course of disease, it was associated with the presence of antiphospholipid antibodies and they had more frequently other CNS manifestations related to SLE activity [14]. Depression, stroke, seizures, cognitive dysfunction, and psychosis have all been associated with antiphospholipid antibodies [14, 32, 33, 64].

Recurrence of acute psychosis was observed in 18 of 59 patients. These patients had also more frequently other CNS events due to SLE activity [14]. Therefore patients with acute psychosis should be followed carefully in order to determine if they develop other primary CNS manifestations secondary to SLE [14].

In our study we observed 38 episodes of corticosteroid induced psychosis in 28 patients during the follow-up period [14]. All patients had active SLE disease and were receiving prednisone in moderate to high doses. As previously described, hypoalbuminemia may be a risk factor for corticosteroid induced psychosis [60, 61, 64-69]. The explanation for these findings may be that corticosteroid binding globulin does not bind to synthetic steroids, whose transport depends on serum albumin which, by contrast, presents low affinity but a great capacity to transport the steroids because of its high plasma concentration. Steroids are biologically inactive when bound to albumin. Therefore, the free (and active) fraction of steroids is higher in patients with low plasma albumin levels, and this will expose the patient to more adverse efects [68]. In patients with SLE, corticosteroid-induced psychiatric events may be difficult to distinguish from primary neuropsychiatric manifestations of SLE. The antiribosomal P antibody is specific for SLE and has been shown to be associated with psychosis related to disease activity and other CNS manifestations, including depression [61, 62, 70-73], but the low sensitivity limits its clinical usefulness for the diagnosis of lupus psychosis [73]. Therefore, a temporal relationship between the beginning of corticosteroid therapy and psychiatric events, and the resolution of symptoms after reduction of corticosteroids is an important feature in diagnosis of corticosteroid induced psychosis in clinical practice.

## Pathogenesis in Psychiatric SLE

### Anti-Neuronal Antibodies

Anti-neuronal antibodies are not well defined, but rather represent a group of antibodies that react to neuronal components [72]. Antineuronal antibodies are detected in the serum in 43 to 95% of SLE patients and in approximately 74% of the CSF. Antineuronal Abs are more predominantly detected in NPSLE patients when compared with SLE patients without neurological manifestations or when compared with patients with other autoimmune diseases [72]. Anti-neuronal antibodies were analyzed in a variety of NP SLE manifestations, rarely in psychosis.

In selected sera from 22 patients with active SLE, 92% of NPSLE indicated definite neuron reactivity, in contrast to only 20% of sera obtained from patients without evidence of NP involvement [74]. Serial studies of 2 SLE patients with transient psychotic episodes revealed a close association between the Ab titers and the appearance of psychosis in 1 patient [74].

Another study evaluated antineuronal antibodies in the CSF from 27 patients with NPSLE and 18 patients with SLE free of CNS disease for antibodies reactivity with the cultured human neuronal cell line SK-N-SH [75]. Whereas 74% of NPSLE CSF samples harbored increased IgG antineuronal activity, only 11% of the CSF samples of non-CNS disease also showed increased antibodies activity. Ninety percent of the patients with psychosis, organic brain syndrome, or generalized seizures had increased IgG antineuronal activity, as compared with only 25% of the patients who had hemiparesis or chorea/hemiballismus. Antineuronal activity per microgram of IgG was concentrated eightfold in the CSF of patients with active CNS disease, as compared with the serum activity. Patients with or without active CNS disease did not differ significantly in the amount of serum antineuronal binding activity.

The results of these studies raise the possibility that the more diffuse CNS manifestations of SLE, such as psychosis may be a result of the interaction of antibodies with neuronal cell membranes.

## Brain-Reactive Antibodies (BRAA)

### *BRAA Are a Subgroup of Antineuronal Antibodies [72, 76, 77]*

One study described BRAA that correlated with psychosis and/or seizures in SLE [77]. Ten percent of 100 lupus patients had NP manifestations. Of those, 60% of the BRAA-positive patients had psychoses and/or seizures compared with 2% of BRAA-negative patients with the same manifestations. These antibodies are specific for neuronal membrane tissues of mammalian origin and are specifically associated with psychosis and/or seizures.

### *Anti-MAP-2*

MAP-2, a cellular protein restricted to neurons, is important in the control of cytoskeletal integrity and other neuronal functions [72]. In 1 study on 100 patients with SLE, 17% of the SLE patients had antibodies to MAP-2, in contrast to 4% of the patients with neurologic injury/disease and 2% of normal controls [78].

Elevated titers of anti-MAP-2 were significantly associated with psychosis, seizure, neuropathy, and cerebritis in 77% of the SLE patients, whereas the absence of anti-MAP-2 Abs was associated with NP symptoms in 20% of the patients.

***Antiphospholipid (aPl) Antibodies***

By far, aPL antibodies, in particular, anticardiolipine (aCL) antibodies and lupus anticoagulant (LAC), have been the most widely investigated antibodies in NPSLE. In an open pilot study of 11 children with NPSLE manifested as encephalopathy with or without grand mal seizures, focal seizures with depression or hallucinations, optic neuritis with transverse myelitis, and psychosis with audiovisual hallucinations, 45% had elevated aCL IgG antibodies [79]. A study evaluated the predictive value of antibodies in determining a relapse in 25 NPSLE patients [37]. The most common antibodies encountered excluding ANA were aPL (defined as aCL or $\beta_2$GPI or LAC), anti-Sm, and anti-Ro antibodies. Six patients with elevated titers of aPL had CVA, seizures, or cognitive dysfunction. The NP manifestations in 3 patients with anti-Sm Abs were seizures or psychosis, and 3 patients with elevated anti-Ro Abs titers had psychosis, myelitis, and cognitive impairment. None of the Abs were significant for CNS lupus when compared with SLE without NP clinical findings. None of the antibodies were predictive of a relapse of CNS disease. Paired measurements of aCL, in the serum and CSF, were performed using the ELISA method in 31 lupus patients and in controls with other diseases. High titers of CSF IgG-aCL were detected in NPSLE patients with lupus headache, acute psychosis, cognitive impairment, high cortical dysfunction, and altered consciousness. Intrathecal synthesis occurred in these NPLE patients, rather than the diffusion of IgG-aCL from serum to CNS compartments [80]. In another small study (n = 5), aCL was not detected in any CSF samples [81].

***IL6***

Although previous studies disclosed that CSF IL-6 was elevated in patients with NP-SLE, including psychosis [82-84], but not in SLE patients without neuropsychiatric manifestations [7], the operating characteristics of CSF IL-6 in the diagnosis of psychosis have not been determined. The results have clearly demonstrated that CSF IL-6 is a useful tool for diagnosis of psychosis. Thus, the sensitivity and specificity of CSF IL-6 for diagnosis of psychosis were 87.5% and 92.3%, respectively, at the cut-off value of 4.3 pg/ml. It should be also pointed out that CSF IL-6 was found to be decreased after successful immunosuppressive therapy [82-84], suggesting that it may be useful for monitoring the effects of treatment. It should be noted that CSF IL-6 is elevated in a variety of conditions, including CNS infections and cerebrovascular diseases [85, 86]. Therefore, it is necessary to rule out these conditions to make a correct diagnosis of psychosis. Careful clinical evaluation as well as MRI scans would be important for differential diagnosis. Of note, CSF IL-6 has been found to be elevated in NP-SLE other than psychosis, including aseptic meningitis and transverse myelitis [87]. Moreover, we have recently reported that CSF IL-6 was elevated in SLE patients with reversible focal neurological deficits, which are possibly caused by vasculitis [88]. Although these conditions rarely result in psychiatric manifestations, it is difficult to make a correct diagnosis of psychosis by CSF IL-6, when SLE patients present both psychiatric manifestations and focal symptoms at the same time.

***Anti-P***

The clinical association between elevated titers of anti-Rib P antibodies and psychosis was originally described by Bonfa and coworkers [89]. In a recent review, 12 of 17 studies showed an association between elevated titers of serum anti-P antibodies and NP lupus, predominantly psychosis and depression [89-102], whereas others refuted the association [90, 103-107]. Our group found that 14% of 44 Israeli SLE patients had elevated titers of anti-P antibodies. Of those, 2/6 patients harbored NPSLE, 1 with psychosis and the other with cognitive dysfunction and depression. Anti-P antibodies are predominantly found in the serum of patients with NP SLE; however,this association remains controversial. After Bonfa [89] observed high titers of anti-P antibodies in lupus psychosis, several studies were performed and published to confirm the possible association between anti-P antibody and psychiatric manifestations, especially psychosis [92, 94, 95, 98, 100]. Reichlin reviewed publications that, despite some existing controversies, suggested a meaningful relationship between anti-P antibodies and central nervous system disease [108]. Yoshio et al. [102] detected a significantly higher frequency of anti-P antibodies in cerebrospinal fluid (CSF) in patients suffering from SLE with serum anti-P antibodies and in those suffering from NPSLE, particularly complex presentations [102]. This observation may confirm the pathogenic role of anti-P antibodies in neuropsychiatric lupus. Although serum (and/or CSF) anti-P antibodies are associated with lupus psychosis, the mechanism by whichthese antibodies lead to the development of the symptom is not understood. The interaction of anti-P antibodies with neurocytes has not been directly evidenced in vivo. However, the results of an international metaanalysis disclosed that the sensitivity and specificity of serum anti-P testing for LP were 24–27% and 80%, respectively (73). Thus, serum anti-P testing has been found to be too less sensitive to be used for the diagnosis of LP, although it appeared to be specific for LP.

### *Anti-Ro*

The predictive value of antibodies in determining relapse in 25 NPSLE patients was evaluated [37]. The most common antibodies encountered excluding ANA were antiphospholipid (defined as aCL, $\beta_2$GPI, or LAC), anti-Sm, and anti-Ro antibodies. The 3 patients with elevated anti-Ro antibodies titers had psychosis, myelitis, and cognitive impairment. Anti-Ro antibodies were not significant for NPSLE when compared with SLE without NP clinical findings nor were they predictive of a relapse of CNS disease. Further investigation is warranted for determining the correlation between anti-Ro antibodies and NPSLE.

### *Anti-Sm Abs*

Four studies refer to the association of anti-Sm antibodies and NPSLE. Serologic studies were performed on 25 patients with SLE during 29 acute episodes of CNS disease. Patients with isolated CNS disease were otherwise in apparent clinical and serological remission. Of special interest was an increased incidence of anti-Sm antibodies in the patients with CNS dysfunction relative to that in a large group of patients without NPSLE [109]. A retrospective analysis of 33 anti-Sm antibodies -positive and 243 anti-Sm antibodies -negative patients with systemic connective tissue diseases including SLE and related disorders (overlap, mixed, and undifferentiated connective tissue diseases) revealed no association between anti-Sm antibodies and NP features [110]. In an open pilot study of 11 children with NPSLE manifest as encephalopathy with or without grand mal seizures, focal seizures with depression or hallucinations, optic neuritis with transverse myelitis, and psychosis with audiovisual hallucinations, 36% had elevated titers of anti-Sm antibodies [79].

The predictive value of Abs in determining relapse in 25 NPSLE patients was evaluated in 1 study [25]. The NP manifestations in 3 patients with anti-Sm antibodies were seizures or psychosis. Antinuclear antibodies, anti-dsDNA antibodies, and anti-Sm antibodies were not predictive of CNS relapse.

### Treatment of Psychiatric Manifestations in SLE

Given the diversity in clinical manifestations, the management is tailored to the specific needs of individual patients. The management of psychiatric lupus manifestations is often frustrating and currently no consensus is available. Counseling and other interventions that assist a person in developing coping skills may be helpful. In the absence of controlled studies, the use of symptomatic therapies, immunosuppressive, anticoagulants and adjunctive psychotropic medication is sup- ported by case series and clinical experience [6, 13]. There is no standardized treatment for lupus psychosis. In our cohort, we have used a variety of therapies. All the patients received corticosteroids and anti-psychotics and 90% of them received an immunosuppressive agent. To the best of our knowledge, there are no controlled trials assessing any treatment strategy in the management of lupus psychosis. Several small studies have reported the benefit of the use of corticosteroids and different immuno-suppressive strategies in patients with NP lupus [13, 14, 111-116]. More recently, one study reported the efficacy and tolerability of rituximab in the treatment of patients with lupus psychosis [117].

Little is known about the outcome of psychosis due to lupus. One year after the diagnosis and treatment, 60 and 40% of our patients with lupus psychosis showed complete resolution of their psychiatric symptoms or chronic psychotic activity, respectively.

## Conclusion

Psychosis has been described to occur between 11-18% of SLE patients, both at disease onset and during follow-up period. Patients with psychosis have to be carefully evaluated, in order to differentiate primary psychotic disorders unrelated to SLE, substance or drug-induced psychotic disorders and psychologically mediated reactions to SLE as a major stressor. Both antibody-mediates and cytokines, especially IL-6 are involved in the pathogenesis of psychosis in SLE. There is no standardized treatment for lupus psychosis and little is known about outcome in SLE patients with psychosis.

## Acknowledgments

Grants: Fundação de Amparo à Pesquisa do Estado de São Paulo (FAPESP 08/020917-0) and Conselho Nacional Pesquisa Desenvolvimento-Brasil CNPq (300447/2009-4).

## REFERENCES


[1] Rahman A, Isenberg DA. Systemic lupus erythematosus. *N. Engl. J. Med.* 2008; 358:929-39.

[2] Kozora E, Arciniegas DB, Filley CM, *et al.* Cognition, MRS neurometabolites, and MRI volumetrics in non-neuropsychiatric systemic lupus erythematosus: preliminary data. *Cogn. Behav. Neurol.* 2005; 18:159-62.

[3] Maneeton B, Maneeton N, Louthrenoo W. Cognitive deficit in patients with systemic lupus erythematosus. *Asian Pac. J. Allergy Immunol.* 2010; 28:77-83.

[4] Adhikari T, Piatti A, Luggen M. Cognitive dysfunction in SLE: development of a screening tool. *Lupus.* 2011.

[5] Hanly JG, Harrison MJ. Management of neuropsychiatric lupus. *Best Pract. Res. Clin. Rheumatol.* 2005; 19:799-821.

[6] Postal M, Costallat LT, Appenzeller S. Neuropsychiatric manifestations in systemic lupus erythematosus: epidemiology, pathophysiology and management. CNS Drugs. 2011; 25: 721-36.

[7] West SG. Neuropsychiatric lupus. *Rheum. Dis. Clin. North Am.* 1994;20:129–58.

[8] Hanly JG, Walsh NM, Sangalang V. Brain pathology in systemic lupus erythematosus. *J. Rheumatol.* 1992; 19:732–41.

[9] Johnson RT, Richardson EP. The neurological manifestations of systemic lupus erythematosus. Medicine Baltimore) 1968; 47:337–69.

[10] Williams TS, Aranow C, Ross GS, *et al.* Neurocognitive impairment in childhood-onset systemic lupus erythematosus: Measurement issues in diagnosis. *Arthritis Care Res. Hoboken*). 2011; 63:1178-87.

[11] Petri M, Naqibuddin M, Carson KA, *et al.* Cognitive function in a systemic lupus erythematosus inception cohort. *J. Rheumatol.* 2008; 35:1776-81.

[12] Purandare KN, Wagle AC, Parker SR. Psychiatric morbidity in patients with systemic lupus erythematosus. *Q J. Med.* 1999; 92:283–6.

[13] Hanly JG. Neuropsychiatric lupus. *Rheum Dis. Clin. North Am.* 2005; 31:273-98

[14] Appenzeller S, Cendes F, Costallat LT. Acute psychosis in systemic lupus erythematosus. Rheumatol Int. 2008;28:237-43.

[15] Stojanovich L, Zandman-Goddard G, Pavlovich S, Sikanich N. Psychiatric manifestations in systemic lupus erythematosus. *Autoimmun. Rev.* 2007; 6: 421-6.

[16] Waterloo K, Omdal R, Husby G, *et al.* Neuropsychological function in systemic lupus erythematosus: a five-year longitudinal study. *Rheumatology* 2002; 41: 411–5.

[17] Brey RL, Holliday SL, Saklad AR, *et al.* Neuropsychiatric syndromes in lupus prevalence using standardized definitions. *Neurology* 2002; 58:1214–20.

[18] Lewis DA, Smith RE. Steroid induced psychiatric syndromes: a report of 14 cases and a review of literature. *J. Affect Disord.* 1983; 5: 319–32.

[19] Ainiala H, Hietaharju A, Loukkola J, *et al.* Validity of the new American College of Rheumatology criteria for neuropsychiatric lupus syndromes: a population-based evaluation. *Arthritis Rheum.* 2001; 45: 419–423.

[20] Afeltra A, Garzia P, Mitterhofer AP, et al. Neuropsychiatric lupus syndromes, relationship with antiphospholipid antibodies. *Neurology.* 2003: 61; 108-10.

[21] Mok CC, Lau CS, Wong RW. Neuropsychiatric manifestations and their clinical associations in southern Chinese patients with systemic lupus erythematosus.*J. Rheumatol.* 2001,28:766–71.
[22] Sanna G, Bertolaccini ML, Cuadrado MJ, et al. Neuropsychiatric manifestations in systemic lupus erythematosus: prevalence and association with antiphospholipid antibodies. *J. Rheumatol*. 2003;30:985-92.
[23] Mikdashi J, Handwerger B. Predictors of neuropsychiatric damage in systemic lupus erythematosus: data from the Maryland lupus cohort. *Rheumatology Oxford*). 2004;43:1555-60.
[24] Appenzeller S, Li LM, Costallat LT, Cendes F. Evidence of reversible axonal dysfunction in systemic lupus erythematosus: a proton MRS study. *Brain*. 2005;128:2933-40.
[25] Shimojima Y, Matsuda M, Gono T, Ishii W, Ikeda S. Relationship between clinical factors and neuropsychiatric manifestations in systemic lupus erythematosus. *Clin. Rheumatol*. 2005;24:469-75.
[26] Robert M, Sunitha R, Thulaseedharan NK. Neuropsychiatric manifestations systemic lupus erythematosus: a study from South India. Neurol India. 2006;54:75-7.
[27] Hanly JG, Su L, Farewell V, et al. Prospective study of neuropsychiatric events in systemic lupus erythematosus. *J. Rheumatol*. 2009;36:1449-59.
[28] Tan EM, Cohen AS, Fries JF, *et al*. The 1982 revised criteria for the classification of systemic lupus erythematosus. *Arthritis Rheum*. 1982; 25: 1271–7.
[29] Ainiala H, Loukkola J, Peltola J, *et al*. The prevalence of neuropsychiatric syndromes in systemic lupus erythematosus. *Neurology*. 2001; 5: 496-500.
[30] Afeltra A, Garzia P, Mitterhofer AP, *et al*. Neuropsychiatric lupus syndromes: relationship with antiphospholipid antibodies. *Neurology*. 2003;61: 108-10.
[31] Hanly JG, Fisk JD, McCurdy G, *et al*. Neuropsychiatric syndromes in patients with systemic lupus erythematosus and rheumatoid arthritis. *J. Rheumatol*. 2005; 32: 1459-6.
[32] Sanna G, Bertolaccini ML, Cuadrado MJ, *et al*. Neuropsychiatric manifestations in systemic lupus erythematosus: prevalence and association with antiphospholipid antibodies. *J. Rheumatol*. 2003;30:985-92.
[33] Mok CC, Lau CS, Wong RW. Neuropsychiatric manifestations and their clinical associations in southern Chinese patients with systemic lupus erythematosus. *J. Rheumatol.* 2001; 28: 766–71.
[34] Hanly JG, McCurdy G, Fougere L, *et al*. Neuropsychiatric events in systemic lupus erythematosus: attribution and clinical significance, *J. Rheumatol.* **2004; 31:** 2156–2162.
[35] Mikdashi J, Handwerger B. Predictors of neuropsychiatric damage in systemic lupus erythematosus: data from the Maryland lupus cohort. *Rheumatology Oxford*). 2004; 43: 1555-60.
[36] Robert M, Sunitha R, Thulaseedharan NK. Neuropsychiatric manifestations systemic lupus erythematosus: a study from South India. *Neurol India*. 2006; 54: 75-7.
[37] Shimojima Y, Matsuda M, Gono T, *et al*. Relationship between clinical factors and neuropsychiatric manifestations in systemic lupus erythematosus. *Clin. Rheumatol.* 2005; 24: 469-75.
[38] American College of Rheumatology ACR) nomenclature and case definitions for neuropsychiatric lupus syndromes. *Arthritis and Rheumatism* 1999; **42**: 599–608.

[39] Ainiala H, Hietaharju A, Loukkola J, *et al.* Validity of the new American College of Rheumatology criteria for neuropsychiatric lupus syndromes: a population-based evaluation. *Arthritis Rheum* 2001; 45: 419–423.

[40] American Psychiatric Association. Diagnostic and statistical manual of mental disorders. Washington, DC: American Psychiatric Association; 1994; 4.

[41] Hirohata S, Kanai Y, Mitsuo A, *et al.* Accuracy of cerebrospinal fluid IL-6 testing for diagnosis of lupus psychosis. A multicenter retrospective study. *Clin. Rheumatol.* 2009; 28: 1319-23.

[42] Jonsen A, Bengston AA, Nived O, *et al.* Outcome of neuropsychiatric systemic lupus erythematosus within a defined Swedish population: increased morbidity but low mortality. *Rheumatology* 2002; 41: 1308-12.

[43] Appenzeller S, Cendes F, Costallat LT. Cognitive impairment and employment status in systemic lupus erythematosus: a prospective longitudinal study. *Arthritis Rheum.* 2009; 61; 680-7.

[44] Feng PH, Cheah PS, Lee YK. Mortality in systemic lupus erythematosus: a 10-year review. *Br. Med. J.* 1973; 4: 772-4.

[45] Cheatum DE, Hurd ER, Strunk SW, Ziff M. Renal histology and clinical course of systemic lupus erythematosus. A prospective study. *Arthritis Rheum.* 1973; 16:670-6.

[46] Lee P, Urowitz MB, Bookman AA, *et al.* Systemic lupus erythematosus. A review of 110 cases with reference to nephritis, the nervous system, infections, aseptic necrosis and prognosis. *Q J. Med.* 1977; 46: 1-32.

[47] Ginzler EM, Diamond HS, Weiner M, *et al.* A multicenter study of outcome in systemic lupus erythematosus. I. Entry variables as predictors of prognosis. *Arthritis Rheum.* 1982; 25: 601-611.

[48] Sibley JT, Olszynski WP, Decoteau WE, Sundaram MB. The incidence and prognosis of central nervous system disease in systemic lupus erythematosus. *J. Rheumatol.* 1992; 19: 47-52.

[49] Sergent JS, Lockshin MD, Klempner MS, Lipsky BA. Central nervous system disease in systemic lupus erythematosus. Therapy and prognosis. *Am. J. Med.* 1975; 58: 644-54.

[50] Feinglass EJ, Arnett FC, Dorsch CA, *et al.* Neuropsychiatric manifestations of systemic lupus erythematosus: diagnosis, clinical spectrum, and relationship to other features of the disease. *Medicine Baltimore*). 1976; 55: 323-39.

[51] Kovacs JA, Urowitz MB, Gladman DD. Dilemmas in neuropsychiatric lupus. *Rheum Dis. Clin. North Am.* 1993; 19: 795-814.

[52] Hanly JG, Su L, Farewell V, *et al.* Prospective study of neuropsychiatric events in systemic lupus erythematosus. *J. Rheumatol.* 2009; 36: 1449-59.

[53] Panopalis P, Julian L, Yazdany J, *et al.* Impact of memory impairment on employment status in persons with systemic lupus erythematosus. *Arthritis Rheum.* 2007; 57: 1453-60.

[54] Hebra F, Kaposi M. On diseases of the skin, including the exanthemata. New Sydenham Society, London 1874; 4: 1866–1880.

[55] Osler W. The visceral lesions of the erythema group. *Br. J. Dermatol.* 1900; 12: 227–245.

[56] Tan EM, Cohen AS, Fries JF, *et al.* The 1982 revised criteria for the classiWcation of systemic lupus erythematosus. *Arthritis Rheum.* 1982; 25: 1271–1277

[57] Kassan SS, Kagan LJ. Central nervous system lupus erythematosus: measurment of CSF cyclic GMP and other clinical markers of disease activity. *Arthritis Rheum.* 1979; 22: 449–457.

[58] Singer J, Denburg JA. Ad Hoc neuropsychiatric lupus workshop group: diagnostic criteria for neuropsychiatric systemic lupus erythematosus: the result of a consensus meeting. *J. Rheumatol.* 1990; 17: 1397–1402.

[59] Kasitanon N, Louthrenoo W, Piyasirisilp S, *et al.* Neuropsychiatric manifestations in Thai patients with systemic lupus erythematosus. *Asian Pac. J. Allergy Immunol.* 2002; 20: 179–185.

[60] Boston Collaborative Drug Surveillance Program. Acute adverse reactions to prednisone in relation to dosage. *Clin. Pharmacol. Ther.* 1972; 13: 694–698.

[61] Lopez-Medrano F, Cervera R, Trejo O, *et al.* Steroid induced psychosis in systemic lupus erythematosus: a possible role of serum albumin level. *Ann. Rheum. Dis.* 2002; 61: 562–563.

[62] Chau SY, Mok CC. Factors predictive of corticosteroid psychosis in patients with systemic lupus erythematosus. *Neurology* 2003; 61:104–107.

[63] Fernández Ga de Las Heras V, Gorriti MA, García-Vicuña R, Santos Ruiz JL. Psychosis leading to the diagnosis of unrecognized systemic lupus erythematosus: a case report. *Rheumatol Int.* 2007; 27: 883-5.

[64] Hanly JG, Urowitz MB, Sanchez-Guerrero J, *et al.* Neuropsychiatric events at the time of diagnosis of systemic lupus erythematosus: an international inception cohort study. Arthritis Rheum 2007; 7: 265–273.

[65] 65.Wysenbeek AJ, Leibovici L, Zoldan J. Acute central nervous system complications after pulse steroid therapy in patients with SLE. *J. Rheumatol.* 1990; 17: 1695–1696.

[66] Lewis GP, Jusko WJ, Graves L, Burke CW. Prednisone side-eVects and serum-protein levels. A collaborative study. *Lancet* 1971; 2: 778–780.

[67] Kohen M, Asherson RA, Gharavi AE, Lahita RG. Lupus psychosis: diVerentiation from the steroid-induced state. *Clin. Exp. Rheumatol.* 1993; 11: 323–326.

[68] Sirois F. Steroid psychosis: a review. *Gen. Hosp. Psychiatry* 2003; 25: 27–33.

[69] Patten SB, Neutel CI. Corticosteroid-induced adverse psychiatric eVects: incidence, diagnosis and management. *Drug Saf.* 2000; 22: 111–122.

[70] Isshi K, Hirohata S. DiVerential roles of the anti-ribosomal P antibody and antineuronal antibody in the pathogenesis of central nervous system involvement in systemic lupus erythematosus. *Arthritis Rheum.* 1998; 41: 1819–1827.

[71] Toubi E, Shoenfeld Y. Clinical and biological aspects of anti-P-ribosomal protein autoantibodies. *Autoimmun. Rev.* 2007; 6: 119– 125.

[72] Zandman-Goddard G, Chapman J, Shoenfeld Y. Autoantibodies involved in neuropsychiatric SLE and antiphospholipid syndrome. *Semin Arthritis Rheum.* 2007; 36: 297-315.

[73] Karassa FB, Afeltra A, Ambrozic A, *et al.* Accuracy of anti-ribosomal P protein antibody testing for the diagnosis of neuropsychiatric systemic lupus erythematosus: an international meta-analysis. *Arthritis Rheum.* 2006; 54:312–324.

[74] Bresnihan B, Oliver M, Williams B, Hughes GR. An antineuronal antibody cross-reacting with erythrocytes and lymphocytes in systemic lupus erythematosus. *Arthritis Rheum.* 1979; 22 :313-20.

[75] Bluestein HG, Williams GW, Steinberg AD. Cerebrospinal fluid antibodies to neuronal cells: association with neuropsychiatric manifestations of systemic lupus erythematosus. *Am. J. Med.* 1981; 70 :240-6.

[76] Hoffman SA, Madsen CS. Brain specific autoantibodies in murine models of systemic lupus erythematosus. *J. Neuroimmunol.* 1990; 30 :229-37.

[77] Tin SK, Xu Q, Thumboo J, *et al.* Novel brain reactive auto Abs: prevalence in systemic lupus erytematosus and association with psychoses and seizures. *J. Neuroimmunol.* 2005; 169 :153-60.

[78] Williams RC Jr, Sugiura K, Tan EM. Antibodies to microtubule-associated protein 2 in patients with neuropsychiatric systemic lupus erythematosus. *Arthritis Rheum.* 2004; 50 :1239-47.

[79] Reiff A, Miller J, Shaham B, *et al.* Childhood central nervous system lupus; longitudinal assessment using single photon emission computed tomography. *J. Rheumatol.* 1997; 24: 2461-5.

[80] Lai NS, Lan JL. Evaluation of cerebrospinal anticardiolipin Abs in lupus patients with neuropsychiatric manifestations. *Lupus* 2000; 9: 353-7.

[81] Fields RA, Sibbitt WL, Toubbeh H, Bankhurst AD. Neuropsychiatric lupus erythematosus, cerebral infarctions, and anticardiolipin Abs. *Ann. Rheum. Dis.* 1990; 49: 114-7.

[82] Hirohata S, Miyamoto T. Elevated levels of interleukin-6 in cerebrospinal fluid from patients with systemic lupus erythematosus and central nervous system involvement. *Arthritis Rheum.* 1990; 33: 644–649.

[83] Trysberg E, Carlsten H, Tarkowski A. Intrathecal cytokines in systemic lupus erythematosus with central nervous system involvement. *Lupus* 2000; 9:498–503.

[84] Fragoso-Loyo H, Richaud-Patin Y, Orozco-Narváez A, *et al.* Interleukin-6 and chemokines in the neuropsychiatric manifestations of systemic lupus erythematosus. *Arthritis Rheum.* 2007; 56: 1242–1250.

[85] Vila N, Castillo J, Davalos A, Chamorro A. Proinflammatory cytokines and early neurological worsening in ischemic stroke. *Stroke* 2000; 31:2325–2329.

[86] Torre D, Zeroli C, Ferraro G, *et al.* Cerebrospinal fluid levels of IL-6 in patients with acute infections of the central nervous system. *Scand. J. Infect. Dis.* 1992; 24:787–791.

[87] Trysberg E, Blennow K, Zachrisson O, Tarkowski A. Intrathecal levels of matrix metalloproteinases in systemic lupus erythematosus with central nervous system engagement. *Arthritis Res. Ther.* 2004; 6:R551–R556

[88] Kimura M, Aramaki K, Wada T, *et al.* Reversible focal neurological deficits in systemic lupus erythematosus: report of 2 cases and review of the literature. *J. Neurol. Sci.* 2008; 272:71–76.

[89] Bonfa E, Golombek SJ, Kaufman LD, Skelly S, Weissbach H, Brot N, *et al.* Association between lupus psychosis and antiribosomal P protein Abs. *N. Eng. J. Med.* 1987; 317: 265-71.

[90] Reichlin M, Wolfson-Reichlin M. Evidence for the participation of anti-ribosomal P Abs in lupus nephritis. *Arthritis Rheum.* 1999; 42: 2728-9.

[91] Schneebaum AB, Singleton JD, West SG, *et al.* Association of psychiatric manifestations with Abs to ribosomal P proteins in systemic lupus erythematosus. *Am. J. Med.* 1991; 90: 54-62.

[92] Arnett FC, Reveille JD, Moutsopoulos HM, *et al.* Ribosomal P auto Abs in systemic lupus erythematosus. Frequencies in different ethnic groups and clinical and immunogenetic associations. *Arthritis Rheum.* 1996; 39: 1833-1839.

[93] Gerli R, Caponi L, Tincani A, *et al.* Clinical and serological associations of ribosomal P autoAbs in systemic lupus erythematosus: prospective evaluation in a large cohort of Italian patients. *Rheumatology Oxford*) 2002; 41:1357-66.

[94] Nojima Y, Minota S, Yamada A, *et al.* Correlation of Abs to ribosomal P protein with psychosis in patients with systemic lupus erythematosus. *Ann. Rheum. Dis.* 1992; 51: 1053-1055.

[95] Massardo L, Burgos P, Martinez ME, *et al.* Antiribosomal P protein Abs in Chilean SLE patients: no association with renal disease. *Lupus* 2002; 11: 379-83.

[96] West SG, Emlen W, Wener MH, Kotzin BL. Neuropsychiatric lupus erythematosus: a 10-year prospective study on the value of diagnostic tests. *Am. J. Med.* 1995; 99: 153-63.

[97] Press J, Palayew K, Laxer RM, *et al.* Antiribosomal P Abs in pediatric patients with systemic lupus erythematosus and psychosis. *Arthritis Rheum.* 1996; 39:671-6.

[98] Watanabe T, Sato T, Uchiumi T, Arakawa M. Neuropsychiatric manifestations in patients with systemic lupus erythematosus: diagnostic and predictive value of longitudinal examination of anti-ribosomal P antibody. *Lupus* 1996; 5: 178-183.

[99] Yoshio T, Masuyama J, Ikeda M, *et al.* Quantification of antiribosomal P0 protein Abs by ELISA with recombinant P0 fusion protein and their association with central nervous system disease in systemic lupus erythematosus. *J. Rheumatol.* 1995; 22:1681-7.

[100] Isshi K, Hirohata S. Association of anti-ribosomal P protein Abs with neuropsychiatric systemic lupus erythematosus. *Arthritis Rheum.* 1996; 39:1483-1490.

[101] Tzioufas AG, Tzortzakis NG, Panou-Pomonis E, *et al.* The clinical relevance of Abs to ribosomal-P common epitope in two targeted systemic lupus erythematosus populations: a large cohort of consecutive patients and patients with active central nervous system disease. *Ann. Rheum. Dis.* 2000; 59: 99-104.

[102] Yoshio T, Hirata D, Onda K, *et al.* Antiribosomal P protein Abs in cerebrospinal fluid are associated with neuropsychiatric systemic lupus erythematosus. *J. Rheumatol.* 2005; 32: 34-9.

[103] Elkon K. Ribosomal RNP. In: van Venrooij WJ, Maini RN, eds. Manual of biological marker of diseases. Dordrecht: Kluwer Academic Publishers, 1994; B2.5:1-11.

[104] Derksen RH, van Dam P, Gmelig Meyling FH, *et al.* A prospective study on antiribosomal P proteins in two cases of familial lupus and recurrent psychosis. *Ann. Rheum. Dis.* 1990; 49: 779-82.

[105] Teh LS, Doherty DG, Williams BD. HLA-DRB genes and antiribosomal P Abs in systemic lupus erythematosus. *B.r J. Rheumatol.* 1994; 33: 1125-6.

[106] van Dam A, Nossent H, de Jong J, *et al.* Diagnostic value of Abs against ribosomal phosphoproteins. A cross sectional and longitudinal study. *J. Rheumatol.* 1991; 18: 1026-34.

[107] Golombek SJ, Graus F, Elkon KB. AutoAbs in the cerebrospinal fluid of patients with systemic lupus erythematosus. *Arthritis. Rheum.* 1986;2 9: 1090-7.

[108] Reichlin M._Ribosomal P antibodies and CNS lupus. *Lupus*. 2003; 12: 916-8.

[109] Winfield JB, Brunner CM, Koffler D. Serologic studies in patients with systemic lupus erythematosus and central nervous system dysfunction. *Arthritis Rheum.* 1978; 21: 289-94.

[110] Singh RR, Malaviya AN, Kailash S, Varghese T. Clinical significance of anti-Sm antibody in SLE and related disorders. *Indian J. Med. Res.* 1991; 94: 206-10.

[111] Boumpas DT, Yamada H, Patronas NJ, *et al.* Pulse cyclophosphamide for severe neuropsychiatric lupus. *Q J. Med.* 1991; 81: 975–84.

[112] Neuwelt CM, Lacks S, Kaye BR, *et al.* Role of intravenous cyclophosphamide in the treatment of severe neuropsychiatric systemic lupus erythematosus. *Am. J. Med.* 1995; 98: 32–41.

[113] Ramos PC, Mendez MJ, Ames PR, *et al.* Pulse cyclophosphamide in the treatment of neuropsychiatric systemic lupus erythematosus. *Clin. Exp. Rheumatol.* 1996; 14: 295–9.

[114] Baca V, Lavalle C, Garcı´a R *et al.* Favorable response to intravenous methylprednisolone and cyclophosphamide in children with severe neuropsychiatric lupus. *J. Rheumatol.* 1999; 26: 432–9.

[115] Takada K, Illei GG, Boumpas DT. Cyclophosphamide for the treatment of systemic lupus erythematosus. *Lupus* 2001; 10: 154–61.

[116] Mok CC, Lau CS, Wong RWS. Treatment of lupus psychosis with oral cyclophosphamide followed by AZA maintenance: an open-label study. *Am. J. Med.* 2003;115: 59–62.

[117] Tokunaga M, Saito K, Kawabata D *et al.* Efficacy of rituximab anti-CD20) for refractory systemic lupus erythematosus involving the central nervous system. *Ann. Rheum. Dis.* 2007; 66: 470–5.

# INDEX

## A

## B



## C

## D

## E

## F



## G



## H

## I

## J



## K



## L



## M

## N



## O



## P

## N



## O



## P

## Q



## R



## S

## T

## U



## V



## W



## Y



## Z